"My mother is 67 years ol... different time in our cultu... hospital for three days with... Her doctor watched over her... having a difficult labor. One day he came into her hospital room and noticed her gazing at her belly button. He asked her "Jerry, why are you looking at your belly button?" She said, "I want to see my baby come out." He took her hand and said "Jerry, that is not how it works."

She was raised to not talk about her body. Her grandmother chastised her because someone had said afterbirth when her grandfather was within earshot and her grandmother thought my mom said it. Women were taught to not discuss female reproductive systems or childbirth. So, my mom has observed the drastic cultural change as she observes her granddaughters discuss pregnancy including the cervix report or dilation reports. My mother agrees that it is better to have good scientific information to empower her granddaughter's and great granddaughter's women's health."

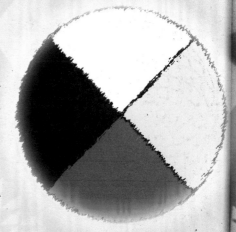

-submitted from a sister
JourneyWoman
Betsy Buckingham

A Woman's Health and Wellness

When a woman is healthy, she has the energy and strength to do her daily work, to fulfill the many roles she has in her family and community, and to build satisfying relationships with others. In other words, a woman's health affects every area of her life. Yet for many years, 'women's health care' has meant little more than maternal health services such as care during pregnancy and birth. These services are necessary, but they only address women's needs as mothers.

Every woman has a right to complete health care, throughout her life. A woman's health care should help her in all areas of life—not just in her role as a wife and mother. A woman's health is influenced not just by the way her body is made, but by the social, cultural, and economic conditions in which she lives.

This larger view helps us understand the underlying (core) causes of women's poor health. Improving women's health includes treating their health problems, but it also requires changing the conditions of their lives so they can gain more power over their own health.

When this happens, everyone—the woman, her family and community—benefits. A healthy woman has a chance to fulfill all of her potential. Plus, she will have healthier babies, be better able to care for her family, and can contribute more to her community. This kind of view also helps us see that a woman's health problem is almost never her problem alone. Women's health is a community issue.

Good health is more than the absence of disease.

Good health means the well-being of a woman's body, mind, and spirit.

Welcome

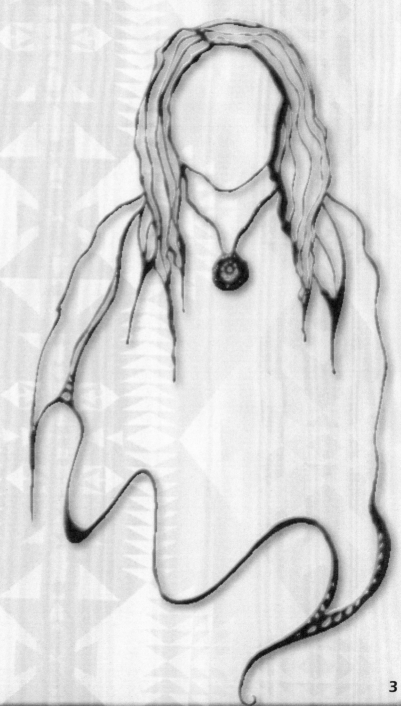

Cover layout and
Design by:
**Travis Warren,
Confederated
Tribes of Siletz**

Acknowledgements

First, we want to acknowledge you, a fellow JourneyWoman (or JourneyMan) for opening this guide. We acknowledge that the power of healing is within each of us. We acknowledge the strength and power of all Native Women to guide us on the right path on our journey to wellness.

JourneyWoman is the result of work, talent, gifts and guidance by Native Women & staff involved in the Women's Wellness Progam at the NARA Indian Health Clinic in Portland, Oregon. The idea for this guide came from the Native Women themselves who recieve services from NARA including their annual woman's exam. They asked for health & wellness information tailored for them, covering topics important to Native Women. We then took the time to travel to three area Tribes including the Cowlitz, Confederated Tribes of Warm Springs and the Burns Paiute Tribe to ask for their advice on what to include and how to create a wellness manual for Native Women.

The annual women's exam, while an important time to screen for cancers that touch women, is also a time for many of us to talk to a trusted health care provider about women's wellness issues such as sexually transmitted infections, abdominal pain, family planning, questions about menopause and other women's issues. We had no single source of information, with a Native face, that talked about many of the wellness concerns important to women. Instead, the providers and outreach staff hand out multiple pamplets, one for each issue.

As women, we know that we get much of our wellness information from sisters, grandmothers, mothers and daughters, between friends and sometimes from a trusted auntie. We hope that you find a sister or auntie in JourneyWoman. We have all faced women's health issues on life's journey. We hope this guide provides you and your sisters with information that will help you on your journey and start the conversation on how we can all find wellness on this journey through the cycle of life.

While this guide may not cover every topic important to Native Women, we hope it starts the discussion. We welcome feedback on this manual and hope to continue on the journey of providing wellness information that speaks to Native Women.

Guides and Reviewers

Cowlitz Tribe
Cecelia Konopski
Wendy Kinswa

Burns Paiute Tribes of SE Oregon
Minerva Soucie
Women of the Burns
Paiute Weavers Group
Twila Teeman
Sally Allen
Cheryl Barney
Myra Peck
Phyllis Miller
Shelly Richards
Roberta Teeman

Sophie Trettevick Indian Health Center/ Makah Tribe
Betsy Buckingham

Confederated Tribes of Warm Springs
Yvonne Iverson
Joy Ramirez
Cassie Katchia
Deborah Scott
Christina Zacairias

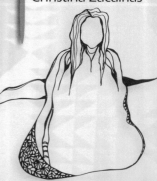

Guides and Reviewers

NARA
Dr. May Wang
Amelia Mainord
Jesse Mainord
Lanya Elliott
Christy Gonzalez
Trysha Foster
Sara Jasper
Lois Jasper
Leah Miller
Linda Drebin
Alison Goerl
Penny Schumacher
Artice Geary
Sheila Heuschkel
Rebecca Wright
Cindy Olson

Cancer Information Service and Spirit of the E.A.G.L.E.S.
Teresa Guthrie
Kathy Bryant

The Choctaw Nation of Oklahoma
Lee Ann Griffin
Bernice Williams
Annette Choate

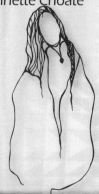

Sponsors and Contributors

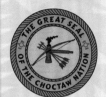

JourneyWoman, a Native Woman's Guide to Wellness, was made possible through funding and support from the:
Center for Disease Control & Prevention,
Choctaw Nation of Oklahoma
California Rural Indian Health Board
Nebraska Urban Indian Health Coalition, Inc.
Aberdeen Area Indian Health Service
Squaxin Island Charitable Fund

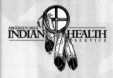

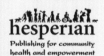

JourneyWoman gives special thanks to the Hesperian Foundation. A significant portion of the content of this manual has been inspired and adapted from the Hesperian publication "**Where Women Have No Doctor**" (3rd revised edition, 2006 www.hesperian.org.)

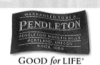

JourneyWoman thanks the **Pendleton Woolen Mills** for allowing us to use Pendleton blanket designs for the beautiful backgrounds for this manual.
In-kind services and resources were provided from several other partners including:
> *National Cancer Institute's Cancer Information Service*
> *National Cancer Institute Visuals Online*
> *The Spirit of the E.A.G.L.E.S.*
> *Our Bodies Our Selves*
> *Cultural Communications*

Additional information and graphics obtained from the National Cancer Institute, National Women's Health Information Center, American Cancer Society, American Heart Association, American Lung Association, Indian Health Service, and other public domain sources.

The contents of JouneyWoman are solely the responsibility of the authors and do not necessarily represent the official views of the sponsors and contributors or the Native American Rahabilitation

5

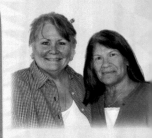

This manual was only made possible because of the vision and unwavering support of Sharon Fleming, Choctaw and the inspiring artistic talents of Az Carmen, Chicasaw.

An additional heart-felt thank you goes to Minerva Soucie, Burns Paiute Tribe, Wendi Kinswa, Cowlitz and the Rev. Anne Scissions of the Rosebud Sioux for contributing to this manual and being "Cancer Warriors" and role models for all Native Women.

Thank you to Chastity Walker and Jackie Mercer for allowing us to "journey" outside the box

Thank you to our JourneyWomen

Az Carmen PhD, Chickasaw, JourneyWoman Artis

Sharon Fleming, Choctaw JourneyWoman Leader

Thank you Jen for the Journey.

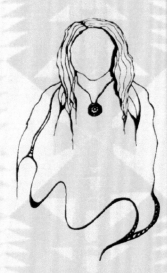

This health guide can be improved with your help. We would like to hear about your experiences, traditions and practices. If you are a midwife, Healer, Community Health Represenetive/Aid, doctor, nurse, mother, or anyone with suggestions for ways to make this book better meet the needs of your community, please write to us. Thank you for your help.

Information gathering, layout and design by Jen Olson

Printed in China by MCRL Overseas Printin

3rd printing of *JourneyWoman: A Native Woman's Guide to Wellness*

The contents of JourneyWoman are solely the responsibility of the authors and do not necessarily represent the official views of the Centers for Disease Control and Prevention, the Native American Rehabilitation Association of the Northwest, Inc. or the Choctaw Nation of Oklahoma.

The views and ideas presented in this guide address many topics for informational purpose only.

This guide is not meant to take the place of advice from your clinic or health care provider.

Contents

Mira's Story

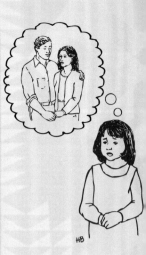

When Mira was a little girl, she dreamed of living in a big house, with nice kitchen and many bedrooms. Her husband would be handsome and kind, and she would be able to do whatever she wished. But Mira's family was poor, and her reservation was located far from any city. When Mira was 15, she got pregnant. She dropped out of school and got married. She didn't see any future for herself besides having children. Mira had no choice in the matter. With the birth of Mira's second child—a son—her husband stopped insisting on sex so often. Mira was very glad for that. Although he did not hurt her, he had warts all over his penis that disgusted her. Over the next 20 years, she had 6 more children, including a little girl who died at age 3, and a boy who died at birth. One day, Mira noticed a bloody discharge coming from her vagina when it wasn't time for her monthly bleeding. She had never gone to the clinic for a "woman's exam". She didn't feel comfortable with her body and didn't want a stranger examining her. Besides, she felt it was selfish to put herself before her family.   Her husband said he didn't trust doctors and told her not to go.

Mira was 40 when she began to suffer constant pain low in her belly. The pain worried her, but she didn't know who to talk to about it. Mira's health continued to worsen, and she became discouraged, realizing that something was still wrong. Some months later, Mira finally decided she had to go against her husband's wishes and get medical help. She was frightened for her life. Finally, Mira became so weak that her husband believed she really was ill, and took her to a hospital in the big city far away. Finally, she was told that she had cancer of the cervix. The doctor said they could remove her womb, but that the cancer had already spread. The doctor asked, "Why didn't you get regular Pap tests? If we had found this earlier, we could have treated it easily." But it was too late for that. Mira went home, and in less than two months, she died.

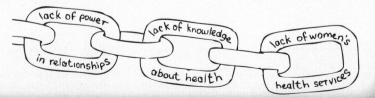

These are some of the links in the chain of causes that led to Mira's death. They are the same links that cause many of women's health problems.

8

Here are some common answers to this question:

A doctor may say...

> Mira died of advanced cervical cancer because she did not get treatment earlier.

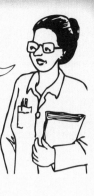

Or a teacher...

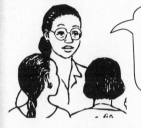

> Mira died because she didn't know she should have a Pap test done.

Or a health worker...

> Mira died because her husband exposed her to genital warts and other STIs. These put her at high risk for developing cancer of the cervix.

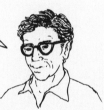

Native Women's Health and Wellness depends not only on the individual, but all of us to make sure the resources, education and awareness, and community & family support are in place so that Native Women's Wellness becomes the priority.

Women are the foundation of our communities. Let's work together to keep our sisters, mothers, daughters healthy.

All these answers are correct. Women who start having sex at a young age and are exposed to genital warts are at a greater risk for cancer of the cervix. And if the cancer is found early (usually by having a Pap test), it can almost always be cured.

Yet these answers show a limited understanding of the problem. Each of them blames one person—either Mira or her husband—and goes no further. Mira was at greater risk of dying of cervical cancer because she did not want to put herself before her family and did not feel comfortable going to the clinic until the disease was advanced. You may think of other reasons why some Native Women do not take the time to get their annual, preventive wellness checkups. As sisters, mothers, daughters, aunties, we need to support one another to put our wellness first.

National Breast and Cervical Cancer Early Detection Program
American Indian/Alaska Native Organizations

Arctic Slope Native
Association Limited
Breast and Cervical Cancer
Early Detection Program
Department of Health and
Social Services
PO Box 69
Barrow, AK 99723
1 (800) 478-6606, Ext. 270
(907) 852-5880
Fax: (907) 852-5882

Cherokee Nation
Breast and Cervical Cancer
Early Detection Program
PO Box 948
Tahlequah, OK 74465
(918) 458-4491
Fax: (918) 458-6267

Cheyenne River Sioux Tribe
Breast & Cervical Cancer
Early Detection Program
2001 Main Street
PO Box 590
Eagle Butte, SD 57625
(605) 964-8917
Fax: (605) 964-1176

Hopi Tribe
Breast and Cervical Cancer
Early Detection Program
PO Box 123
Kykotsmovi, AZ 86039
(928) 734-1150
Fax: (928) 734-1158

Kaw Nation Programs and
Services
http://www.kawnation.com/
Programs/proghome.html
Kanza Health Clinic
PO Box 474
Newkirk, OK 74647
(580) 362-1039 Ext. 228
Fax: (580) 362-1467

Native American Rehabilitation
Association of the Northwest,
Inc.
Women's Wellness Program
15 N. Morris Street
Portland, OR 97227
(503) 230-9875
Fax: (503) 230-9877

Navajo Nation
Breast and Cervical Cancer
Early Detection Program
PO Box 1390
Window Rock, AZ 86515
(928) 871-6249 Ext. 23
Fax: (928) 871-6255

Poarch Band of Creek Indians
Breast and Cervical Cancer
Early Detection Program
5811 Jack Springs Road
Atmore, AL 36502
(850) 476-5128 (Home)
Fax: (850) 478-0832

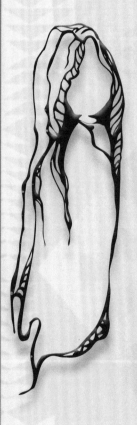

National Breast and Cervical
Cancer Early Detection Program

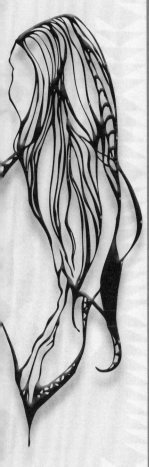

National Breast and Cervical er Early Detection Program

South East Alaska Regional
Health Consortium
Breast and Cervical Cancer Early
Detection Program
222 Tongass Drive
Sitka, AK 99835
(888) 388-8782

South Puget Intertribal Planning
Agency
Breast and Cervical Cancer Early
Detection Program
3104 Old Olympic Hwy SE
Shelton, WA 98584
(360) 462-3222
Fax: (360) 427-1625

Southcentral
Foundation
Breast and Cervi-
cal Cancer Early
Detection Pro-
gram
4320 Diplomacy
Drive, Suite 2360
Anchorage, AK
99508
(907) 729-8891
Fax: (907) 729-
3265

Yukon-Kuskokwim Health
Corporation
Breast and Cervical Cancer
Early Detection Program
700 Chief Eddy Hoffman Hwy
PO Box 287, Pouch 3000
Bethel, AK 99559
(907) 543-6996
Fax: (907) 543-6561

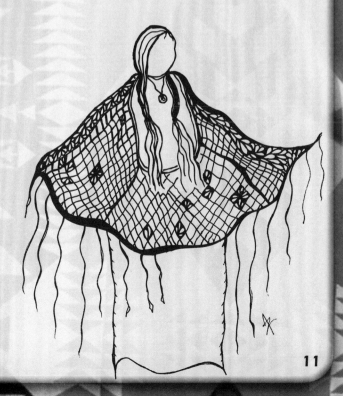

Welcome to this first chapter in JourneyWoman. We start our journey with "the Medical System". Health and wellness comes from many directions including our own intuition, the support from our family, community, healers and the Medical System. All women need to find affordable medical care and a doctor and clinic we trust as the starting point for wellness and self-care. As women, we need to have an exam every year for wellness. Some women may need medical care more often. You may need to meet several health providers before you feel comfortable. That's ok. Sometimes your clinic, friends and sisters can help you find medical care that is best for you.

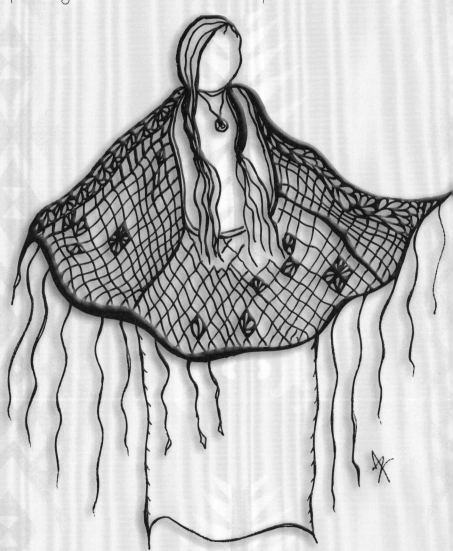

As women, we also need to help our daughters, mothers and sisters make sure they get a wellness exam at least once a year as part of our journey to wellness.

The Health System

Most areas of the United States have several different kinds of health care. For example, there are community health representatives, midwives and traditional healers, doctors and nurses. Some women may have access to a Tribal, Village, Urban Indian or Indian Health Service (IHS) clinic, Some women may have a private doctor. Some may have health care through the Veteran's Administration. Some women, who do not have public or private medical insurance, nor access to an IHS sponsored clinic, may not have any access to health care beyond the emergency room at the nearest hospital. Some health care facilities have the latest modern equipment and testing "cutting edge" treatment—and sometimes they are working focused more on community-based health care. Together they are called the medical system. Most people use some combination of modern medicine and traditional remedies to treat their health problems themselves. This is often all they need to do. But sometimes they need to seek care from the medical system.

Unfortunately, many Native Women have problems getting good health care. They may not have enough money or insurance coverage to visit a clinic or buy medicine. Or maybe they are in a rural community and have to travel far for medical services. Even if women can go to a clinic, it can be difficult to talk with health providers about their problems. Sometimes the clinic or hospital does not offer the services they need. This chapter gives some ideas about how women can get better health advice and better medical care.

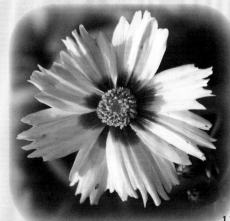

Important Health Services

The medical system offers many different kinds of services. Some services, like surgery, x-rays or ultrasounds are usually only available in hospitals. But the following services that women need should be offered at low cost at the community level:

- health information so that everyone can make better decisions about their health, treat health problems correctly, and prevent illness.
- immunizations or vaccinations that can prevent many diseases, including tetanus, measles, diphtheria, whooping cough, polio, tuberculosis, rubella, and hepatitis.
- care during pregnancy (prenatal care) that can help a woman find and treat problems affecting her or her unborn baby before they become serious.
- family planning services and supplies.
- health exams to help find and treat problems such as diabetes, high blood pressure, cancer screening and sometimes sexually transmitted infections (STIs).

Some health centers have laboratories with the equipment needed to get the results of different tests. However, often a woman will need to go to a hospital or speciality clinic to be tested or get diagnostic or follow up tests.

Other services are only available in hospitals. If a woman has a serious illness, or if she needs an operation, she will probably need to go to a hospital.

If you are an enrolled American Indian or Alaska Native you can access health care.

In 2003 Forty-nine percent of American Indian/Alaska Natives have private insurance coverage as compared to 83% of Caucasians.

The Medical System

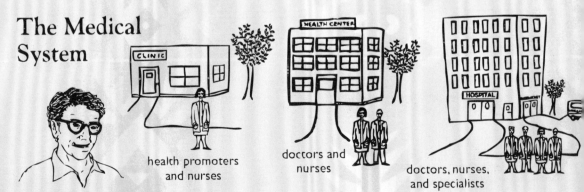

health promoter
(Community Health Representative (CHR) or Community Health Aide (CHA), Outreach Worker)

health promoters and nurses

doctors and nurses

doctors, nurses, and specialists

In many parts of the United States, American Indians and Alaska Natives have great access to health care through an IHS hospital, Tribal Clinic or Urban Indian Clinic. However, health care services do not reach all Native women and their families. Many urban centers do not have an Urban Indian Clinic, many tribal clinics have limited funds for preventive care and those Native Women without private health insurance may have to wait or be denied services due to lack of IHS or other public funds. Even where health services do exist, there are many barriers that keep women from using them, such as limited clinic hours, historical mistrust of western medicine, fear of getting an unwelcome diagnosis or not feeling comfortable with a non Native clinic or health care provider. One way to make sure everyone has good medical services is by discussing the health care problems that affect people in your community—including lack of access to good care—with other women and men.

I would like the clinic to be open in the evenings, after I have finished my work.

I can't tell my doctor I'm also using traditional medicine, he will look down on me. I wish the clinic would honor traditional ways of healing.

There is always such a long wait. If someone asked right away what each person needed then the really sick people could be treated sooner.

I don't like having a man examine me. I wish there were women health care providers.

I wish they explained what was wrong. This is the 4th time this year I've had pain when I passed urine. Why does this keep happening?

I wish they didn't run out of diabetes supplies. I wasn't able to test my blood sugar because the clinic ran out, and I can't afford to buy a lot on my own.

Those doctors from the hospital look down on us. I would feel better if Native people helped run the clinic.

15

Who Pays for Health Care

Finding out how to pay for health care, especially if you or your family does not have private insurance, can keep some people from seeking health care. Many feel they may have to pay for the health care themselves. There are a number of ways to have your health care covered. Below are examples:

Private Insurance

If you have priviate insurance or are a member of an Health Maintenance Organization (HMO) most of your health care is paid through your insurance. You may still have to pay a co-pay for each office visit. A co-pay is what is due after the insurance company pays it's portion of the medical services.

Public Insurance

Medicaid pays for health care services for eligible low-income people, children, pregnant women and others including some people with disabilities. Whether or not a person is eligible for Medicaid will depend on the state where he or she lives. Most States have additional "State-only" programs to provide medical assistance for eligible poor persons who do not qualify for the Medicaid program. Here are some resources to find out more information on Medicaid and links to your state's Medicaid program:
www.govbenefits.gov
www.cms.hhs.gov/home/medicaid.asp

Medicare is a Federal Health Insurance Program for people 65 years of age and older, some disabled people under 65 years of age, and people with End-Stage Renal Disease (permanent kidney failure treated with dialysis or a transplant).
www.medicare.gov   OR 1-800-MEDICARE

Veteran's Administration Benefits. Eligibility for most veterans' health care benefits is based solely on active military service in the Army, Navy, Air Force, Marines, or Coast Guard (or Merchant Marines during WW II), and discharged under other than dishonorable conditions. Others may be eligible for limited services. Find out more:
http://www.va.gov/healtheligibility
VA Benefits: 1-800-827-1000
Health Care Benefits: 1-877-222-8387
Mammography Helpline: 1-888-492-7844

Tribal or State Breast and Cervical Cancer Screening Programs offer women's annual exams and mammograms for women with no insurance or limited insurance. To find out about a program in your area see:
national website: http://apps.nccd.cdc.gov/cancercontacts/nbccedp/contacts.asp
national phone contact: 1-(800) CDC-INFO

16

The Indian Health Care System:

If you are an enrolled American Indian or Alaskan Native, you may be eligible for direct health care services through the Indian Health Care system. Due to limited budgets, many clinics may only provide services within their clinic and cannot cover other medical services such as hospital care, medicines, or wellness checks when you are not yet sick. Many IHS/Tribal/Urban (I/T/U) clinics may have staff that can help you find additional services such as those listed on the previous page.

Indian Health Service (IHS) direct health care services.

IHS services are administered through a system of 12 Area offices & 163 IHS and tribally managed service units across the nation.

Tribally-operated health care services.

Tribal facilities are operated under the authority of the Indian Self-Determination and Education Assistance Act (Public Law 93-638, as amended), Titles I and V. These compacts represent 322 Tribes, more than half of all the federally recognized Tribes. There are also approximately 241 Tribes and tribal organizations that contract under Title I. Overall, approximately 54% of the IHS budget authority appropriation is administered by Tribes, primarily through Self-Determination contracts or Self-Governance compacts. Each Tribally-operated health care system determines who is eligible for advanced levels of services, such as non-tribal hospital care and medicines.

Urban Indian health care services and resource centers.

There are 34 urban programs, ranging from community health to comprehensive primary health care services.

> **IHS Population Served (2007):**
> Members of 561 federally recognized Tribes in 35 States 1.9 million American Indians and Alaska Natives residing on or near reservations and 600,000 American Indians in urban clinics.
>
> Per Capita Personal Health Care Expenditures Comparisons:
> IHS user population: $2158
> Total U.S. population: $5921

The most common standard applied for eligibility for health services from the Indian Health Service is that the individual is an enrolled member of a Federally recognized Tribe.

resource: www.ihs.gov (phone numbers for IHS Area Offices listed at end of chapter)

The Medical System

No matter where you go for health care, it is your right to be treated with respect. All people who care for your health should do their best to provide you with:

1. Access. Everyone who needs medical care should be able to have it. It should not matter where you live, how much money you have, what your religion is, how much status you have in the community, the color of your skin, your political beliefs, or what health problem you have.

2. Information. You should be told about your problem and about what the different possible treatments mean for you. The person caring for you should make sure you understand what you need to do to get better, and how to prevent the problem from happening again.

3. Choice. You should be able to choose whether or not you are treated, and how. Also, you should be able to choose where to go for treatment.

4. Safety. You should be given the information you need to avoid harmful side effects or results of treatment. You should also be told how to prevent dangerous health problems in the future.

5. Respect. You should always be treated with respect and courtesy.

6. Privacy. Things that you say to a doctor, nurse or other health care worker should not be overheard by others or repeated to anyone else. Exams should be given in a way that other people cannot see your body. If there are other people who need to be in the room, you should be told who they are and why they are there. You have the right to tell them to leave if you do not want them there.

7. Comfort. You should be made as comfortable as possible during an exam. You should also have a good place to wait and not have to wait too long.

8. Follow-up care. If you need more care, you should be able to go back to the same person, or be given a written record of the care you have received to take to a new doctor, nurse, or health worker.

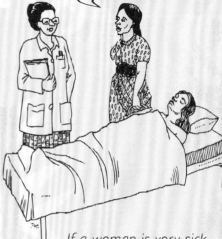

I am her mother. I can answer some of your questions.

If a woman is very sick, someone who can give information should go with he

The Patient's Bill of Rights

The following was adopted by the US Advisory Commission on Consumer Protection and Quality in the Health Care Industry in 1998. Many health plans have adopted these principles.

Information Disclosure. You have the right to accurate and easily understood information about your health plan, health care professionals, and health care facilities. If you speak another language, have a physical or mental disability, or just don't understand something, assistance will be provided so you can make informed health care decisions.

Choice of Providers and Plans. You have the right to a choice of health care providers that is sufficient to provide you with access to appropriate high-quality health care.

Access to Emergency Services. If you have severe pain, an injury, or sudden illness that convinces you that your health is in serious jeopardy, you have the right to receive screening and stabilization emergency services whenever and wherever needed, without prior authorization or financial penalty.

Participation in Treatment Decisions. You have the right to know your treatment options and to participate in decisions about your care. Parents, guardians, family members, or other individuals that you designate can represent you if you cannot make your own decisions.

Respect and Nondiscrimination. You have a right to considerate, respectful and nondiscriminatory care from your doctors, health plan representatives, and other health care providers.

Confidentiality of Health Information. You have the right to talk in confidence with health care providers and to have your health care information protected. You also have the right to review and copy your own medical record and request that your physician change your record if it is not accurate, relevant, or complete.

Complaints and Appeals. You have the right to a fair, fast, and objective review of any complaint you have against your health plan, doctors, hospitals or other health care personnel. This includes complaints about waiting times, operating hours, the conduct of health care personnel, and the adequacy of health care facilities.

Who can care for My Woman's Health Needs?

Caring for your reproductive health is an important part of growing up. If you notice body changes that you are not sure are normal, ask one of your parents or a trusted adult to make an appointment for you with a health care provider. You can see:

A Gynecologist
A gynecologist is a doctor who focuses on women's reproductive health. You may need to visit a gynecologist as you get older.

A Nurse Practitioner (NP)
A nurse practitioner is a registered nurse with special training. If your clinic or doctor's office has a NP, he or she can do many of the things a doctor can and will work with the doctor if you need special tests or medicines.

A Physician's Assistant (PA)
A physician assistant is a health care professional licensed to practice medicine with the supervision of a licensed physician.

A Family Practitioner or General Practitioner
This is a doctor whose practice does not focus on a specific medical specialty, but instead covers varied medical problems in patients of all ages.

Routine Health Care Includes An Annual Women's Exam

(even if you feel fine)

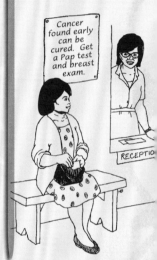

Cancer found early can be cured. Get a Pap test and breast exam.

RECEPTION

Bring a friend or family member

Many people feel worried about seeking medical care—even for illnesses that are not serious. And when a person is sick, it can be even harder for them to demand the care they need. If another person can go along, it can help.

A friend can:

- watch the woman's children.
- help think of questions to ask, remind the woman to ask them, and make sure they are answered.
- answer questions if the woman is too sick to talk.
- keep the woman company while she waits.
- stay with the woman while she is being examined, to support her and make sure the doctor acts in a respectful way.
- be another set of ears to hear what the heath care provider is saying

The Exam

In order to know what is wrong with you and how serious your problem is, you may need an examination. Most exams include looking at, listening to, and feeling the part of your body where the problem is. For most problems you need to undress only that part of your body. If you would feel more comfortable, ask a friend or female health care worker to be in the room with you during the exam.

Tests

Tests can give more information about a health problem. Many tests are done by taking a small amount of urine or stool and sending it to a laboratory. Or, a needle is used to take a small amount of blood from your finger or arm. Other common tests include:

> X-rays are safe if they are used properly. A lead apron should be used to protect your reproductive organs.

- taking some fluid from your vagina to test for sexually transmitted infections (STIs).
- scraping cells from the opening of your womb (cervix) to test for cancer. (This is called a Pap test. See the "Cervical Cancer" chapter).
- taking tissue from a growth to test for cancer (biopsy).
- using X-rays or ultrasound to see inside your body. X-rays may be used to find broken bones, severe lung infections, and some cancers. Try not to be X-rayed during pregnancy. Ultrasound can be used during pregnancy to see the baby inside your womb. Neither of these tests causes any pain.

Before you have any test, discuss the cost. Ask the doctor, nurse, or health worker to explain what he or she will learn from the test, and what would happen if the test was not done.

Many doctors and nurses may not be used to giving information in a way that is easily understood, or they may be busy and not take the time to answer your questions. Be respectful, but firm! They should answer your questions until you understand. If you do not understand, it is not because you are stupid, but because they are not explaining well.

If You Need to Go to the Hospital

If you need to have an operation or you have a serious illness, this advice may help:

• Bring someone with you who can help you get the attention you need and help you make decisions.

• Different people may examine you. Each one should write down what he or she did in your medical chart. This way the next person who cares for you will know what has already been done.

• Before anyone begins a test or treatment, it is very important to ask what they are going to do and why. This way you can decide if you want them to do it or if you want to get another opinion before you decide.

• Ask what medicines you are being given and why.

• Ask for a copy of your records when you leave.

• If you are unsure of how your treatment will be paid for, you can ask to talk to the hospital social worker to find out resources to help pay for your care.

• Keep a journal or ask your friend/family member to keep notes on the procedures you are having, the medications you are given and recommendations of the doctor or nurse at the hospital. This may come in handy when you talk to your doctor back at your community and as you recover.

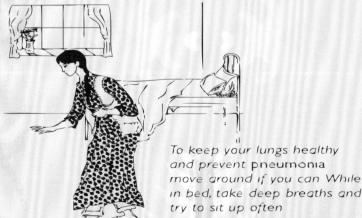

To keep your lungs healthy and prevent pneumonia move around if you can While in bed, take deep breaths and try to sit up often

An operation is sometimes the only answer to a serious health problem. During many operations, a doctor makes a cut in the skin in order to fix problems inside the body or to change the way the body functions. Here are some of the operations women commonly have:

Common Operations for Women

- Emptying the womb by either scraping or suctioning (D and C, or MVA). Sometimes the lining of the womb must be removed—either during or after an abortion or miscarriage, or to find the cause of abnormal bleeding from the vagina.

- Birth by operation (cesarean section or c-section). When complications make it dangerous for a woman or her baby to go through normal labor and birth, a cut is made in a woman's belly so her baby can be born. C-sections can be necessary, but too often they are done for the benefit of the doctor, not the woman. See the chapter on "Pregnancy.

- Removing the womb (hysterectomy). A hysterectomy is a serious operation, so it should be done only when there is no better way to solve your health problem. Ask if you can have your ovaries left in.

After you have an operation

Before you leave the hospital, ask:
- What should I do to keep the incision (cut) clean?

- What should I do about pain?

- How long should I rest?

- When can I have sex again? (If you feel too shy to ask this, perhaps the doctor or health worker can talk to your partner.)

- Do I need to see a doctor again? If so, when?

Eat soft, mild foods that are easy to digest. Rest as much as you can. If you are at home, ask your family to take care of your daily chores. A few days spent taking care of yourself can help you get better faster. Watch for signs of infection: yellow discharge (pus), a bad smell, fever, hot skin near where you were cut, or more pain. See a health provider if you have any of these signs.

If your operation was in the abdomen, try not to strain the area that was cut. Press against it gently with a folded cloth, blanket, or pillow whenever you move or cough.

It's Your Choice

There are many decisions to make when you have a health problem. One decision is whether to see a health worker, and what kind of health worker you think you need. If there is more than one way to treat a problem, you will need to consider the risks and benefits of each kind of treatment before you make a decision. You will be able to make the best decisions—and get the best care—if you can take an active role in working with your doctor, nurse, or health worker to solve your health problem.

Questions about your health

It is best to learn as much as you can about your health problem before you use the medical system. Reading this book may help you understand your health problem and the possible causes. For help thinking about health problems, see "Solving Health Problems."

The doctor, nurse, or health worker who sees you should ask about the problem you are having now and about your past health. Try to give complete information, even if you feel uncomfortable, so that the person asking the questions can learn as much as possible about your health. Always tell about any medication you are taking, including aspirin or family planning methods.

You should also have a chance to ask any questions you may have. It is very important to ask as many questions as you need to make a good decision about how to solve your health problem. If these questions have not already been answered, you may want to ask:

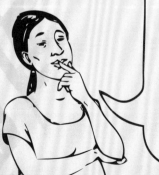

- What are the different ways this problem can be treated?
- What will the treatment do? Are there any dangers?
- Will I be cured? Or will the problem come back?
- How much will the tests and treatment cost?
- When will I get better?
- Why did the problem happen and how can I keep it from happening again?

Know what to expect
You will be best able to take an active role in your health if you are prepared and know what to expect when you seek medical care.

It often helps to think of the questions you want to ask before you go for medical care. Write them down and take with you.

IHS Area Offices

Breast and Cervical Cancer Early Detection Programs

The Centers for Disease Control and Prevention (CDC) provides low-income, uninsured, and underserved women access to timely, high-quality screening and diagnostic services, to detect breast and cervical cancer at the earliest stages, through the National Breast and Cervical Cancer Early Detection Program (NBCCEDP).

If you want to find out more about the IHS services, including IHS, Tribal and Urban Indian Health resources in your location, contact the Area office in you state:

Aberdeen (States of ND, SD, NE, IA) 605-226-7581

Alaska (All Alaska Tribes and locations) 907-729-3686

Albuquerque (States of NM, CO, TX) 505-248-4102

Bemidji (States of MI, MN, WI, and IN) 218-444-0458

Billings (States of MT, WY) 406-247-7107

California (All California Tribes and locations) 916-930-3927

Nashville (States of TX, MO, AR, LA, MS, AL, GA, FL, SC, NC, TN, KY, VA, WV, IL, OH, PA, MD, DE, NJ, NY, CT, RI, MA, VT, NH, ME) 615-467-1500

Navajo (Navajo Nation Reservation) 928-871-5811

Oklahoma (States of OK, KS, TX) 405-951-3768

Phoenix (States of NV, UT, AZ) 602-364-4123

Portland (States of WA, OR, ID) 503-326-2020

Tucson (The Tohono O'odham Nation & Pascua Yaqui Tribe of Arizona) 520-295 -2405

Urban Indian Health Centers

National Council of Urban Indian Health
www.ncuih.org/programsarial.html

Breast and Cervical Cancer Early Detection Programs

The CDC contracts with states and tribal organizations to provide these services. For breast and cervical cancer screening services in your area call: 1 (800) CDC-INFO or go to:
http://apps.nccd.cdc.gov/cancercontacts/nbccedp/contacts.asp

National Breast and Cervical Cancer Early Detection Program

25

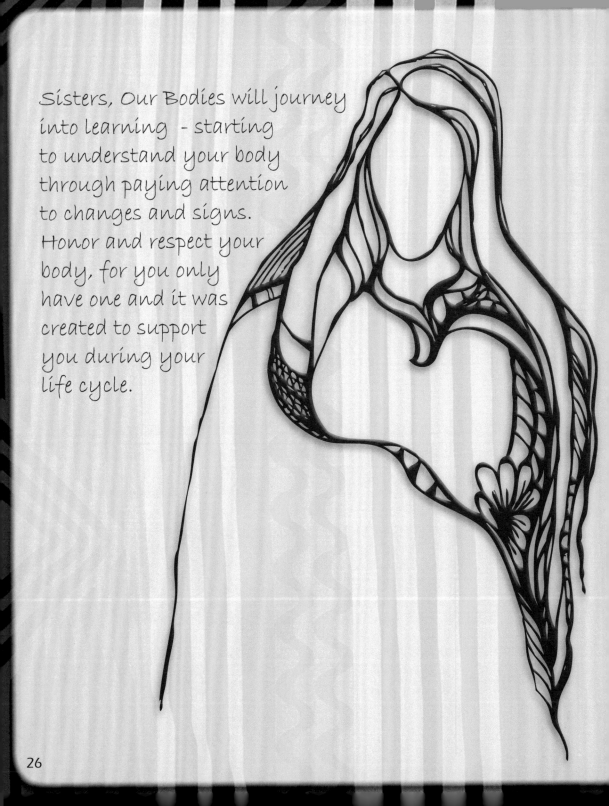

Sisters, Our Bodies will journey
into learning - starting
to understand your body
through paying attention
to changes and signs.
Honor and respect your
body, for you only
have one and it was
created to support
you during your
life cycle.

Understanding Our Bodies

In many ways, a woman's body is no different from a man's. For example, women and men both have hearts, kidneys, lungs, and other parts that are the same. But one way they are very different is in their sexual or reproductive parts. These are the parts that allow a man and a woman to make a baby. Many of women's health problems affect these parts of the body. This chapter gives an introduction to women's bodies, our cycles and changes that are unique to women. The chapters that follow will give even more information on health and wellness issues for women.

Women are the strength and the foundation of our communities. We can keep ourselves strong by seeking balance between the mind, body and spirit. Understanding our bodies is the first step. Through life's journey we learn to be aware of change, pleasure as well as pain, cyles, gain and loss. This is our journey towards understading our bodies.

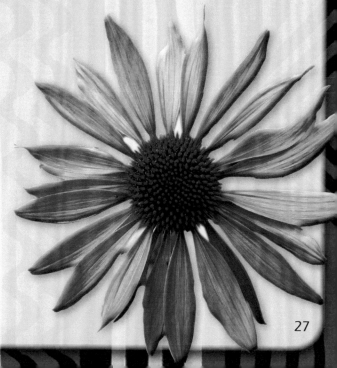

A Woman's Body

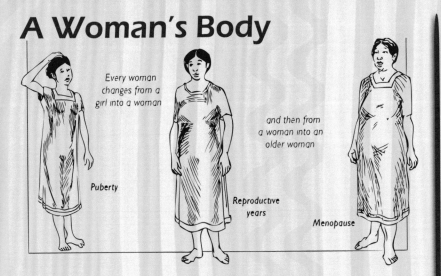

Every woman changes from a girl into a woman

and then from a woman into an older woman

Puberty

Reproductive years

Menopause

Sometimes talking about the sexual parts of our bodies can be difficult, especially if you are shy, or do not know what different parts of the body are called. In many places, the reproductive parts of the body are considered 'private'.

But knowing how our bodies work means we can take better care of them. We can recognize problems and their causes and make better decisions about what to do about them. The more we know, the more we will be able to decide for ourselves if the advice that others give us is helpful or harmful.

Since different communities sometimes have their own words for parts of the body, in this book we often use medical or scientific names. This way, women from many different regions will be able to understand the words.

A woman's body goes though many important changes during her life—at puberty, during pregnancy and breastfeeding, and when she stops being able to have a baby (menopause). In addition, during the years she can have a baby, her body changes every month—before, during, and after the time of her monthly bleeding. The parts of the body where many of these changes happen are the vagina, womb, ovaries, fallopian tubes, and the breasts, also called the reproductive system. Many of the changes are caused by special chemicals called hormones.

Puberty

As a young girl blossoms into womanhood, a variety of changes happen to her body and spirit. As the body nears adulthood, young woman may experience body changes, new thoughts, emotions and desires.

Reproductive years

A woman's body is at her prime. She is ready to nuture a family. Her body, mind and spirit are strong. She is the foundation of the family.

Becoming an Elder

We are living longer than ever before, and many Elders are living active, healthy, and productive lives. Taking good care of our body, spirit, and mind will help us enjoy these golden years.

Hormones

Hormones are chemicals the body makes that control how and when the body grows. A little while before a girl's monthly bleeding first starts, her body begins to produce more estrogen and progesterone, the main female hormones. These hormones cause the changes in her body known as puberty.

During the years when she can have a baby, hormones cause a woman's body to prepare for possible pregnancy each month. They also tell her ovaries when to release an egg (an egg every month). So hormones determine when a woman can get pregnant. Many family planning methods work to prevent pregnancy by controlling the hormones in a woman's body (see "Family Planning" chapter). Hormones also cause changes during pregnancy and breastfeeding. For example, hormones keep a pregnant woman from having her monthly bleeding, and after childbirth they also tell the breasts to make milk. When a woman is near the end of her reproductive years, her body slowly stops producing estrogen and progesterone. Her ovaries stop releasing eggs, her body stops preparing for a pregnancy, and her monthly bleeding stops forever. This is called menopause. The amount and kind of hormones produced by a woman's body can also affect her moods, sexual feelings, weight, body temperature, hunger, and bone strength.

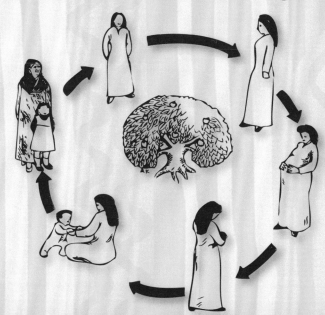

The Breasts

Breasts come in all shapes and sizes. They start to grow when a girl is between 10 and 15 years old, when she changes from a girl to a woman (puberty). They make milk for babies after pregnancy. When they are touched during sexual relations, a woman's body responds by making her vagina wet and ready for sex.

Inside the breasts:

The **areola** is the dark and bumpy skin around the **nipple**. The bumps make an oil that keeps the nipples clean and soft. The nipple is where milk comes out of the breast. Sometimes they stick out. Sometimes they are flat. **Sinuses** store the milk until the baby drinks it. **Ducts** carry the milk to the nipple. **Glands**, also called **lobules**, make the milk.

Inside the breasts:

Glands *make the milk.*

Ducts *carry the milk to the nipple*

Sinuses *store the milk until the baby drinks it*

The **nipple** *is where milk comes out of the breast Sometimes they stick out Sometimes they are flat*

The **areola** *is the dark and bumpy skin around the nipple The bumps make an oil that keeps the nipples clean and soft*

Early detection of Breast Cancer includes:
• Self Breast Exams
• Annual Clinical Breast Exams (CBE)
• Annual mammograms starting at age 40

Talk to your health care provider about how to screen for breast cancer.

Lymph nodes and Lymph vessels carry waste materials from the cells

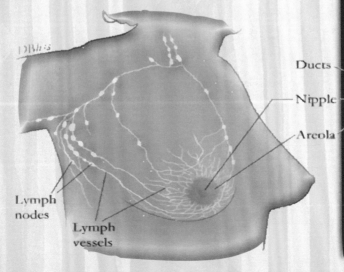

Lymph nodes

Lymph vessels

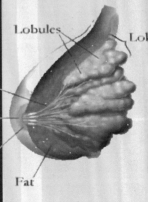

Lobules

Lob

Ducts

Nipple

Areola

Fat

and size

Measure around the
est directly under the
east. Add 5 inches to
at measurement. This
mension is your bra/
nd size

up Size

Now measure
ound the chest at the
ight of the fullest part
the breast. Find the
ference between step
nd step 1

lf inch	AA cup
e inch	A cup
o inches	B cup
ree inches	C cup
ur inches	D cup
e inches	DD or E cup
inches	F cup
ven inches	G cup

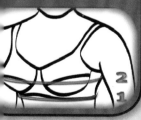

gerie manufacturer
derick's of
lywood reports that
996, the average
of bras they sold
34B.

A Bra That Fits

Eight out of ten women may be wearing a bra that doesn't fit. A woman's breasts change significantly over time, particularly during and after pregnancy. Weight loss, gain and monthly cycle variations can also have an effect on the fit of your bra. Check your bra size once or twice a year or as necessary due to significant weight changes.

The Band

The back and front of your bra band should be level and parallel to the floor when you look at yourself from the side in a mirror. If the band is too tight, digs into your flesh or is just plain uncomfortable, it's too small.

The Cup

Your bra cups should be large enough to prevent breast tissue from bulging or spilling out over the neckline or armhole edges. You'll know if your bra cups are too large if they have wrinkling, or are clearly larger than both of your breasts.

The Straps

Shoulder straps on a bra should rest flat on your shoulders. They shouldn't cause dents or fall off your shoulders. Shoulder straps are designed to carry minimal breast weight (10% or less). If your shoulders have dents from your straps, then your straps are working too hard - you probably need a smaller band size to give your bra more support. If your straps keep slipping, there are several possible causes:

- The straps could also be sewn too far apart on the back of your bra.
- If your cup size is too large, there will not be enough breast tissue to fill out the top of your cup and this will cause your straps to slide down your shoulders.
- If the strap in front and/or back is attached to a ring this ring allows the strap to swivel and could cause the strap to fall off your shoulder.

A Woman's Reproductive System

A woman has sexual parts both outside and inside her body. They are called the reproductive organs, or genitals. The outside parts are called the vulva. Sometimes people may use the word vagina for the whole area. But the vagina is the part that begins as an opening in the vulva and leads inside to the womb. The vagina is sometimes called the 'birth canal'.

The Reproductive Parts on the Outside

Vaginal opening: The opening of the vagina.

Vulva: All the sexual parts you can see between your legs.

Mons: The hairy, fatty part of the vulva.

Clitoris: The clitoris is small and shaped like a flower bud. It is the part of the vulva that is most sensitive to touch. Rubbing it, and the area around it, can make a woman sexually excited and cause climax.

Urinary opening: The outer opening of the urethra. The urethra is a short tube that carries urine from where it is stored in the bladder to the outside of the body.

Anus: The opening of the intestine, where waste (stool) leaves the body.

Hymen (hi-mun)**:** The thin piece of skin just inside the vaginal opening. A hymen may stretch or tear and bleed a little because of sports or other activities. This can also happen when a woman has sex for the first time. All hymens are different. Some women do not have a hymen at all.

Outer folds: The fatty lips that close up when the legs are together. They protect the inner parts.

Inner folds: These flaps of skin are soft, without hair, and are sensitive to touch. During sex, the inner lips swell and turn darker.

Every woman's body is different. There are differences in the size, shape, and color of the parts, especially of the outer and inner folds.

The Reproductive Parts on the Inside

Vagina or birth canal:

The vagina leads from the vulva to the womb. The vagina is made of a special kind of skin that stretches easily during sex and when giving birth. The vagina makes a fluid or wetness (discharge) that helps it keep itself clean and prevents infection.

Cervix:

This is the opening or 'mouth' of the womb, where it opens into the vagina. Sperm can enter the womb through the small hole in the cervix, but it protects the womb from other things, like a man's penis.

Fallopian tubes:

The fallopian tubes connect the womb with the ovaries. When an ovary releases an egg, it travels through the fallopian tubes into the womb.

Womb (uterus):

The womb is a hollow muscle. Monthly bleeding comes from the womb. The baby grows here during pregnancy.

Ovaries:

The ovaries release one egg into a woman's fallopian tubes each month. When a man's sperm joins the egg, it can develop into a baby. A woman has 2 ovaries, one on each side of the womb. Each ovary is about the size of an almond or grape. The ovaries are also part of the endocrine system because they produce female sex hormones such as estrogen (pronounced: es-truh-jun) and progesterone (pronounced: pro-jes-tuh-rone).

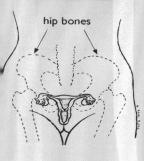

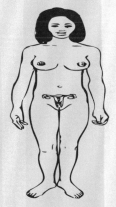

hip bones

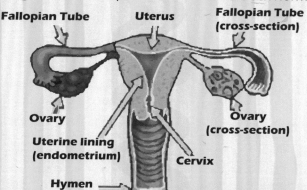

Fallopian Tube

Uterus

Fallopian Tube (cross-section)

Ovary

Ovary (cross-section)

Uterine lining (endometrium)

Cervix

Hymen

Vagina

33

Monthly Cycle (menstrual cycle)

The monthly cycle is different for each woman. It begins on the first day of a woman's monthly bleeding. Most women bleed every 28 days. But some bleed as often as every 20 days or as little as every 45 days. The amount of the hormones estrogen and progesterone produced in the ovaries changes throughout the monthly cycle.

During the first half of the cycle, the ovaries make mostly estrogen, which causes a thick lining of blood and tissue to grow in the womb. The body makes the lining so a baby would have a soft nest to grow in if the woman became pregnant that month.

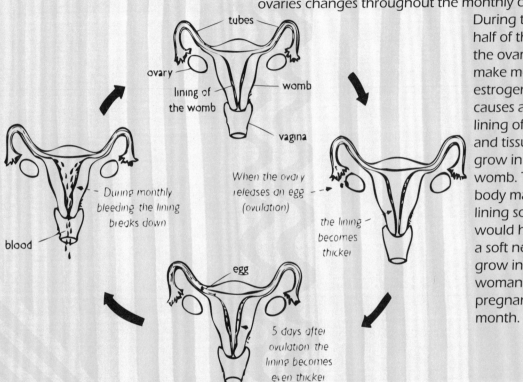

tubes

ovary

lining of the womb

womb

vagina

During monthly bleeding the lining breaks down

blood

When the ovary releases an egg (ovulation)

the lining becomes thicker

egg

5 days after ovulation the lining becomes even thicker

Natural options to alleviate cramping:

- Increase exercise. This will improve blood and oxygen circulation throughout the body, including the pelvis.
- Use a heating pad on your tummy - or fill a sock with uncookedrice and microwave for 2-3 minutes, this will keep warm and can be used as a "heating pad".
- Avoid red meat, refined sugars, milk, and fatty foods.
- Eat lots of fresh vegetables, whole grains (especially if you experience constipation or indigestion), nuts, seeds and fruit.
- Avoid caffeine. It constricts blood vessels and increases tension.
- Drink ginger root tea (especially if you experience fatigue).
- Put cayenne pepper on food. It is a vasodilator and improves circulation.
    Breathe deeply, relax, notice where you hold tension in your body and let it go.

Most women think of their monthly bleeding as a normal part of their lives. But often they do not know why it happens or why it sometimes changes. Differnt communities and women have many different names for their monthly bleeding.

- I have a visitor
- It's that time for me
- I have my period
- A friend is visiting
- I have my monthly bleeding
- My monthly habit is here
- Aunt Flo is visiting
- I'm on my cycle
- I'm on my moon
- Menses

A woman may find that the time between each monthly bleeding changes as she grows older, after she gives birth, or because of stress.

About 14 days before the end of the cycle, when the soft lining is ready, an egg is released from one of the ovaries. This is called ovulation. The egg then travels down a tube into the womb. At this time a woman is fertile and she can become pregnant. If the woman has had sex recently, the man's sperm may join with her egg. This is called fertilization and is the beginning of pregnancy. During the last 14 days of the cycle—until her next monthly bleeding starts—a woman also produces progesterone. Progesterone causes the lining of the womb to prepare for pregnancy. Most months, the egg is not fertilized, so the lining inside the womb is not needed. The ovaries stop producing estrogen and progesterone, and the lining begins to break down. When the lining inside the womb leaves the body during the monthly bleeding, the egg comes out too. This is the start of a new monthly cycle. After the monthly bleeding, the ovaries start to make more estrogen again, and another lining begins to grow.

More information on our monthly cycle is in the chapter called "Our Moon".

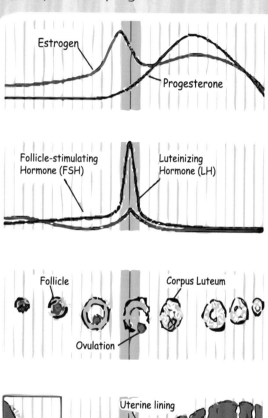

Estrogen

Progesterone

Follicle-stimulating Hormone (FSH)

Luteinizing Hormone (LH)

Follicle

Corpus Luteum

Ovulation

Uterine lining

Menstruation

Follicalar Phase

Luteal Phase

Ovulatory Phase

1 2 3 4 5 6 7 8 9 10 11 12 13 14 15 16 17 18 19 20 21 22 23 24 25 26 27 28

Day of Cycle

Tobacco Use and Impact on Wellness

In some regions of the United States over 50% of Native women use and abuse tobacco. Decreasing or eliminating the non-tradition use of tobacco by Native Women is way to respect our bodies and improve overall wellness.

Tobacco is a sacred plant to many Native Peoples, yet tobacco use in a non-traditional manner leads to many health problems for ourselves and those around us.

Health problems from smoking

Persons who smoke become addicted to a drug in tobacco called nicotine. Without a cigarette, they may feel sick or nervous. It is very hard to stop smoking, because nicotine is a very addictive drug.

In both men and women, smoking can cause:

Serious diseases of the lungs, including chronic bronchitis and emphysema.

- severe colds and coughs.
- cancer of the lung, mouth, throat and neck, and bladder.
- heart attack, stroke, and high blood pressure.

Some of these problems can cause death. In fact, 1 out of 4 people who smoke will die from a health problem connected to smoking.

Smoking is worse for women

In addition to the problems above, women who smoke have a greater risk of:

- difficulty getting pregnant (infertility).
- miscarriage, and babies born too small or too soon.
- problems when using birth control pills.
- monthly bleeding that ends earlier in life (menopause).
- weaker bones that break more easily during mid-life and old age (osteoporosis).
- cancer of the cervix and womb.

A woman who is pregnant should try to avoid other people who are smoking, so that the smoke will not harm her baby.

Children whose parents smoke have more lung infections and other lung and breathing health problems than children whose parents do not smoke.

Two out of five American Indians and Alaska Natives who smoke will die from a health problem connected to smoking.

Smoking can cause disease in those around you who do not smoke.

36

Resources:

Make sure to have an ANNUAL Women's Wellness Exam!

The best gift you can give yourself and your loved ones is health and wellness.

An annual Women's Wellness exam will help screen for and prevent diseases such as breast and cervical cancers and will give you a chance to talk to your health care provider about other women's issues.

Many women find it is easiest to get their annual exam during the same month as their birthday.

A gift to yourself and those you love: *Your wellness.*

www.ourbodiesourselves.org/

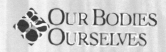

National Women's Health Information Center
The Office on Women's Health

www.4women.gov/
1-800-994-9662 or 1-888-220-5446 for the hearing impaired.
Monday through Friday, 9AM to 6PM EST.

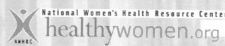

National Women's Health Resource Center (NWHRC) .

www.healthywomen.org/
Call Us: 1-877-986-9472 (toll-free)

www.girlshealth.gov/

Girl Power!,
www.girlpower.gov/

www.cdc.gov/women/

www.ihs.gov/MedicalPrograms/MCH

The Women's Health Center
www.mayoclinic.com/health/womens-health/WO99999

MayoClinic.com
Tools for healthier lives

eHEALTH INFORMATION RESOURCES
TRIBAL CONNECTIONS

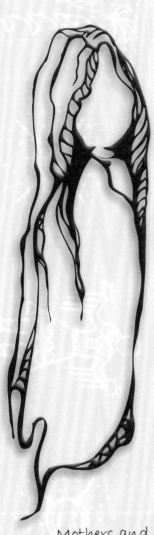
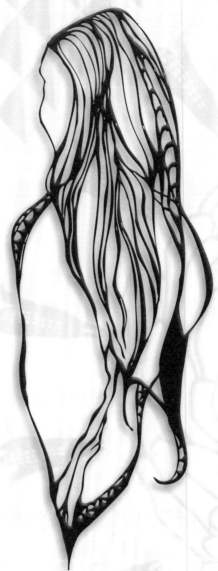

Mothers and Grandmothers, this section will help you discuss, provide encouragement, and support little girls becoming young women. It is a difficult journey to leave childhood behind, so please prepare in a warm and gentle environment, involve them, and answer ALL questions honestly. Journey Woman was born in an age when growing up was not discussed and she does not want to see any daughter raised like she was.

From Girl to Woman

Throughout Native American culture, the transition from girl to womanhood is celebrated in a highly symbolic ceremony that teaches the adolescent girl of her heritage, emphasizing her physical and spiritual transformation into an individual with responsibilities within the tribe. This is also time for inner reflection.

The AWAKENING design on the blanket in the background of this chapter draws its inspiration from the Navajo Kinalda Ceremony, which incorporates song, dance and rituals emphasizing the tribes traditions.

Corn grinding and the baking of a large corn cake in a corn husk basket teaches the girl to understand and cater to her people. The sprinkling of corn pollen on the baked cake symbolizes fertility, nourishment and beauty. The washing of the girl's hair and painting of her body are designed to aid her walk through womanhood.

Traveling in the four directions each day attunes the girl to her physical strength and endurance emphasizing the cycles of the days, seasons and life.

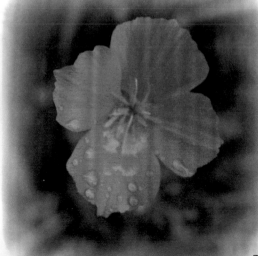

Each of these rituals prepares her for the role she will take upon rejoining the tribe as a woman.

Growing Into Your Woman Body

Sometime between the ages of 10 and 15, a girl's body begins to grow and change into an adult body. These can be exciting and difficult years. A young woman may not feel exactly like a girl or a woman—her body is somewhere in between and is doing new things she is not used to. What can make it harder is when no one talks about the changes, and so a girl may not know what to expect. This chapter describes these changes, tells a girl how she can stay healthy as she grows, and gives information to help her make the right decisions for a healthy life.

All girls go through changes in their bodies, but the changes happen differently for each girl. So do not worry if your body does not look exactly like your sister's or friend's.

Growing

Your first change will probably be that you grow fast. You may be taller than all of the boys your age for a while. You will usually stop growing 1 to 3 years after your monthly bleeding starts. Besides growing fast, your body will begin to change. There are natural chemicals in the body called hormones that tell your body to grow and that make these changes happen.

You grow taller and rounder

- Your face gets oily and pimples or spots may grow.
- You sweat more.
- Hair grows under your arms and on your genitals.
- Your breasts grow as they become able to make milk. As they get larger, it is common for the nipples to hurt sometimes. One breast may begin to grow before the other, but the smaller breast almost always catches up.
- Wetness (discharge) starts to come out of your vagina.
- Your monthly bleeding starts (menstruation).

Changes Inside Your Body

Changes are going on inside your body. As you go through these changes you become more aware of your body. You may also become more interested in boys, and in your friends. There may be times when your feelings are hard to control. In the days before monthly bleeding, it is even more common to have strong feelings of all kinds—joy, anger, and worry, for example. There are other changes that you cannot see. The womb (uterus), tubes, ovaries, and vagina grow and change position.

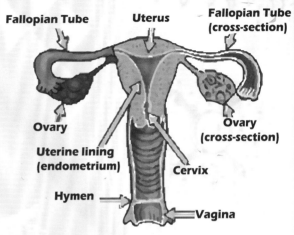

Fallopian Tube Uterus Fallopian Tube (cross-section)

Ovary Ovary (cross-section)

Uterine lining (endometrium) Cervix

Hymen Vagina

As a teen girl, you start developing breasts. You may wish your breasts were bigger, or you may wish they were smaller. The important thing to keep in mind is that every woman is different in the shape and size of her breasts. Your breasts don't need to look like your friend's breasts or a magazine model's breasts. It is very common for your two breasts to be different sizes – especially as you first start developing.

In girls, the breasts may form a mass, or "bud", directly behind the nipple a year or two before your moon starts. As the years go by, the ductal tissue in the bud grows out into fatty tissue. Most of the growth happens early in puberty (between 8 and 13), but slower growth continues during the teen years.

Throughout puberty, you might see or feel lumps and other changes in your breasts. During your period, they may even feel a little tender or sore. Most of the changes your breasts will go through are normal. To get used to these normal changes, you can do regular breast self-examinations (BSE). See the "Breast Cancer" chapter to learn how to correctly do your breast self-exam.

Monthly Bleeding (period, menstruation)

During puberty, hormones are released from the brain that stimulate the ovaries. The ovaries then produce estrogen and progesterone – hormones that cause the eggs in the ovaries to mature so the woman can become pregnant when she chooses to. Here's how the process goes: Every month, one egg leaves one of the ovaries on its way to the uterus via the fallopian tubes. Meanwhile, in preparation for the egg, the uterus starts to develop a thicker lining and it's walls become cushiony (the endometrial lining). If the egg reaches the uterus and is fertilized by a sperm cell, it attaches to this cushiony wall.

Most of the time the egg just passes right through without fertilization. Since the uterus no longer needs the extra blood and tissue which made the walls thick, it sheds them by way of the vagina. This cycle will happen nearly every month until the ovaries stop releasing eggs, usually several decades later. (Menopause).

Your Moon

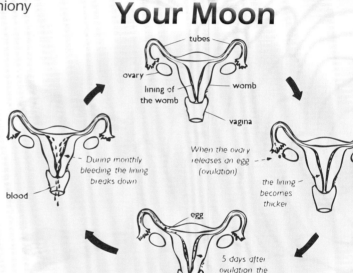

tubes

ovary

lining of the womb

womb

vagina

When the ovary releases an egg (ovulation)

the lining becomes thicker

During monthly bleeding the lining breaks down

blood

egg

5 days after ovulation the lining becomes even thicker

How do I take care of my period?

There are three types of products you can use for your period: sanitary pads, tampons, and menstrual cups. You might decide one is best for you, or you may want to use a combination. No one can see that you are wearing a tampon, pad, or menstrual cup, although you may find some pads to feel a little bulky. You just have to find the right products for you. Whichever ones you use, it is important to follow the instructions on the packaging and wash your hands before and after use.

What to expect with your period

Periods are different for every woman. Some girls start menstruation when they're 9 or 10; some in their late teens. The length of the cycle also varies. Some periods last longer than 28 days, some shorter. If you have just begun your menstruation, your body will need time to regulate itself to these changes. The number of days between your periods may be different each time at first. You may have two cycles in one month and miss having one the next month. How long your period lasts also varies. Some girls have their periods for only 3 or 4 days, others as long as a week. The menstrual flow of blood can vary from woman to woman also.

Some girls may have body and or mood changes around the time of their period. Menstrual cramps are pretty common during the first few days of your period. These are most likely caused by prostagladins (hormones). Prostaglandins causes the muscles of the uterus to contract. These cramps tend to become less uncomfortable and sometimes even disappear completely as a girl gets older. Over-the-counter pain medication like ibuprofen or acetaminophen can often give relief; if not, a health care provider can help. If your cramps are severe, tell your health care provider.

Monthly bleeding is a sign that your body can become pregnant.

No girl can know exactly when she will get her first monthly bleeding. It usually happens after her breasts and the hair on her body start to grow. Several months before her first monthly bleeding, she may notice some wetness coming from the vagina. It may stain her underclothes. This is normal. Some girls are happy when they have their first monthly bleeding, especially if they know what to expect. Girls who were never told about it often worry when the bleeding starts. It is something that happens to all women, and you can feel accepting and even proud of it. It is not something to feel shameful about, it is a natural part of becoming a woman.

Menstruation is the outward proof that a girl is becoming a woman. Having a period is your body's way of saying it's functioning properly.

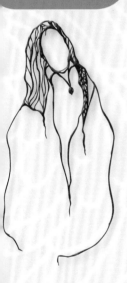

See chapter called "Our Moon" for more information on monthly bleeding.

Your Skin

Your skin is just one more thing that changes when you go through puberty. Acne often starts in your early teen years because your body is making more oil glands, which is normal. A few different skin problems are a part of acne: 1)whiteheads, 2)blackheads, and 3)cystic acne.

1.   **Whiteheads** are made when a hair follicle (root) is plugged with oil and skin cells.

2.   If this plugged up stuff comes up to the surface of the skin and the air touches it, it turns black and becomes a blackhead. So, **blackheads** are not caused by dirt.

3.   If a plugged follicle breaks, the area swells and becomes a red bump. If this happens close to the surface of the skin, the bump most often becomes a pimple. If it breaks deep inside in the skin, nodules or cysts can form, which can look like larger pimples. This is **cystic acne**.

Acne is common among teens, but not everyone will have the same troubles. It may be worse in boys because they have more oils in their skin. Also, it can run in the family. If your mother or father had bad acne, the same may happen for you. Some people also just have more sensitive skin.

How do I know if I'm not getting enough sleep?

Did you know that teens need 8.5 to 9 hours of sleep a night? But research shows that, on average, teens get just 7 to 7.5 hours a night. If you don't get enough sleep, you may have problems paying attention in class or doing your homework. Or you could become moody, irritable, or depressed.

What does not cause acne? Dirt, fried foods or chocolate, and sexual activity do **not** cause acne. These are myths

You may not be getting enough sleep if you:

• have a hard time getting up in the morning
• can't focus
• fall asleep during class
• feel moody or very sad

Sweating

You might think that you are only supposed to sweat when you are hot, but once you hit puberty, you will also sweat when you are nervous. Your sweat glands (which make sweat) become more active during the teen years, causing both more sweat and also some smell. You actually have two to four million sweat glands all over the body. Most are on the soles of the feet, the palms, forehead, cheeks, and in the armpits. Don't panic, though. Sweat and smell are normal parts of becoming an adult. Sweating also does an important job – it helps to cool your body down when you are hot.

You are what you eat!

A lot of the foods that we like to eat don't have much nutritional value. These foods are referred to as "junk food" = empty calories, because while they provide calories that can be turned into energy, they don't provide much else in the way of things our bodies can use.

One of the most important things a girl can do to stay healthy is to eat well. Your body needs to get enough protein, vitamins, and minerals during years of growth. To prevent weak blood (anemia), you will need to replace the lost blood by eating foods with iron in them. Also, girls and women both need foods with calcium to help their bones grow strong.

There are six types of nutrients: protein, carbohydrates, fats, vitamins, minerals, and water. In simple terms, nutrients are the chemicals that your body gets from food. The New Food Pyramid below gives some ideas of types and amounts of food recommended by nutritionists for a healthy, well balanced diet.

New Food Pyramid
www.Stanford.edu

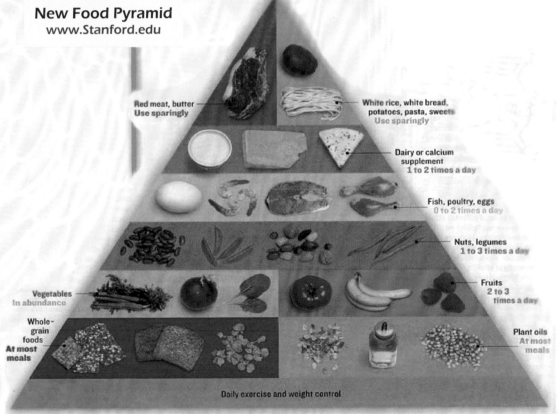

Red meat, butter — Use sparingly

White rice, white bread, potatoes, pasta, sweets — Use sparingly

Dairy or calcium supplement 1 to 2 times a day

Fish, poultry, eggs 0 to 2 times a day

Nuts, legumes 1 to 3 times a day

Fruits 2 to 3 times a day

Vegetables In abundance

Whole-grain foods At most meals

Plant oils At most meals

Daily exercise and weight control

What Happens at a Women's Health Visit?

When you talk with a doctor or nurse about reproductive health issues, he or she may want to do a pelvic exam or a Pap test, particularly if you are sexually active or having physical problems. Keep in mind, it's normal to be nervous before your first pelvic exam. But don't let that stop you from making an appointment! A check-up is one important way to keep yourself healthy.

What questions will the doctor or nurse ask me?
When you talk to any doctor or nurse about your reproductive health, she or he will ask you questions about your general health and any problems you may be having. The questions may be about:

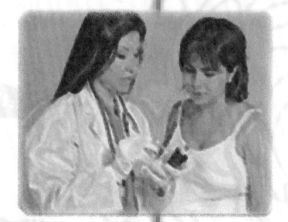

• allergies, medicines you are taking, and any concerns you have about your general health

• your period, such as how long it normally lasts, how old you were when you first got it and the first day of your last period, when your breasts started to develop

• whether you have ever had sex

• your vagina, such as if you have had any unusual discharge (fluid), itching, or odor It is important to be honest so that they have all the right information about your health and body

• questions you may have such as maintaining a healthy diet, how to keep from getting pregnant if you are sexually active, changes in your body and new emotions you may be having

Ask about your doctor or nurse's confidentiality (privacy) policy before you begin. Your doctor might not test you for STIs. If you are sexually active, ask to be tested for all STIs.

e Pap test checks
abnormal cells
your cervix
ening to the
mb). Abnormal
l changes can be
used by the Human
pallomavirus, also
lled HPV.

vaccine to
REVENT the
pes of HPV
at can cause
rvical cancer is
ow available to
rls ages 9-12.

lk to your health
re provider for more
ormation and see
e chapter called
ervical Cancer".

Part of your first visit may be just to talk so you can get to know each other. Your doctor may ask a lot of questions about you and your family. You can also ask the doctor any questions you have. You don't have to be scared or embarrassed.

Many teens have the same questions and concerns. You can also talk to your doctor about:

- cramps and problem periods
- acne
- weight issues
- sexually transmitted diseases
- having the blues or depression

During your visit, your doctor will check your height, weight, and blood pressure. He or she may also do the following exams:

Breast exam – It is really common for young women to have some lumpiness in their breasts, but your doctor will check your breasts to make sure you don't have strange lumps or pain.

Pelvic exam – The doctor will examine inside your pelvic area to make sure your reproductive organs are healthy. The doctor will check out the outside of your genital area (the vulva) and will then use a tool called a speculum to look inside your vagina to see your cervix. Try to relax and breath. Finally, the doctor will feel inside to make sure your internal organs feel okay. There will be pressure, and is not painful for many women. However, this can be painful or uncomfortable for women especiallly those who are not sexually active.

Pap test – If you are 21 or older OR within three (3) years of your first sexual experience, you should have a Pap test. This test is done to make sure the cells in your cervix are normal. The doctor will lightly swab your cervix during your pelvic exam to gather cells that can be looked at on a slide at a lab. It is best to have a Pap test when you don't have your period. If there are any problems with your cells, you should be contacted but it is always a good idea to call your doctors office for the results if you have not heard from them.

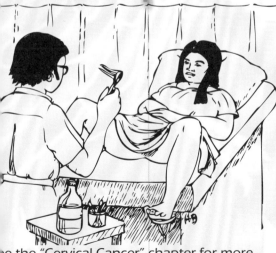

e the "Cervical Cancer" chapter for more
formation on getting your Pap test.

Emotional Wellbeing

As you go through the changes to become a woman you become more aware of your body. You may also become more interested in boys, and in your friends. There may be times when your feelings are hard to control. In the days before monthly bleeding, it is even more common to have strong feelings of all kinds—joy, anger, and worry, for example.

Talking with your mother or father can be hard sometimes.

Your parents may want you to live by tradition, but you feel that times are changing. You may feel that your parents do not listen or try to understand you. Or you may be afraid they will get angry. Your family can love you without agreeing with everything you say. They may get angry because they care —not because they do not like you. Try to talk with them respectfully and help them to understand you better.

How mothers can help their daughters

You may have grown up in a time when girls were not allowed to have an education, plan their families, or make decisions about their lives. Life can be different for your daughter. If you listen to her, share your own experiences, and give her useful information, you can help her make her own good decisions. You can help her to see the good things about being a girl and a woman.

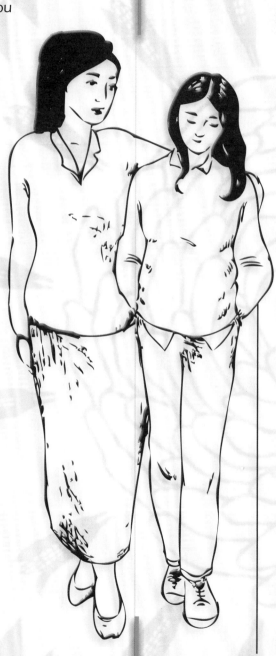

48

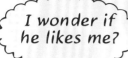

I wonder if he likes me?

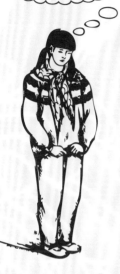

Deciding About Boyfriends and Sex

Decisions about boys and men are difficult. Most young people begin to have loving or sexual feelings as they get older. Thinking about touching or being touched by someone in a sexual way is not unusual. (Girls may even think about another girl or woman in this way.) But people often have these feelings before they are ready to act on them. Young women have sex for many different reasons. Some do it because they want to have a baby. Others do it because it makes them feel good or wanted. Some women feel they have very little choice because it is their duty as a wife. Others have sex because they think it will make a man love them more. Sometimes a friend or a boyfriend can make a girl feel that she should have sex when she is not ready. No one should have sex when she does not want to. Only have sex when you decide you are ready. Sex can be enjoyed by both people, but it is difficult to enjoy something when you feel fear or shame. If you are ready for a sexual relationship, always protect yourself against disease and consider whether you want to take precautions to avoid pregnancy.

Only have sex when you decide that you are ready and know how to protect yourself from harm. Sex can be enjoyed by both people, but not if there is fear or shame.

What Girls Should Know About Having Sex

• You can get pregnant the first time you have sex.

• You can get pregnant any time you have sex without a family planning method (even if it is only once).

• You can get pregnant even if the man thinks he did not let his seed (sperm) come out.

• You can get an STI or HIV/AIDS if you do not use a condom when you have sex with an infected person. And you cannot always tell by looking at a person if he is infected.

• It is easier for a girl to get a sexually transmitted infection (STI) or HIV from a boy or man than it is for her to give these diseases to him. This is because of the way sex works—because she is the 'receiver'. It is also harder to know if a girl has an infection because it is inside her body.

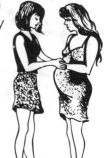

49

Having a Relationship With No Sex

Building a loving relationship takes time, caring, respect, and trust from both sides. Sex is not the only way of showing someone that you care. Having sex does not mean that you will fall in love. You can spend personal time together without having sex. By talking and sharing experiences you can learn something more important about each other—how you view life, decisions you would make together, what kind of partner and parent you would each make, and how you feel about each other's plans for life. Touching each other (without sexual intercourse) can be satisfying by itself, and is not dangerous as long as it does not lead you to lose control and to have sex when you are not ready.

Talk to your boyfriend. If you are sure he is right for you, but you are not sure you want to have sex, talk about ways to wait. You may find that he is not ready for sex, either. If you respect each other, you will be able to decide together. Talk to your friends. You may find that some girl friends are facing the same difficult choices. You can help each other find ways to have good relationships without sex. But think twice about advice from a friend who is already having sex. A friend may try to convince you to do something she is doing to make herself feel better about doing it. This is called 'peer pressure'. Always use a condom for protection against STIs and HIV/AIDS. But the most certain way to avoid pregnancy, STIs, and HIV/AIDS is to not have sex.

Two-Spirit

Two-Spirit are a third gender people (for example, woman-living-man) that are among many American Indian and Canadian First Nations indigenous groups. It can mean having a masculine spirit and a feminine spirit living in the same body. It is also used by some contemporary gay, lesbian, bisexual, transgender, queer, same-sex attracted and intersex Native Americans to describe themselves.

Traditionally, two-spirits were highly regarded and respected as artisans, craftspeople, child rears, couples counselors and tribal arbiters, and yet, one of the reasons they got respect was out of fear, because two-spirits were considered to be touched by the spirits and considered to have powers on the order of a shaman in some tribes.

Protecting Yourself if You Are Ready for Sex

When you decide you are ready for a sexual relationship, you must protect yourself against pregnancy and disease. There are many ways to make sex safer. This means you have to plan before you have sex.

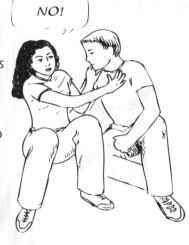

NO!

Many communities have people who are trained to provide condoms and other family planning methods. Talk to them or ask a health provider where to get a method of protection. If you feel embarassed to ask, find someone you trust to help you. Some family planning clinics have special services for teenagers and may have trained teenagers as peer counselors who can give you information.

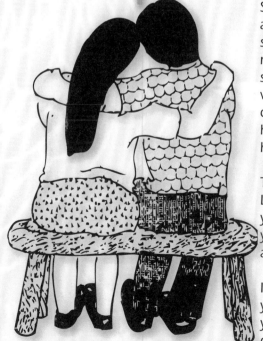

Since you cannot tell by looking if a man has a sexually transmitted infection or AIDS, sex is safer only if you use a condom every time. If a man has a discharge coming from his penis or a sore somewhere on it, he has an infection and will almost certainly give it to you! If he really cares about you, he will want to protect you. If he is pushing for sex, he may care only about himself.

Talk to your boyfriend before you have sex. Let him know how important it is to protect yourself. If you find it hard to discuss, perhaps you can first pretend you are talking about another couple.

If you had sex and notice a new discharge from your vagina, sores on your genitals, or pain in your lower belly, you could have an STI. See the chapter on "Sexually Transmitted Infections."

Healthy Habits for a Lifetime

Starting healthy habits when you are young is the best way to ensure maintain health, preventing diseases such as diabetes, heart disease and sometimes cancer as a woman. Here are some tips:

Avoid non-traditional uses of Tobacco!

Not smoking may be the single most important thing you can do for yourself and your loved ones. Smoking leads to heart disease, cancer, diabetes complications, anxiety, depression, birth defects, asthma, ulcers...the list goes on.

Be aware of what you drink!

It's amazing how many extra calories are in the sodas, juices, and other drinks. Cutting out soda completely can save you 360 calories or more each day. AVOID diet soda too, the artificial sweeteners are probably not good very good for you & they tend to make some people hungry. Drink a lot of water. Switching from whole to nonfat or low fat milk is also a good idea, or switching to soy milk is even a better idea.

Move your body!

You may find that you don't need to give up calories as much as you need to get off your behind. Not a jock, you say? Find other ways to fit activity into your day: walk to school, jog up and down the stairs a couple of times before your morning shower or take a stroll with your friends - anything that gets you moving. Your goal should be to work up to 30 minutes of aerobic exercise at least 3 to 5 times a week - but it's fine to start out by simply taking a few turns around the block before bed. This may also help you to avoid becoming a TV, video game, or Internet junkie!

Stop eating when you're full!

Lots of teens (and adults) eat when they're bored, lonely, or stressed or keep eating long after they're full out of habit. Slowing down can help because it takes about 20 minutes for your brain to recognize how much is in your stomach. Sometimes taking a break before going for seconds can keep you from eating them. Avoid eating when you feel upset or bored.

Five a day (fruits and vegetables)!

Trash the junk food and buy lots of fruits and vegetables! Five or more servings of fruits and veggies aren't just a good idea to help you lose weight - they'll help keep your heart and the rest of your body healthy. Other suggestions for eating well: exchange white bread for whole-wheat; drink lots of water and make sure you eat a healthy breakfast. Don't skip breakfast. (Having low fat cereal and milk and a piece of fruit is a much better idea than inhaling a donut as you run to the bus stop or eating no breakfast at all!)

Do you want more information? Resources :

This site was created to help girls (ages 10-16) learn 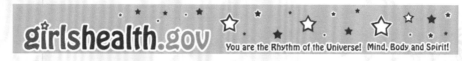 about health, growing up, and issues they may face. It focuses on health topics that girls are concerned about and helps motivate them to choose healthy behaviors by using positive, supportive, and non-threatening messages. The site gives girls reliable, useful information on the health issues they will face as they become young women and tips on handling relationships with family and friends, at school and at home.

http://www.girlshealth.gov/

Girl Power!, the national public education campaign sponsored by the U.S. Department of Health and Human Services to help encourage and motivate 9- to 13- year-old girls to make the most of their lives. Girls at 8 or 9 typically have very strong attitudes about their health, so Girl Power! seeks to reinforce and sustain these positive values among girls ages 9-13 by targeting health messages to the unique needs, interests, and challenges of girls.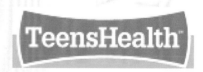

http://www.girlpower.gov/

TeensHealth was created for teens looking for honest, accurate information and advice about health, relationships, and growing up. We offer a safe, private place that's accessible 24 hours a day to get the doctor-approved info you need to understand the changes that you (or your friends) may be going through - and to make educated decisions about your life.

http://www.kidshealth.org/teen

http://www.nlm.nih.gov/medlineplus/teenhealth.html

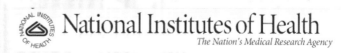

National Institutes of Health
The Nation's Medical Research Agency

Sisters, as we age, wrinkles will start to appear, your moon will stop coming, your breasts may drop, veins may appear on your arms and legs, and your hair will start turning gray, but don't be afraid, ahhhhhhhhhh, you're coming to the best part of your life cycle and you have earned every wrinkle and gray hair.
ENJOY.

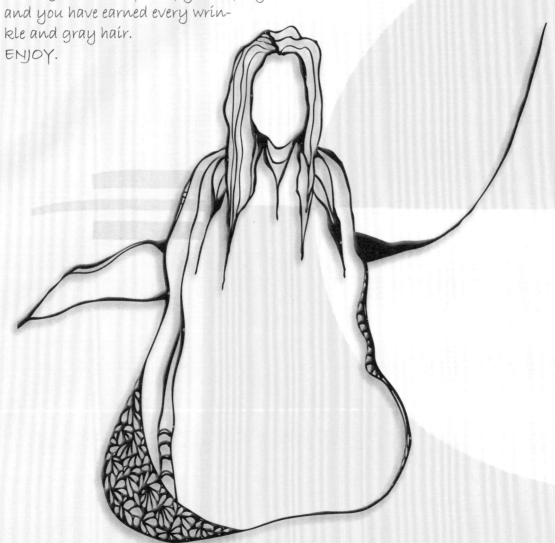

Elder's Journey

Today more and more people are living longer. Cleaner living conditions, vaccinations and better nutrition help prevent many diseases and modern medicines cure others. But longer life has also brought difficulties. First, older people tend to have more health problems than younger people. Although most of these problems are not caused by age itself, the changes age makes in a person's body can make the problems more serious or difficult to treat. Second, as the world changes and younger family members move away from their communities to earn a living, many older people are left to care for themselves. Older women are more likely to face these problems than older men, because women usually live longer and often reach old age without a partner. So in this chapter we describe how older women can take care of their health, treat common health problems of aging, and celebrate becoming an Elder.

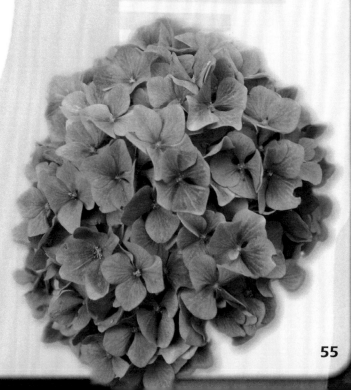

Taking Care of Your Health

Eating Well

As a woman grows older she still needs nutritious food to keep her body strong and to fight disease. Her need for certain kinds of food also increases. Because her body makes less estrogen, it helps to eat foods high in plant estrogens, such as soy beans, tofu (bean curd), lentils, and other beans. Since her bones become less dense as she ages, it helps to eat foods high in calcium, a mineral that makes strong bones. Sometimes older people feel less like eating than they used to. This may be caused by changes in taste and smell, which make eating less pleasurable. Or changes in the body that come from aging can make a person quickly feel full after starting to eat. But this does not mean that older people need less nutritious food. They need encouragement to continue to eat well, and to eat a variety of foods.

Drinking a Lot of Liquids.

As a person ages, the amount of water in the body decreases. Also, some older people drink less to avoid having to pass urine during the night or because they are afraid of leaking urine. All these things can cause dehydration. To prevent this, drink 8 glasses or cups of liquid every day. To avoid getting up at night to pass urine, try not to drink anything for 2 to 3 hours before going to sleep. Just as a girl's body changes when she becomes a woman, so a woman's body changes when her childbearing years end. Menopause and aging cause changes in bone strength, muscle and joint strength and flexibility, and overall well-being. A woman can make a big difference in living her later years with energy and good health by:

Getting regular exercise. Everyday activities, such as walking, playing with grandchildren, going to the grocery store, cooking, and farming can all help keep a woman's muscles and bones strong, and prevent stiff joints. Regular exercise will help maintain weight and prevent heart disease.

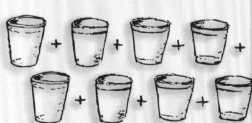

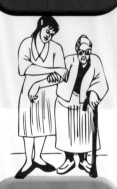

Staying active

A woman will stay healthier and happier if she is active and productive. Try to take up an activity, join a group, or work on a community project. This may be a good time for a woman to work for better conditions in the community.

Treating illness early

Some people think that getting older means being sick much of the time. But this is not true. If a woman does not feel well, she may have an illness that can be treated, and that has nothing to do with age. She needs treatment as soon as possible.

I Was Young Once and Always Will Be

Growing up on a tiny Indian community in Southeastern Oregon and being with older relatives when I was a little girl, I did not look or think of them as being ancient. I saw them as people who had a wealth of knowledge about everything, and I was happy to be around them. Listening to their stories about the "Old days" was listening to history first hand of course it was all in Paiute. These "old ladies" were in their 20's, 30's and maybe the really old ladies were in their 40's! But they were special Indian women to me.

I did not realize at the time that I would someday, be older. Going into my sixties and drawing my "old age pension" were foreign to me as a young person. But, now that I am at that stage of my life and being called an Elder, I reflect on my young life age about how I viewed older people, and ask myself this question, did I pass on the same wisdom and cultural sharing of my people, as my older relatives did for me?

Life for Indian children is so different today, than in the days when I grew up. At an early age I was taught how to find the right plants to dig, pound chokecherries in the fall and gather willow for basketry with my elders. Those were activities that were set in place as children and we did not question why, we just did it. My children were taught by their grandmother early on and today my grandchildren do the same and look forward to it each year.

I teach and share with my grandchildren and others. Because being an Elder, I realize that we have much to offer our Indian people, especially our children. We are the keepers of culture, many of our elders are; the historians of our tribe, many of us speak our tribal language, many of us spend days digging roots and gathering, and many of us are called on to make those special prayers for the sick and to talk on behalf of Indian people. The teachings of our Elders have given us that gift to pass on.

When young people ask me questions about the "old days", I tell them stories about Rock & Roll, of watching the Beatles coming to America, staying up all night to watch "Sputnik and Mission Control", living through the Viet Nam War, and working to get our Paiute people recognized as Indians. Those were the "old days" to me. I smile when I think of the memories with my friends.

I am honored to be called an Elder today I have earned that right in a respectful way by passing on knowledge. Many people just get older.

       -Minerva Soucie

       Enrolled Burns Paiute -Wada Tika

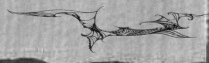

Common Health Problems with Aging

The following pages describe some of the most common health problems of older women. For other problems, like gallbladder problems, heart trouble, stroke, thyroid gland problems, sores on the legs from poor blood flow, and difficulty sleeping, talk to your doctor or contact your clinic. For information on diabetes, see the "Diabetes" chapter or call your local clinic.

High blood pressure

High blood pressure can cause many problems, like heart disease, kidney disease, and strokes. High blood pressure at first causes no signs. It should be lowered before danger signs develop. People who are overweight or who think they might have high blood pressure should have their blood pressure checked regularly.

Weak bones (osteoporosis)

After menopause, a woman's body starts to make less estrogen, and her bones become weaker. Weak bones break easily and heal slowly.

A woman is more likely to get weak bones if she:

- is over 70 years old.
- is thin.
- does not exercise.
- does not eat enough foods rich in calcium.
- has been pregnant many times.
- drinks a lot of alcohol.
- smokes or chews tobacco.

See the "Healthy Bones" chapter to find out more information on maintaining healthy bones.

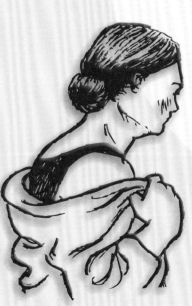

If you are visiting a clinic for any reason try to have your bloo pressure checked at the same time.

If your blood pressure is very high, you may also need to take medicine.

Both exercise and calcium make the bones stronger.

- Walk for 20 to 30 minutes every day
- Eat foods rich in calcium.

Weak bones are a major cause of disability for older women.

Swollen Veins in the Legs (varicose veins)

Varicose veins are veins that are swollen and often painful. Older women who have had many children are most likely to suffer from this problem.

Treatment:

There is no medicine for varicose veins, but the following can help:

- Try to walk or move your legs at least 20 minutes every day.

- Try not to spend much time standing or sitting with your feet down, or with your legs crossed.

- If you have to sit or stand for a long time, try to take breaks to lie down with your feet above the level of your heart. Do this as often as possible during the day.

- When you have to stand for a long time, try to walk in place.

- Sleep with your feet up on pillows or on a bundle of cloth.

- To help hold in the veins, use elastic stockings, elastic bandages, or cloth that is not wrapped too tightly. But be sure to take them off at night.

Joint pain (arthritis)

Many older women suffer from joint pain caused by arthritis. Usually it cannot be cured completely, but the following treatment may help.

Treatment:

- Rest the place that hurts.

- Soak cloths in hot water and place them on the painful areas. Be careful not to burn your skin. (Some people with joint pain lose their sense of feeling from the skin on the painful areas.)

- Keep your joints moving by gently rubbing and stretching them every day.

- Take a mild pain medicine. Aspirin works best for arthritis. Talk to your doctor about using medicine to treat arthritis.

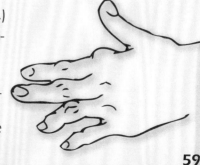

Seeing and Hearing

As they get older, many women are not able to see and hear as well as they used to. Women with seeing or hearing problems are more likely to have accidents, and less likely to work outside the home or to take part in community life.

Problems with seeing

After the age of 40, it is common to have problems seeing close objects clearly. This is called being farsighted. Often eye glasses will help.

A woman should also watch for signs of too much pressure from fluid in the eye (glaucoma), which can damage the inside of her eye and lead to blindness. Acute glaucoma starts suddenly, with severe headache or pain in the eye. The eye will also feel hard to the touch. Chronic glaucoma usually is not painful, but a woman slowly starts to lose vision to the side. If possible, older women should get their eyes checked at a health center for these problems.

Women with diabetes should get their eyes checked for retinopathy every year. For more information, see your doctor at your clinic.

Problems with hearing

Many women over the age of 50 have hearing loss. Other people may overlook the problem since they cannot see it. Or they may start to leave the person out of conversations and social activities.

If you notice that you are losing your hearing, here are some things you can do:

- Sit facing the person you are talking to.

- Ask family members and friends to speak slowly and clearly. But tell them not to shout. Shouting can make words even more difficult to understand.

- Turn off radios or televisions when participating in conversations.

- Ask your health provider if your hearing loss can be treated with medicines, surgery, or by using a hearing aid.

Diabetic Retinopathy

is a leading cause of blindness in American adults. It caused by changes the blood vessels of the retina.

In some people with diabetic retinopathy blood vessels may swell and leak fluid. In other people, abnormal new bloo vessels grow on the surface of the retina A healthy retina is necessary for good vision.

If you have diabetic retinopathy, at first you may not notice changes to your vision. But over time, diabetic retinopathy can get worse and cause vision loss. Routine eye exams can find diabetic retinopathy early.

Mental Confusion (dementia)

Some older people have difficulty remembering things and thinking clearly. When these problems become severe, it is called dementia.

Signs:

- difficulty concentrating, or getting lost in the middle of a conversation.

- repeating the same thing over and over. The person will not remember having said the same thing before.

- difficulty with daily tasks. The person may have trouble knowing how to dress or prepare food.

- behavior changes. The person may become irritable, angry, or do sudden, unexpected things.

Treatment:

There is no special treatment or cure for dementia. Caring for someone who is confused can be very hard on family members. It helps to share the responsibility of care and get support from people outside the family when possible.

To help the person with dementia, try to:

- make her surroundings as safe as possible.

- keep daily routines regular so she knows what to expect.

- keep familiar objects around the house.

- talk to her in a calm, slow voice. Give her plenty of time to answer.

- set clear limits without a lot of choices. Ask questions that can be answered "yes" or "no." These signs are caused by changes in the brain, and usually develop over a long period of time. If the signs begin suddenly, the problem probably has other causes, such as too much medicine in the body (toxicity), a serious infection, malnutrition, or severe depression. The confusion will often go away if these problems are treated.

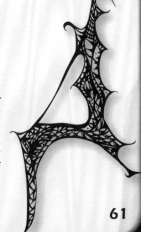

Anxiety and depression

Older women sometimes feel anxious or depressed because their role in the family and community has changed, because they feel alone or worried about the future, or because they have health problems that cause pain and discomfort. For more information on anxiety and depression, see the chapter on "Emotional Well-being."

61

The End of Monthly Bleeding

One of the main signs of growing older is that a woman's monthly bleeding ends. It may end suddenly, or it may stop gradually over 1 to 2 years. For most women this change happens between the age of 45 and 55.

Try to see a health provider at your clinic if you feel ill and have been unable to treat the problem yourself.

Signs:

• Your monthly bleeding changes. It may just stop, or you may bleed more often for a while. Or you may stop bleeding for a few months and then bleed again.

• At times you may suddenly feel very hot or sweaty (this is also called having 'hot flashes'). This can wake you up at night.

• Your vagina becomes smaller and less wet.

• Your feelings change easily.

Hormones

These signs happen because a woman's ovaries stop making eggs, and her body makes less of the hormones estrogen and progesterone. The signs will start to go away as her body gets used to less estrogen. How a woman feels about the end of her monthly bleeding sometimes depends on how she is affected by the changes in her body. It also depends on how her community thinks about and treats older women. She may be relieved not to have her monthly bleeding every month. But she may also feel sad that she cannot have any more children.

Post-menopausal women, in some cultures, were often viewed as the wisest because they retained their "wise blood." In the 17th century these Elder women were constantly persecuted for witch craft because it was thought their menstrual blood remained in their veins.

Journey Woman's husband, a Cherokee, calls himself a "Menopause Survivor." While I was going through changes in my body, I sometimes would become hateful to him for no reason. If he took a shower when I didn't think he should, I cried and yelled, "Why are you taking a shower?" And if he decided to buy chips or something in the store, I cried, "Why do you want chips?" It is funny now, but back then, it was not, at least to him. He would very politely inform those around us that his wife was having "a moment", as he calls it. He would say to me as well, "Is this a moment?" Or, I think you are having "a moment". All in all, he did pretty well and is still with me. I am planning on having a t-shirt made with "Menopause Survivor" on it.

What to do During Menopause

Menopause is a normal part of life. Most women will be able to feel better by following some of the suggestions below. In the past, doctors used to recommend that women take medicines containing estrogen and progesterone to relieve the most severe symptoms of menopause. This is called "Hormone Replacement Therapy" (HRT). Unfortunately, HRT has now been shown to increase women's risk of breast cancer, heart disease, blood and stroke. So a woman should talk to her doctor or nurse about using these medicines.

If you are having signs that make you uncomfortable, try the following:

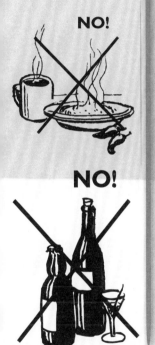

NO!

NO!

- Dress in clothes that you can take off easily when you begin to sweat.

- Avoid hot or spicy foods or drinks. They can cause hot flashes.

- Get regular exercise.

- Do not drink much coffee or tea. They contain caffeine, which can make you feel nervous and prevent you from sleeping.

- Explain to your family that your feelings may change easily. It may also help to discuss how you feel with other women who are going through menopause.

- Ask about the use of traditional remedies in your community. Often women who have already been through menopause will know ways to help you feel better.

- If you drink alcohol, drink only small amounts. Alcohol can increase bleeding and hot flashes.

- Stop smoking or using tobacco in a non-traditional way. It can cause unusual bleeding and make problems with weak bones much worse.

Heavy monthly bleeding

Between the ages of 40 and 50, many women have changes in their monthly bleeding. Some have heavier bleeding, or bleeding that lasts longer. Heavy bleeding that goes on for months or years can cause anemia. The most common causes of heavy monthly bleeding and bleeding that lasts longer are:

- hormone changes
- growths in the womb (fibroids or polyps)

63

Historically, menopause was called many other names, including The Curse, The Change, and women were even locked up in insane asylums. Journey Woman can remember when the word was spoken in a hush, like a bad thing, but we know better. Our life cycle is only taking on another phase of life; that of enjoying life, experiencing new feelings and ideas, making time for us, and living.

When I was going through this cycle, I prepared myself in advance, but still I did not know all of the physical, mental, and spiritual side effects. Sisters, to help prepare you and your daughters, here are a few of the important lessons I learned and from my sisters:

- You may loose some of your hair on your head and eye lashes, but you may also grow hair in other places, such as above your upper lip, on your chest, breasts, and chin.
- Suffer from depression or feeling "blue." This is natural, but if you find you are depressed all of the time or more than every once in a while, please see your health care provider.
- Mood swings; at the drop of a hat.
- Lack of sexual drive or desire and dryness. This is common. Please see your health care provider or talk to a friend or family member. For dryness, there are oils we can use. Remember, talk to your partner and include them. This too will pass if you are open, don't be shy, we are still alive with feelings, express them with love.

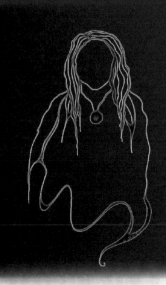

- Insomnia happens to all of us, but if it occurs quite frequently, see you health care provider.
- Weight gain. This gets harder after menopause, has to do with hormones.
- Hormone Replacement Therapy. Be careful here.
- Hot flashes; becoming very hot all of a sudden. I was lucky, but some are not and experience hot flashes for years. There are herbs that can help, but talk to your health care provider as well.

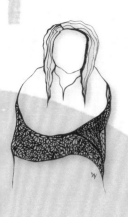

Guess what -

starting at age 50 for most of us, we need to start being screened for a couple of other things including:

•Osteoporosis (see more information in this chapter)

•Colorectal cancer. Talk to your health care provider and find out more about this preventable cancer in the "Other Cancer"chapter.

JourneyWoman's tips To help you prepare for this cycle of life (Menopause):

• Get plenty of exercise, fresh air and sleep.

• Take your vitamins and minerals, eat fruit, vegetables, and high fiber.

• Continue breast screening yearly, remember, as we age, our risk of breast cancer increases. Also, remember to get a complete physical once a year as part of your screenings. Your physical may now include colorectal cancer and osteoperosis screening.

• Continue to get screened for cervical cancer. If you have had 3 normal Paps and haven't change partners, you can have this test less frequently.

• Don't be shy to ask questions from your family, friends, and heath care system.

• Today's pre and post menopausal topics can be confusing, I know I get confused with all of the new terminology. Pay attention to HRTs and ask your health care provider if you have questions.

• Confide in your partner, let them be a part of this wonderful cycle.

• Menopause knows no age limit, sometimes, women in their 30s go through the cycle.

• Pay attention of your body, she will talk to you if you listen.

• Take a breath and smile. Keep laughing, stay strong, and love.

Sexual Relations

For some women, menopause means freedom from the sexual demands of marriage. Other women become more interested in sex because they no longer fear an unwanted pregnancy. All women, though, continue to need love and affection. As a woman grows older, some of the changes in her body may affect her sexual relations:

- She may take longer to become excited during sex (this also happens to men).

- Her vagina may be more dry, which can make sex uncomfortable, or make her get an infection of the vagina or the urine system more easily.

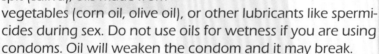

What to do:

- Try to take more time before having sex, so your vagina can make its natural wetness. You can also use spit (saliva), oils made from vegetables (corn oil, olive oil), or other lubricants like spermicides during sex. Do not use oils for wetness if you are using condoms. Oil will weaken the condom and it may break.

> Do not use petroleum gel or oils that contain perfumes to increase wetness in the vagina. These can cause irritation.

> There is no reason based on age alone that a woman cannot enjoy sex for as long as she lives.

Protecting yourself against pregnancy and sexually transmitted infections (STIs)

You can still become pregnant until your monthly bleeding has stopped for one full year. To prevent unwanted pregnancy, you should continue to use a family planning method during that time (see "Family Planning" chapter).

If you are using a hormonal method of family planning (the pill, injections, or implants), stop using it around the age of 50 to see if you are still having monthly bleeding. Use another method of family planning until you have no monthly bleeding for one whole year (12 months). Unless you are certain neither you nor your partner has an STI, including HIV/AIDS, be sure to use a condom each time you have sex—even if you can no longer become pregnant (see "Sexually Transmitted Infections" chapter).

Resources

National Resource Center on Native American Aging (NRCNAA)
The National Resource Center on Native American Aging serves the elderly Native American population of the United States. The Center is committed to increasing the awareness of issues affecting American Indian, Alaskan Native, and Native Hawaiian Elders and being a voice and advocate for their concerns.

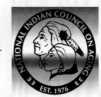

http://ruralhealth.und.edu/projects/nrcnaa/

The National Indian Council on Aging (NICOA) has served as the leading aging organization for American Indian and Alaska Native Elders for over 30 years.

www.nicoa.org/

The goal of the Elder Care Initiative is to promote the development of high-quality care for American Indian and Alaska Native Elders by acting as a consultation and liaison resource for IHS, tribal, and urban Indian health programs.

www.ihs.gov/MedicalPrograms/Elder-Care/

National Association of Area Agencies on Aging

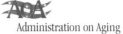
Administration on Aging

www.n4a.org/

www.mayoclinic.com/health/menopause/DS00119

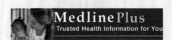
MayoClinic.com
Tools for healthier lives

www.nlm.nih.gov/medline-plus/menopause.html

MedlinePlus
Trusted Health Information for You

www.4women.gov/FAQ/menopaus.htm
1-800-994-9662

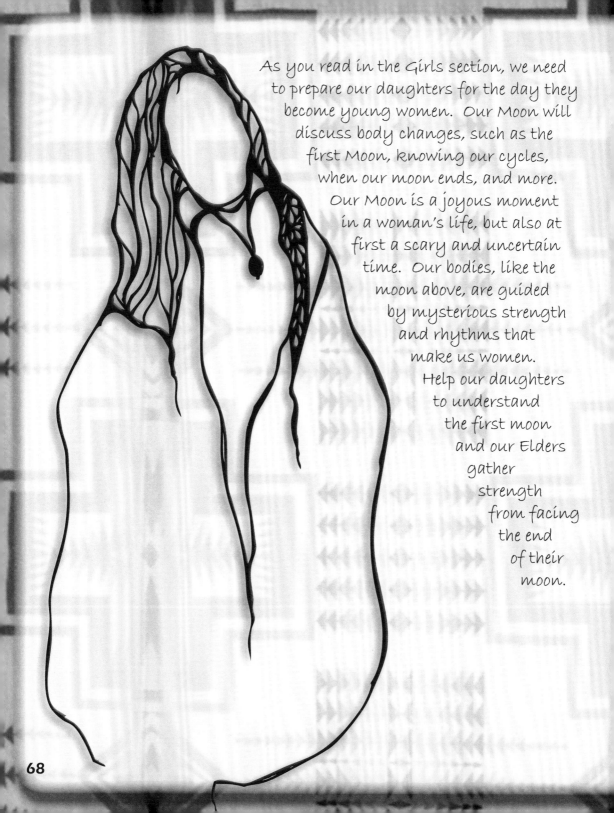

As you read in the Girls section, we need to prepare our daughters for the day they become young women. Our Moon will discuss body changes, such as the first Moon, knowing our cycles, when our moon ends, and more. Our Moon is a joyous moment in a woman's life, but also at first a scary and uncertain time. Our bodies, like the moon above, are guided by mysterious strength and rhythms that make us women. Help our daughters to understand the first moon and our Elders gather strength from facing the end of their moon.

Our Moon

Menstruation has many names – your moon, period, monthly cycle, Aunt Flo. Regardless of what you call it, menstruation is vaginal bleeding that occurs approximately every 28 days in adolescent girls and premenopausal women.

During the monthly menstrual cycle, female sex hormones prepare the uterus to support a pregnancy. If pregnancy takes place, menstruation usually does not return until after childbirth. If pregnancy does not occur, the endometrial lining (the lining of the uterus) sheds during menstruation. Menstrual blood and tissues leave the body through the vagina and it usually lasts from three to seven days.

"Follow your Grandmother Moon. Her illuminating cycles will transform your spirit." Begin with the Grandmother Moon at her brightest and most open. This is a time of outward activity and high energy. Sleep where the moonlight touches you. Walk outside where there are no artificial lights. Feel joy and creativity. As the Grandmother begins to cover her face, begin to withdraw into a quieter, less social place. Move to that inward place that is more about "being" than "doing." In the dark of the moon, when bleeding, the veil between you and the Great Mystery is the thinnest. Be receptive to visions, insights, intuitions. Go to a quiet separate place such as a Moon Lodge. Later, come out of the dark, a woman with a cleansed body. As the moon returns, come back out into the world, carrying your vision."

(from Lakota tradition)

Monthly Cycle (menstrual cycle)

Most women think of their monthly bleeding as a normal part of their lives. But often they do not know why it happens or why it sometimes changes. Different communities and women have many different names for their monthly bleeding.

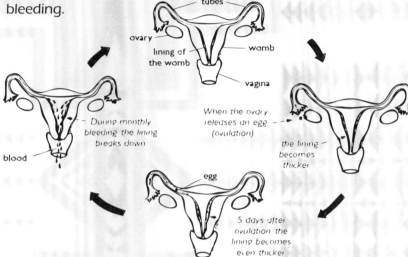

tubes

ovary

lining of the womb

womb

vagina

During monthly bleeding the lining breaks down

blood

When the ovary releases an egg (ovulation)

the lining becomes thicker

egg

5 days after ovulation the lining becomes even thicker

The monthly cycle is different for each woman. It begins on the first day of a woman's monthly bleeding. Most women bleed every 28 days. But some bleed as often as every 20 days or as little as every 45 days. The amount of the hormones estrogen and progesterone produced in the ovaries changes throughout the monthly cycle. During the first half of the cycle, the ovaries make mostly estrogen, which causes a thick lining of blood and tissue to grow in the womb. The body makes the lining so a baby would have a soft nest to grow in if the woman became pregnant that month.

- I have a visitor
- It's that time for me
- I have my period
- A friend is visiting
- I have my monthly bleeding
- My monthly habit is here
- I see the moon
- Aunt Flo is visiting
- Its shark week on the Discovery Channel
- I'm on my cycle
- I'm on my moon
- Menses

Natural options to alleviate cramping:
- Increase exercise. This will improve blood and oxygen circulation throughout the body, including the pelvis.
- Avoid red meat, refined sugars, milk, and fatty foods.
- Eat lots of fresh vegetables, whole grains (especially if you experience constipation or indigestion), nuts, seeds and fruit.
- Avoid caffeine. It constricts blood vessels and increases tension.
- Drink ginger root tea (especially if you experience fatigue).
- Put cayenne pepper on food. It is a vasodilator and improves circulation.
- Breathe deeply, relax, notice where you hold tension in your body and let it go.

What's Happening During Your Cycle

About 14 days before the end of the cycle, when the soft lining is ready, an egg is released from one of the ovaries. This is called ovulation. The egg then travels down a tube into the womb. At this time a woman is fertile and she can become pregnant. If the woman has had sex recently, the man's sperm may join with her egg. This is called fertilization and is the beginning of pregnancy.

During the last 14 days of the cycle—until her next monthly bleeding starts—a woman also produces progesterone. Progesterone causes the lining of the womb to prepare or pregnancy. Most months, the egg is not fertilized, so the lining inside the womb is not needed. The ovaries stop producing estrogen and progesterone, and the lining begins to break down. When the lining inside the womb leaves the body during the monthly bleeding, the egg comes out too. This is the start of a new monthly cycle. After the monthly bleeding, the ovaries start to make more estrogen again, and another lining begins to grow.

> A woman may find that the time between each monthly bleeding changes as she grows older, after she gives birth, or because of stress.

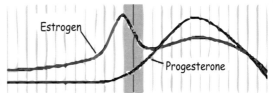

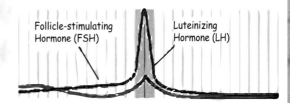

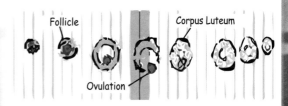

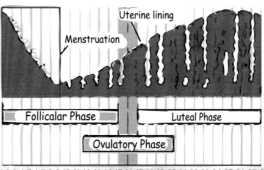

1 2 3 4 5 6 7 8 9 10 11 12 13 14 15 16 17 18 19 20 21 22 23 24 25 26 27 28

Day of Cycle

Pre-Menstrual Syndrome (PMS)

Some women and girls feel uncomfortable a few days before their monthly bleeding begins. They may have one or more of a group of signs that are known as pre-menstrual syndrome (PMS).

Women who have PMS may notice:

- sore breasts
- a full feeling in the lower belly
- constipation (when you cannot pass stool)
- feeling extra tired, irritable or depressed
- sore muscles, especially in the lower back or belly
- a change in the wetness of the vagina
- oiliness or spots (pimples) on the face
- feelings that are especially strong or harder to control

Many women have at least one of these signs each month & some women may have all of them. A woman may have different signs from one month to the next. For many women, the days before their monthly bleeding starts are a time of unrest. But some women say they feel more creative and better able to get things done.

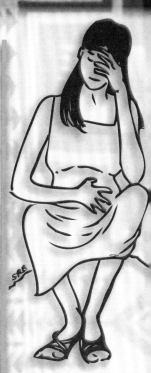

What to do:

What helps with PMS is different for each woman. To find out what will help, a woman should try different things and notice what makes her feel better. First, try following the suggestions for pain with monthly bleeding.
These ideas may also help:

- Eat less salt. Salt makes your body keep extra water inside, which makes the full feeling in your lower belly worse.
- Try to avoid caffeine (found in coffee, tea and some soft drinks like cola).
- Try eating whole grains, peanuts, fresh fish, meat and milk, or other foods that are high in protein. When your body uses these foods, it also gets rid of any extra water, so your belly feels less full and tight. Try plant medicines. Ask the older women in your community which ones work.

Some women have PMDD (Premenstrual dysphc disorder). Th is a severe form of PMS. If you feel like your symptoms are severe, you may wan to talk to your health care provider as there are medications that can help.

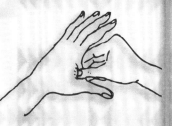

-Acupressure-
Pressing hard on the tender place be-tween your thumb and first finger can ease many kinds of pain.

72

If you have problems with your monthly bleeding, try to talk with your mother, sisters or friends. You may find that they have them too and they may be able to help you.

Pain with monthly bleeding

During monthly bleeding the womb squeezes in order to push out the lining. The squeezing can cause pain in the lower belly or lower back, sometimes called cramps. The pain may begin before bleeding starts or just after it starts.

What to do:

- Rub your lower belly. This helps the tight muscles relax.
- Fill a plastic bottle or some other container with hot water and place it on your lower belly or lower back. Or use a thick cloth you have soaked in hot water.
- Drink tea made from raspberry leaves, ginger, or chamomile. Women in your community may know of other teas or remedies that work for this kind of pain.
- Keep doing your daily work.
- Try to exercise and walk.
- Take a mild pain medicine. Ibuprofen works very well for the pain that comes with monthly bleeding.
- If you also have heavy bleeding and nothing else works, taking a low-dose birth control pill for 6 to 12 months may help (see "Family Planning" chapter).

Changes in bleeding

Sometimes the ovary does not release an egg. When this happens, the body makes less progesterone, which can cause changes in how often and how much a woman bleeds. Girls whose monthly bleeding has just begun—or women who have recently stopped breastfeeding—may only bleed every few months, or have very little bleeding, or too much bleeding. Their cycles usually become more regular with time. Women who use hormonal family planning methods sometimes have bleeding in the middle of the month. See "Family Planning" chapter for more information about changes in bleeding caused by hormonal family planning methods. Older women who have not yet gone through menopause may have heavier bleeding or bleed more often than when they were younger. As they get closer to menopause, they may stop having monthly bleeding for a few months and then have it again.

If you are over 18 and have never had a monthly period, talk to your health provider.

If monthly bleeding suddenly changes, always think about the possibility of pregnancy—even if a family planning method is being used.

Exercise can help with both the signs of PMS and pain with monthly bleeding.

73

Problems with Monthly Bleeding

Heavy monthly bleeding, or bleeding that lasts a long time

- Monthly bleeding is heavy if a pad or cloth is soaked through in less than 1 hour.
- Monthly bleeding is long if it lasts for more than 8 days.
- Blood clots (soft, dark red, shiny lumps in the blood that look like liver) are also a sign of heavy bleeding.
- Heavy bleeding that goes on for many weeks, months or years can cause weak blood, also know as anemia.

Causes:

- The hormones may be out of balance so the ovary does not release an egg. This is common for women under 20 and women over 40 years of age.
- An intra-uterine device (IUD) may be making monthly bleeding more heavy.
- Miscarriage, even if you did not think you were pregnant.

Causes:

- The *hormones* may be out of balance so the *ovary* does not release an egg. This is common for women under 20 and women over 40 years of age

- An *intra-uterine device (IUD)* may be making monthly bleeding more heavy

- *Miscarriage,* even if you did not think you were pregnant

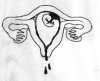

- If you have pain in the abdomen with bleeding, you may have a pregnancy outside the womb in the tube. URGENT. Go to a hospital right away

- You may have a problem with the *thyroid gland.*

- You may have growths (*fibroids* or *polyps*) or *cancer* in your *womb*

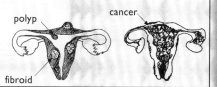

polyp

cancer

fibroid

Danger signs
If a woman has any of these danger signs, she may need medical help right away. See your health care provider if you experience any of these:

- bleeding and pain in the abdomen when regular monthly bleeding has been missed

- bleeding in late pregnancy

- heavy bleeding after childbirth, miscarriage, or abortion

See your doctor if you have heavy bleeding and:
- blood gushes from your vagina.
- monthly bleeding has been heavy and long for 3 months.
- you think you might be pregnant.
- you have severe pain with the bleeding.

Hormonal family planning methods such as pills, implants, or injections, can change monthly bleeding.

Monthly bleeding usually comes about every 21 to 35 days. It may be normal to have an even longer time between bleeding. But something may be wrong, or you may be pregnant, if your monthly bleeding does not come at all.

When monthly bleedings come too far apart, or have stopped

ght bleeding each onth is not a health oblem.
auses:
Some family anning methods— e injections, nplants, and the ll—can make you eed less after ou have been using em for some time. Your ovaries may ot have released an gg.

Causes:

- You may be pregnant.
- You may be pregnant and having a miscarriage.
- The ovary may not have released an egg.
- Stess
- Weight loss.
- If you are over 40 or 45, you may be nearing menopause.
- Some family planning methods—like the pill, injections, and implants—can make monthly bleedings come far apart.

As a woman grows older, her monthly cycle changes.

If you have any of the following problems, tell your doctor right away:

- itching in and near your vagina
- burning or pain in your vagina
- pain when you go to the bathroom
- discharge, or fluid, from your vagina that is not normal, such as thick and white (like cottage cheese) or yellowish-green
- discharge that is foul smelling

75

Other Kinds of Bleeding Problems

BLEEDING DURING PREGNANCY OR AFTER CHILDBIRTH		
Bleeding problem	**May be caused by**	**What to do**
Bleeding during the first 3 months of pregnancy with constant pain or pain that comes and goes	*pregnancy in the tube*	URGENT! Go to a hospital right away.
Bleeding during the last 3 months of pregnancy	the afterbirth (*placenta*) is coming off the wall of the *womb* the placenta is covering the *cervix*	URGENT! Go to a hospital right away.
Bleeding during the first 6 months of pregnancy	may be a *miscarriage* (especially if you also have *cramping* pains like birth pains)	Watch and wait. If bleeding becomes heavy, go to a hospital.
Heavy bleeding during or just after childbirth	pieces of the placenta are left in the womb the womb is too tired to squeeze or tighten	URGENT! go to a hospital if bleeding is heavy.
Light, pink bleeding during the first 3 months of pregnancy without pain	this can be normal, or it may be a sign of early miscarriage	
Spotting or light bleeding instead of your normal monthly bleeding	the developing baby (*fetus*) is attaching to the wall of the womb (*implantation*). This is normal.	

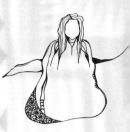

Mothers, this is why it is so important that you have an open-relationship with your daughter and/or niece based upon sharing and respect. Mothers, your little girl is looking to you to guide her in

BLEEDING AFTER AN ABORTION OR MISCARRIAGE

Bleeding problem	May be caused by	What to do
Heavy bleeding, or bleeding that lasts longer than 15 days, or bleeding with pain or fever	pieces of the pregnancy may still be in the womb *infection* in the womb	Go to a hospital or clinic right away.
Bleeding like a normal monthly bleeding, but lasting 5 to 15 days, getting lighter and lighter	this is normal	

BLEEDING AFTER SEX

Bleeding problem	May be caused by	What to do
Bleeding during or after sex	*sexually transmitted infection (STI)* *pelvic inflammatory disease* forced sex growths or cancer of the cervix or womb	See 'gonorrhea and chlamydia'. See 'PID'. See "Rape." See 'cancer of the cervix' and 'problems of the womb'.

BLEEDING AFTER MENOPAUSE

Bleeding problem	May be caused by	What to do
Bleeding that begins 12 months or more after menopause	growths or cancer of the womb growths or cancer of the cervix	See a health worker trained to do a pelvic exam. You may need to have a Pap test or a D and C.

Pain in the Lower Abdomen

Most women have pain in the lower belly or abdomen at some time in their lives. Often women are taught that this pain is normal for them, and that they should endure such pain in silence. Some people think that a woman's pain is not serious until she cannot stand, walk or talk. But when a woman waits that long to seek care for pain, the result could be serious infection, infertility, loss of a pregnancy, or worse..

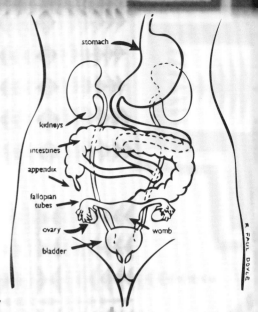

The reproductive organs are in a woman's lower abdomen along with internal organs

This chapter describes different kinds of pain in the lower abdomen (below the navel), and what might be causing the pain. Some pain in the lower abdomen spreads above the navel and could have other causes. Some problems of the lower abdomen will also cause pain in the low back. If the pain seems different from what is described in this chapter, see a health provider trained to give an abdominal exam.

Pain in the lower abdomen can have many causes. It can be difficult to find the cause because so many organs in the abdomen are close together.

Sudden, Severe Pain in the Abdomen

Some lower abdominal pain is an emergency. If you have any of the following danger signs, go to the nearest hospital. A trained health worker will need to do an examination of your abdomen, a pelvic exam, and perhaps special tests. .

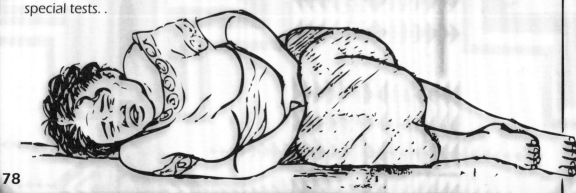

Common growths of the womb

Fibroid tumors

Fibroids are growths of the womb. They can cause abnormal bleeding from the vagina, pain in the lower belly, and repeated miscarriage (losing a pregnancy). They are almost never cancer. Signs:

- heavy monthly bleeding or bleeding at unusual times of the month
- pain or a heavy feeling in the lower belly
- deep pain during sex

Finding and treating fibroids

Fibroids are usually found during a pelvic exam. The womb will feel too large or be the wrong shape. A test called an ultrasound, if it is available, can show how large the fibroids are. If fibroids cause problems, they can be removed with surgery. Sometimes the whole womb is removed. But most of the time, surgery is not necessary because fibroids usually become smaller after menopause and stop causing problems. If monthly bleeding is heavy because of fibroids, anemia may develop. Try to eat foods rich in iron.

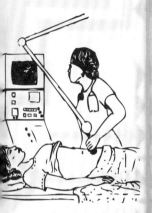

An ultrasound test can show how large fibroids are.

Polyps

Polyps are dark red growths that can grow inside the womb or at the cervix. They are rarely cancer.

Signs:

- bleeding after sex
- heavy monthly bleeding or bleeding at unusual times of the month

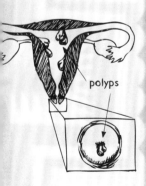

polyps

Finding and treating polyps

Polyps at the cervix can be seen and removed easily and painlessly during a pelvic exam by someone who has been trained. To find polyps inside the womb, the inside of the womb must be scraped out (this is called a D and C). The D and C also removes the polyps. The growth is sent to a laboratory to make sure there is no cancer. Once polyps are removed, they usually do not grow back.

Cysts on the ovaries

These cysts are fluid-filled sacks that women can get on their ovaries. They happen only during the reproductive years, between puberty and menopause. A cyst can cause pain on one side of the lower abdomen and irregular monthly bleeding. But most women only find out they have a cyst if a health care provider feels one during a pelvic examination.

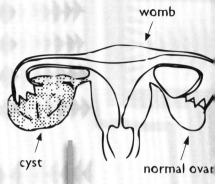

womb

cyst

normal ovar

Most cysts last only a few months and go away on their own. But some can grow very large and must be removed by surgery. If you have severe pain, see a health care provider right away.

Endometriosis

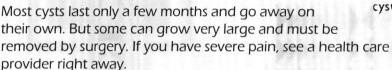

Endometriosis is a condition where tissue similar to the lining of the uterus (womb) is found in other areas in the body near the uterus.

Pain is one of the most common symptoms of endometriosis. Usually the pain is in the abdomen, lower back, and pelvis. The amount of pain a woman feels does not depend on how much endometriosis she has. Some women have no pain, even though their disease affects large areas. Other women with endometriosis have severe pain even though they have only a few small growths. Symptoms of endometriosis include:

- Very painful menstrual cramps
- Pain with periods that gets worse over time
- Chronic pain in the lower back and pelvis
- Pain during or after sex
- Intestinal pain
- Painful bowel movements or painful urination during menstrual • periods
- Heavy and/or long menstrual periods
- Spotting or bleeding between periods
- Infertility (not being able to get pregnant)
- Fatigue

Cancer of the womb

(endometrial cancer, cancer of the uterus)

Cancer of the womb usually starts in the lining inside the womb (the endometrium). If it is not treated it can spread to the womb itself and to other parts of the body. This cancer happens most often to women who:

- are over 40 years old, especially if they have gone through menopause.
- are overweight.
- have diabetes.
- have taken the hormone estrogen without also taking progesterone.

Signs:

- heavy monthly bleeding
- irregular monthly bleeding, or bleeding at unusual times of the month
- bleeding after menopause

Finding and treating cancer of the womb

To find out if a woman has cancer of the womb, a trained health care provider must scrape out the inside of the womb with a D and C, or do a biopsy, and send the tissue to a laboratory to be checked for cancer. If cancer is found, it must be treated as soon as possible with an operation to remove the womb (hysterectomy). Radiation therapy may also be used.

Hysterectomy

In a hysterectomy, sometimes only the womb is removed and sometimes the tubes and ovaries are also removed. Since your ovaries make hormones that help protect you against heart disease and weak bones, it is always better to leave them in, if possible. Talk to a doctor about this.

Important: If you have any bleeding at all, even light spotting, after you have finished menopause (12 months without monthly bleeding), get checked by a health provider to make sure you do not have cancer.

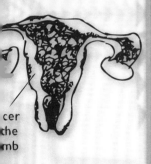

cancer of the womb

If cancer of the womb is found early, it can be cured. If it is more advanced, curing it is more difficult.

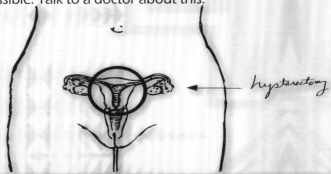

hysterectomy

Describing Pain

Many women may not be used to admitting to others and using words to describe pain. Some women can endure amazing amounts of pain while no one around them knows. If possible, it is important to talk to your doctor about any pain a woman may be having. Pain in the abdomen can mean many things. Here are some ideas on how to best describe the pain a woman may be having. This will help your doctor make a correct diagnosis and find help with the pain.

Sometimes a doctor v give you a diagram the body so you ca mark the areas whe you have pain

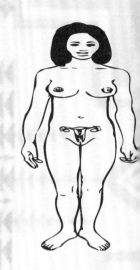

- Where is the pain?

- When describing pain, which words best describe what you experience.

☐ burning, ☐ stabbing, ☐ gnawing, ☐ cramping,

☐ jabbing, ☐ throbbing, ☐ cold, ☐ sharp,

☐ aching, ☐ pressure ☐ other_____.

- Do you have pain with your menstrual periods?

- Do you have painful bowel movements?

- Do you have pain during or after sexual intercourse?

- Tell your physician if you're missing work or school or avoid outings due to your symptom The doctor will also ask if the pain is preventing you from engaging in sports or exercise.

- From the time the pain started until now, has it gotten worse? If so, double? Triple? More

- How bad is your pain?

☐ Pain free.
☐ Very minor annoyance - occasional minor twinges.
☐ Minor annoyance - occasional strong twinges.
☐ Annoying enough to be distracting.
☐ Can be ignored if you are really involved in your work, but still distracting.
☐ Can't be ignored for more than 30 minutes.
☐ Can't be ignored for any length of time, but you can still go to work and participate in social activities.
☐ Makes it difficult to concentrate, interferes with sleep You can still function with effort. Stronger painkillers are only a little effective.
☐ Physical activity severely limited. You can read and have conversation with effort. Pain causes nausea and dizziness..
☐ Unable to speak, crying out or moaning uncontrollably, near delirium.
☐ Unconscious. Pain makes you pass out.

Pain should not be a normal part of a woman's life—it is a sign that something is wrong. Seek care before you are so ill that you cannot stand, walk, or talk.

Kinds of Pain in the Lower Abdomen

If your pain does not fit one of the kinds described in the following tables, these questions may help to learn more about it. What is the pain like? Is it sharp and severe—or dull, achy, and not so bad? Does it come and go, or is it constant?

- Terrible pain that comes and goes could be from a kidney stone. Severe grabbing, clenching, or cramping pain could be from an intestinal problem.

- Sharp, severe pain, especially just in one place, could be appendicitis or a pregnancy outside the womb in the tube.

How long has the pain lasted?
- Sudden, severe pain that does not get better is probably serious. It could be from a pregnancy in the tube, appendicitis or other gut problems, something wrong with the ovary, or pelvic inflammatory disease (PID).
- Pain that lasts for many days or weeks, especially if it is not severe, may be caused by scars from an old infection, indigestion, or nerves. It may be possible to treat this at home.

Does the pain affect your hunger?
- If you have pain in the abdomen and you DO NOT want to eat anything, you may have a serious infection in your intestines, or appendicitis.
- If you have pain and you do feel like eating, you probably do not have one of these problems.

For more information on pain in the lower abdomen, talk to you clinic or doctor or refer to another general medical book.

Kind of pain	May be caused by	What to do
Severe, unusual pain during monthly bleeding or after a monthly bleeding was missed	pregnancy in the tube	URGENT! Go to hospital right away
Ongoing pain during monthly bleeding	fibroids	See 'pain with monthly bleeding' and 'problems of the womb' Use a mild pain medicine.
Cramps during monthly bleeding	normal squeezing of the womb. Some kinds of intra-uterine devices (IUDs) may make the pain worse.	See 'pain with monthly bleeding'
If the monthly bleeding is late	miscarriage	If pain becomes severe, go to a hospital.

Kind of pain	May be caused by	What to do
Pain during sex	pelvic inflammatory disease (PID), or scars from an old pelvic infection	See 'PID'.
	a growth on an ovary (ovarian cyst)	See 'problems of the ovaries'.
	fibroids	See 'problems of the womb'.
	unwanted sex	See 'if sex is painful'.
Pain when moving, walking, or lifting	old pelvic infection, or any of the reasons listed above	Use mild pain medicine if needed.
Pain that lasts only a few hours in the middle of your *monthly cycle*	the lining of the abdomen gets irritated when the ovary releases an egg (ovulation) because there is a small amount of blood blood	Use mild pain medicine if needed.
Pain within 3 weeks of getting an intra-uterine device (IUD)	infection with an IUD is most common soon after the IUD is put in	See a health worker right away.
Pain without other signs	pelvic infections, which can cause constant or on-and-off pain in the abdomen or lower back that lasts for months or years	See a health worker trained to do a pelvic exam.
	intestinal infection from *bacteria* or *parasites*	
	tumor or growth on the womb or ovary	See a health worker trained to do a pelvic exam.

For more information on pain in the lower abdomen, talk to you clinic or doctor or refer to another general medical book.

Kind of pain	May be caused by	What to do
Pain after childbirth, miscarriage, or abortion	infection from pieces of afterbirth (placenta) left in the *womb*, or *germs* that got into the womb during the birth or abortion	See a health worker right away.
Severe pain with or without fever (infection) with or after having a sexually transmitted infection or pelvic infection	another pelvic infection, or a pocket of *pus* in the abdomen (pelvic abcess)	URGENT! Go to a hospital right away.
on one side of the abdomen, with or without *fever, nausea, vomiting,* and no appetite	*appendicitis* or other *intestinal* infection	URGENT! Go to a hospital right away.
	kidney infection	See 'bladder and kidney infections'
Pain with *diarrhea*	intestinal infection from bacteria or parasites	See 'diarrhea'.
Severe pain in the first 3 months of pregnancy, often with bleeding that comes and goes	pregnancy in the tube	URGENT! Go to a hospital right away.
Severe pain in the last 3 months of pregnancy, with or without bleeding	placenta has pulled away from the wall of the womb	URGENT! Go to a hospital right away.
Mild, occasional pain during pregnancy	probably normal	No treatment needed.
Pain with frequent or painful urination	*bladder* or *kidney* infection	See 'bladder and kidney infections'.
Pain with blood in the urine	kidney stone	See 'kidney or bladder stones'.
Pain with *discharge* or light bleeding from the *vagina,* sometimes with fever	pelvic infection which may be caused by a *sexually transmitted infection (STI)*, or by infection after miscarriage, *abortion,* or childbirth	See 'pelvic inflammatory disease',

Resources:

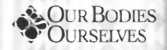

www.ourbodiesourselves.org/

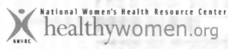

National Women's Health
Information Center
The Office on Women's Health

www.4women.gov/

1-800-994-9662 or 1-888-220-5446 for the hearing impaired.
Monday through Friday, 9AM to 6PM EST.

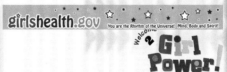

National Women's Health
Resource Center (NWHRC) .

www.healthywomen.org/

Call Us: 1-877-986-9472 (toll-free)

www.girlshealth.gov/

Girl Power!,
www.girlpower.gov/

www.cdc.gov/women/

www.ihs.gov/MedicalPrograms/MCH

The Women's Health Center
www.mayoclinic.com/health/womens-health/WO99999

Moon Calendar

You can use this calendar to help keep track of your cycle. You can circle the first and last days of your moon for each month so you will know your own body's rhythm.

January	February	March	April	May	June	July	August	September	October	November	December
1	1	1	1	1	1	1	1	1	1	1	1
2	2	2	2	2	2	2	2	2	2	2	2
3	3	3	3	3	3	3	3	3	3	3	3
4	4	4	4	4	4	4	4	4	4	4	4
5	5	5	5	5	5	5	5	5	5	5	5
6	6	6	6	6	6	6	6	6	6	6	6
7	7	7	7	7	7	7	7	7	7	7	7
8	8	8	8	8	8	8	8	8	8	8	8
9	9	9	9	9	9	9	9	9	9	9	9
10	10	10	10	10	10	10	10	10	10	10	10
11	11	11	11	11	11	11	11	11	11	11	11
12	12	12	12	12	12	12	12	12	12	12	12
13	13	13	13	13	13	13	13	13	13	13	13
14	14	14	14	14	14	14	14	14	14	14	14
15	15	15	15	15	15	15	15	15	15	15	15
16	16	16	16	16	16	16	16	16	16	16	16
17	17	17	17	17	17	17	17	17	17	17	17
18	18	18	18	18	18	18	18	18	18	18	18
19	19	19	19	19	19	19	19	19	19	19	19
20	20	20	20	20	20	20	20	20	20	20	20
21	21	21	21	21	21	21	21	21	21	21	21
22	22	22	22	22	22	22	22	22	22	22	22
23	23	23	23	23	23	23	23	23	23	23	23
24	24	24	24	24	24	24	24	24	24	24	24
25	25	25	25	25	25	25	25	25	25	25	25
26	26	26	26	26	26	26	26	26	26	26	26
27	27	27	27	27	27	27	27	27	27	27	27
28	28	28	28	28	28	28	28	28	28	28	28
29	29	29	29	29	29	29	29	29	29	29	29
30		30	30	30	30	30	30	30	30	30	30
31		31		31	31		31		31		31

Raising children is not an easy task, it is not like television or movies; it is real. You will be a parent the rest of your life and responsibilities do not end when the child is 18 years. When planning your family, think about, are you ready? A good job and education to provide for a child? Have you traveled and done all you want to as a single person? And, do you have a strong family support system? Mothers and Grandmothers, it is important for you to help your daughters make good choices that will effect their health and happiness for years to come.

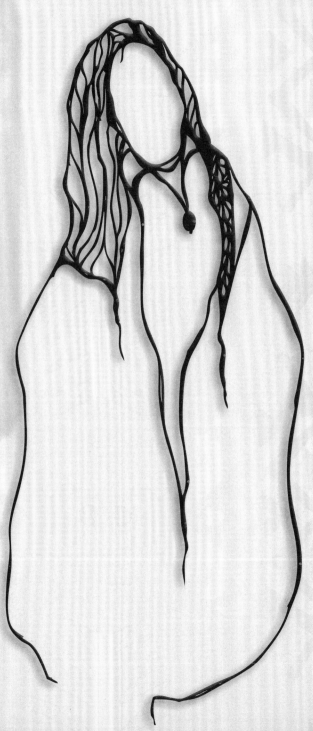

Family Planning

Having the number of children you want, when you want them, is called family planning. If you decide to wait to have children, you can choose one of several methods to prevent pregnancy. These methods are called family planning methods, child spacing methods, or contraception.

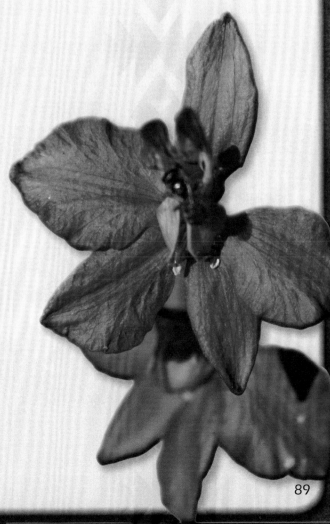

Choosing a Family Planning Method

Once you have decided to use family planning, you must choose a method. To make a good decision you must first learn about the different methods, and their advantages and disadvantages.

There are 5 main types of family planning methods:

1. **Barrier methods,** which prevent pregnancy by keeping the sperm from reaching the egg.

2. **Hormonal methods,** which prevent the woman's ovary from releasing an egg, make it harder for the sperm to reach the egg, and keep the lining of the womb from supporting a pregnancy.

3. **IUDs, (intra-uterine device)** which prevent the man's sperm from fertilizing the woman's egg.

4. **Natural methods**, which help a woman know when she is fertile, so that she can avoid having sex at that time.

5. **Permanent methods.** These are operations which make it impossible for a man or a woman to have any children.

It may also help to talk with your partner, other women, or a health care provider about different methods. Only you can decide which family planning method is best for you.

These methods of family planning are described on the following pages. As you read about each method, here are some questions you may want to consider:

- How well does it prevent pregnancy (its effectiveness)?

- How well does it protect against STIs, if at all?

- How safe is it? If you have any of the health problems mentioned in this chapter, you may need to avoid some types of family planning methods.

- How easy is it to use?

- Is your partner willing to use family planning?

- What are your personal needs and concerns? For example, do you have all the children you want, or are you breast-feeding your baby?

- How much does the method cost?

- Is it easy to get? Will you need to visit a health center often?

- Will the side effects (the problems the method may cause) create difficulties for you?

The information in this table is a general comparison of family planning methods.

Make sure to talk to your health care provider for more information. Some methods may vary in side effects dependant on the dose or device used. For example, one type of IUD may cause heavy and painful bleeding and another brand/type may cause your period to be lighter or even go away.

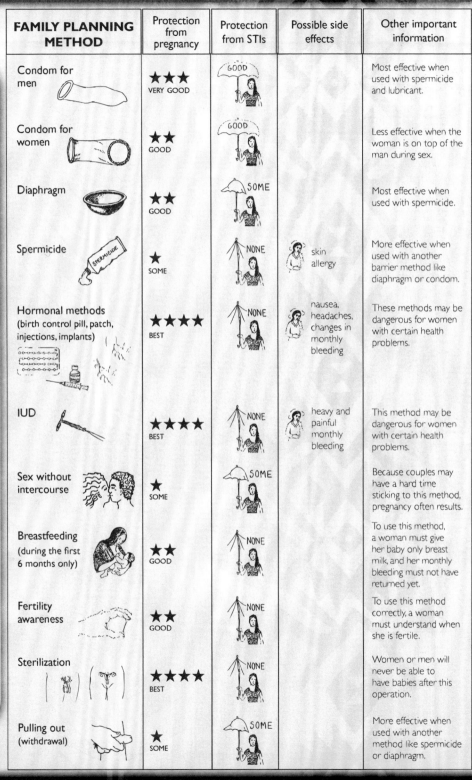

FAMILY PLANNING METHOD	Protection from pregnancy	Protection from STIs	Possible side effects	Other important information
Condom for men	★★★ VERY GOOD	GOOD		Most effective when used with spermicide and lubricant.
Condom for women	★★ GOOD	GOOD		Less effective when the woman is on top of the man during sex.
Diaphragm	★★ GOOD	SOME		Most effective when used with spermicide.
Spermicide	★ SOME	NONE	skin allergy	More effective when used with another barrier method like diaphragm or condom.
Hormonal methods (birth control pill, patch, injections, implants)	★★★★ BEST	NONE	nausea, headaches, changes in monthly bleeding	These methods may be dangerous for women with certain health problems.
IUD	★★★★ BEST	NONE	heavy and painful monthly bleeding	This method may be dangerous for women with certain health problems.
Sex without intercourse	★ SOME	SOME		Because couples may have a hard time sticking to this method, pregnancy often results.
Breastfeeding (during the first 6 months only)	★★ GOOD	NONE		To use this method, a woman must give her baby only breast milk, and her monthly bleeding must not have returned yet.
Fertility awareness	★★ GOOD	NONE		To use this method correctly, a woman must understand when she is fertile.
Sterilization	★★★★ BEST	NONE		Women or men will never be able to have babies after this operation.
Pulling out (withdrawal)	★ SOME	SOME		More effective when used with another method like spermicide or diaphragm.

91

Barrier Methods of Family Planning

Barrier methods prevent pregnancy by blocking the sperm from reaching the egg. They do not change the way the woman's or man's body works, and they cause very few side effects. Barrier methods are safe if a woman is breastfeeding. Most of these methods also protect against STIs, including HIV/AIDs. When a woman wants to become pregnant, she simply stops using the barrier method. The most common barrier methods are the condom, condoms for women, the diaphragm, and spermicides.

The condom

The condom is a narrow bag of thin rubber that the man wears on his penis during sex. Because the man's semen stays in the bag, the sperm cannot enter the woman's body. Condoms made

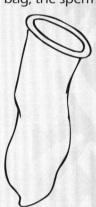

of latex are the best protection against STIs and HIV/AIDS. They can be used alone or along with any other family planning method. Condoms can be bought at many pharmacies and grocery stores, and are often available at health clinics and through AIDS prevention programs. Be careful not to tear the condom as you open the package. Do not use a new condom if the package is torn or dried out, or if the condom is stiff or sticky. The condom will not work. The condom must be put on the man's penis when it is hard, but before it touches the woman's genitals. If his penis touches the woman's genitals or goes into her vagina, he can make the woman pregnant or can give her an STI, even if he does not spill his sperm (ejaculate).

How to us a condom

1. If the man is not circumcised, pull the fore skin back. Squeeze the tip of the condom and put it on the end o the hard penis.

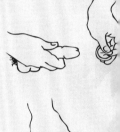

3. After the man ejaculates, he should hold on to the rim of the condom and withdraw from the vagina while his penis is still hard.

Lubricants

Lubricants make the vagina or the condom wet and slippery. They help to keep condoms from breaking and can make sex safer and more enjoyable. Lubricants should be water based, such as spit (saliva), spermicide, or K-Y Jelly. Rub the lubricant on the sides of the condom after it is on the hard penis. Don't use anything with an oil base like baby oil, mineral oil, petroleum gel or skin lotion. They can make the condom break easily.

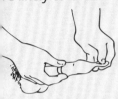

eep squeezing the
while unrolling the
ndom, until it cov-
all of the penis. The
se part at the end
hold the man's
rm. If you do not
ve space for the
rm when it comes
, the condom is
re likely to break.

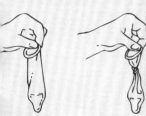

Take
the
ndom.
not let
rm spill
eak.

5. Tie the
condom
shut and
dispose
of it away
from chil-
dren and
animals.

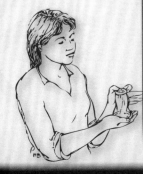

Remember:
• Use a condom every time you have sex.
• If possible, always use condoms made of latex. They give the best protection against HIV. Condoms made of sheepskin may not protect against HIV.
• Keep condoms in a cool, dry place away from sunlight. Condoms that are from old or torn packages are more likely to break.
• Use a condom only once. A condom that has been used before is more likely to break.
• Keep condoms within arm's reach. It is less likely that you will use them if you have to stop what you are doing to look for them.

Question: Which one of these effectively protects you against pregnancy and sexually transmitted infection?

A.   B.

Don't leave your health to luck. Condoms significantly reduce your risk of pregnancy and sexually transmitted infection.

At first, many couples do not like to use condoms. But once they get used to it, they may even recognize benefits besides protecting against unwanted pregnancies and STIs. For example, condoms can help some men last longer before they come.

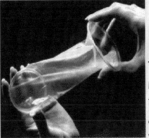

Condoms for women (female condoms)

The female condom is a reversible barrier method of birth control. It is a polyurethane (plastic) pouch with flexible rings at each end. It is inserted deep into the vagina like a diaphragm. The ring at the closed end holds the pouch in the vagina. The ring at the open end stays outside the vaginal opening. A female condom, which fits into the vagina and covers the outer lips of the vulva, can be put in the vagina any time before sex. Female condoms are larger than condoms made for men and are less likely to break.

How the Female Condom Works: The female condom collects semen before, during, and after ejaculation and keeps sperm from entering the vagina.

The female condom is the most effective of the methods controlled by women in protecting against both pregnancy and STIs, including HIV/AIDS.

93

The diaphragm

The diaphragm is a shallow cup made of soft rubber that a woman wears in her vagina during sex. The diaphragm covers the cervix so that the man's sperm cannot get into her womb. The diaphragm should be used with spermicide. If you do

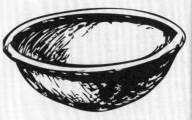

not have spermicide, you can still use the diaphragm, but it may not work as well to prevent pregnancy. Diaphragms come in different sizes, and are available at some health posts and family planning clinics. A health worker who has been trained to do pelvic exams can examine you and find the right size diaphragm. Diaphragms can get holes, particularly after being used for more than a year. It is a good idea to check your diaphragm often. Replace it when the rubber gets dry or hard, or when there is a hole in it. You can put the diaphragm in just before you have sex or up to 6 hours before. If you have sex more than one time after you put the diaphragm in, put more spermicide in your vagina each time before you have sex.

How to use a diaphragm:

1. If you have spermicide, squeeze it into the center. Then spread a little bit around the edge with your finger.

2. Squeeze the diaphragm in half.

3. Open the lips of your vagina with your other hand. Push the diaphragm into your vagina. It works best if you push it toward your back.

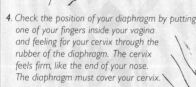

4. Check the position of your diaphragm by putting one of your fingers inside your vagina and feeling for your cervix through the rubber of the diaphragm. The cervix feels firm, like the end of your nose. The diaphragm must cover your cervix.

5. If the diaphragm is in the right place, you will not be able to feel it inside you.

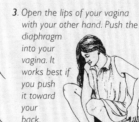

6. Leave the diaphragm in place for at least 6 hours after sex.

You can leave the diaphragm in for up to 24 hours. It is OK to use the diaphragm during monthly bleeding, but you will need to remove it and clean it as often as you would change a cloth or pad.

To remove the diaphragm:

Put your finger inside your vagina. Reach behind the front rim of the diaphragm and pull it down and out. Wash your diaphragm with soap and water, and dry it. Check the diaphragm for holes by holding it up to the light. If there is even a tiny hole, get a new one. Store the diaphragm in a clean, dry place.

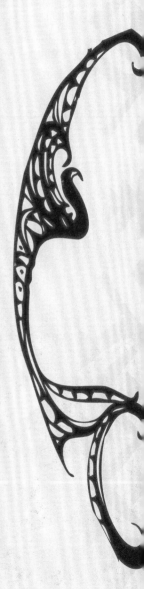

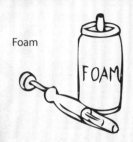

Foam

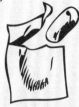

Tablets

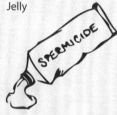

Cream or
Jelly

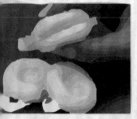

The
sponge is
placed in the vagina
in front of the cervix.

Spermicide comes in many forms—foam, tablets, and cream or jelly—and is put into the vagina just before having sex. Spermicide kills the man's sperm before it can get into the womb. If used alone, spermicide is less effective than some other methods. But it is helpful when used as extra protection along with another method, like the diaphragm or condom.

Spermicides can be bought in many pharmacies and grocery stores. Some women find that some types of spermicides cause itching or irritation inside the vagina. No spermicide provides protection against any STI. Because spermicides can irritate the walls of the vagina, they may cause small cuts that allow HIV to pass more easily into the blood.

Spermicide

When to insert spermicide:

Tablets or suppositories should be put in the vagina 10 to 15 minutes before having sex. Foam, jelly, or cream work best if they are put in the vagina just before having sex. If more than one hour passes before having sex, add more spermicide. Add a new tablet, suppository, or applicator of foam, jelly, or cream each time you have sex.

The sponge is a soft round piece of polyurethane foam containing several different spermicides. It can stay in your vagina up to 12 hours. The sponge absorbs and traps sperm using spermicide to kill sperm . The sponge sits in front of the cervix making it more difficult for sperm to enter. The sponge is 75 to 90 percent effective when used alone. It may be more effective when combined with another method of birth control like a condom. Even alone, the sponge provides some protection against sexually transmitted infections.

A cervical cap is a latex, thimble-shaped device that is inserted into the vagina and fits snugly over the cervix. Suction keeps

Cervical Cap

the cap in place. A cervical cap provides a barrier to block sperm from entering the uterus and prevents fertilization. After intercourse, it should be left in place for 8 hours. A cervical cap is used with spermicidal jellies or creams that kill sperm. As birth control, cervical caps are 84-91% effective for women who have never given birth. They are 68-74% effective for women who have given birth.

Hormonal Methods of Family Planning

These methods contain hormones, called estrogen and progestin, that are similar to the estrogen and progesterone a woman makes in her own body. Hormonal methods include:

> **Important**
> Hormonal methods do not protect against STIs, or HIV/AIDS.

- **implants,** which are put into a woman's arm and last for several years.
- **pills**, which a woman takes every day.
- **injections**, which are given every few months.
- **patches**, which are worn daily
- **vaginal ring**, which last one month to one year.

Hormonal methods work by preventing the woman's ovaries from releasing an egg. The hormones also make the mucus at the opening of the womb very thick, which helps stop the sperm from getting inside the womb.

Most birth control pills and some injections contain both estrogen and progestin. These are called 'combination' pills or injections. The two hormones work together to give excellent protection against pregnancy. However, some women should not use pills or injections with estrogen for health reasons, or because they are breastfeeding. 'Progestin-only' pills (also called mini-pills), implants, and some injections contain only one hormone—progestin. These methods are safer than combined pills or injections for women who should not use estrogen, or are breastfeeding.

Types of Hormonal Birth Control Methods

- implants, which are put into a woman's arm and last for several years.

- injections, which are given every few months.

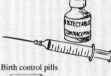

Birth control pills

Vaginal ring

Birth control patch

These women should avoid any kind of hormonal method:

- Women who have breast cancer, or a hard lump in the breast. Hormonal method do not cause cancer. But if a woman already has breast cancer, these methods can make it worse.

- Women who might be pregnant or whose monthly bleeding is late.

- Women who have abnormal bleeding from the vagina during the 3 months befo starting hormonal methods. They should see a health worker to find out if there is a serious problem.

Some hormonal methods are harmful for women with other health problems. Be sure to check each method to see if it is safe for you. Talk to your health care provider.

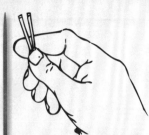

Implants are small, soft tubes that are placed under the skin on the inside of a woman's arm. These tubes contain the hormone progestin and work like mini pills. They prevent pregnancy for 3 years.

Implants

If you are bothered by any body changes after starting birth control pills, talk to a health provider. She might suggest a different pill.

To stop using implants:

Implants can be removed at any time. After removal, you can get pregnant right away, so use another family planning method if you do not want to become pregnant.

Implants can be used by women who are breastfeeding and others who have problems with estrogen. Women should not use implants if they have any of the conditions described on page 97, if they have heart disease, or if they want to become pregnant in the next few years. If you are taking medicines for seizures, you will need to use a backup method, like a condom or a diaphragm, as well as the implants.

Many women want their implants removed early because they do not like the side effects. The most common concern is irregular bleeding.

Common side effects of implants:

During the first months, the implants may cause irregular bleeding (in the middle of your monthly cycle) or more days of monthly bleeding. Or you may have no bleeding at all. This does not mean that you are pregnant or that something is wrong. These changes will go away as your body becomes used to having more progestin. If this irregular bleeding causes problems for you, a health worker may have you take low-dose combined birth control pills along with the implants for a few months. You may also have occasional headaches and the same side effects common with progestin-only injections.

Implants:

A trained health provider makes a small cut in the skin to insert and remove the implants. This is usually done at a clinic or family planning center.

97

The Pill

The Pill is the most popular type of birth control. There are many different brands of The Pill and they come in packs of 21 or 28 pills. One pill is taken every day. The first 21 pills have a combination of synthetic estrogen and progesterone hormones. The Pill stops ovulation, preventing the ovaries from releasing eggs. The Pill also thickens cervical mucus, making it harder for sperm to enter the uterus. The hormones in the Pill prevent fertilization. The last 7 pills of a 28-day pack have no hormones and are called spacer pills. The Pill is 92-99.7% effective as birth control. It does not pro-tect against sexually transmitted infections, including HIV/AIDS.

pills, which a woman takes every day.

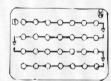

Combined Birth Control Pills - Birth control pills with estrogen and progestin

If you take birth control pills every day, they will protect you from pregnancy for your entire monthly cycle. These pills are usually available at family planning clinics, health clinics. There are many different brands of pills. The pill you get should be what is called a 'low-dose' pill. This means it has about 20 micrograms (mcg or µcg) of the estrogen. (Mini-pills and low-dose pills are different—lowdose pills have both estrogen and progestin, while the mini pill has only progestin.) Never use a method with more than 50 mcg of estrogen. Once you start taking pills, you should try to stick with one brand. If you must change brands, try to get another with the same hormone names and strength. You will have fewer side effects and bet-ter protection.

Birth Control Pills

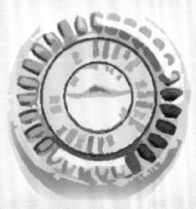

Some women find that taking the pill helps their monthly bleeding to be more regular, with less bleeding and less pain.

Warning signs for problems with combined pills

STOP taking the pill and see a health care provider if you:

• have severe head-aches with blurred vision (migraines) that begin after you start taking the pill.

• feel weakness or numbness in your arms or legs.

• feel severe pain in your chest and short ness of breath.

• have severe pain in one leg.

If you must change to a lower dose pill use a barrier method of family planning or do not have sex during the first month.

These women should avoid combined birth control pills:
If you have any of the following health problems, try to use a method other than combined birth control pills. Try not to take combined pills if you:

- **smoke and are over 35 years old**. You have a greater chance of having a stroke or heart attack if you take combined pills.

- **have diabetes or epilepsy**. If you are taking medicine for seizures ("fits"), you will need to take a stronger (50 micrograms of estrogen) birth control pill. Get medical advice from your doctor.

- **have high blood pressure (more than 130/80)**. If you have ever been told you have high blood pressure or think you might have it, have your blood pressure checked by a health provider. If you weigh too much, have frequent headaches, get out of breath easily, feel weak or dizzy often, or feel pain in the left shoulder or chest, you should be tested for high blood pressure.

Common side effects of combined pills

- **irregular bleeding or spotting** (bleeding at other times than your normal monthly bleeding). Combined pills often make your monthly bleeding shorter and lighter. It is also normal to sometimes skip your monthly bleeding. This is the most common side effect of combined birth control pills. To reduce spotting, be extra careful to take the pill at the same time every day. If the spotting continues, talk with a health worker to see if changing doses of progestin or estrogen will help.

- **nausea.** Nausea, the feeling that you want to throw up, usually goes away after 1 or 2 months. If it bothers you, try taking the pills with food or at another time of day. Some women find that taking the pill just before going to sleep at night helps.

- **headaches.** Mild headaches in the first few months are common. A mild pain medicine should help.

The Mini Pill or Progestin-only Pills

Because this pill does not contain estrogen, it is safer for women who should avoid combined birth control pills (see pages 208 and 209) and for women who have side effects from combined pills. But this pill is less effective than combined birth-control pills.

The mini pill is also a better choice for women who are breast-feeding because it does not cause a decrease in the milk supply. The mini pill is very effective for most breastfeeding mothers. Like the combined pill, it is usually available at family planning clinics, health posts, pharmacies, and through health workers.

Women who are taking medicine for seizures should not take the mini pill. The medicine makes the mini pill less effective.

Common side effects of the mini pill:
- **irregular bleeding or spotting**. This is the most common side effect. If it becomes a problem, taking ibuprofen may help stop spotting.
- **no monthly bleeding.** This is fairly common, but if you go more than 45 days without bleeding you may be pregnant. Keep taking your pills until you can see a health worker to find out if you are pregnant.
- **occasional headaches.**

How to take the mini pill:
- Take your first pill on the first day of your monthly bleeding.
- Take one pill at the same time each day, even if you do not have sex. If you take a pill even a few hours late or forget only one day's pill, you can become pregnant.
- When you finish a packet, start your new packet the next day, even if you have not had any bleeding. Do not skip a day.

Stopping the mini pill:
You can stop taking the pill any time. You can get pregnant the day after you stop, so be sure to use another family planning method right away if you do not want to become pregnant.

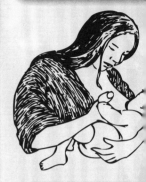

The mini pill is safe and effective durin breastfeeding.

If you are breast-feeding and have not started your monthly bleeding, you can start taking the pills any day. You may not begin bleeding. This is normal.

What to do if you miss a mini pill:
Take it as soon as you remember. Take the next pill at the regular time, even if it means taking 2 pills in one day. You may have bleeding if you take your pill at a later time than usual.

You must take one pill every day, even if you do not have sex. Try to take your pill at the same time every day. It may help to remember that you will always start a new packet on the same day of the week.

Keep the packet where you can see it every day. If you still forget to take your pills often (more than once a month), think about changing to a different method of birth control.

If your monthly bleeding does not come at the normal time and you have missed some pills, continue to take your pills but see a health care provider to find out if you are pregnant.

With both 21-day and 28-day packets, take the first pill on the first day of your monthly bleeding. This way you will be protected right away. If it is after the first day, you can start taking a pill on any of the first 7 days of your monthly cycle. But you will not be protected right away, so for the first 2 weeks you are taking the pill you should also use another family planning method or not have sex.

If you forget to take pills

If you miss pills you could get pregnant. If you forget one pill, take it as soon as you remember. Then take the next pill 12 hours later until you get caught up. This may mean that you take 2 pills in one day.

If you forget to take 2 pills in a row, take emergency contraception if you have had sex during these days. Restart taking your pill the next day. If you do not take Emergency Contraception, skip your missed pills and complete the rest of the pack, use a barrier method of birth control until the next period starts. Late or missed pills may cause some bleeding, like a very light monthly bleeding.

If you have trouble remembering to take pills, try taking a pill when you do a daily task, like preparing the evening meal. Or take the pill when you see the sun go down or before you sleep.

If you vomit within 3 hours after taking your pill or have severe diarrhea, your birth control pill will not stay in your body long enough to work well. Use condoms, or do not have sex, until you are well and have taken a pill each day for 7 days.

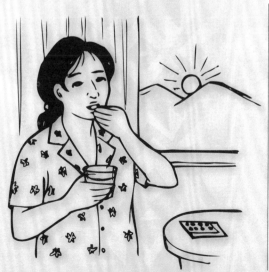

Continous Oral Contraceptives

Birth Control Pills may be prescribed to be taken in cycles or continuously.

This means either:

1 cycle = 21 days on, 7 days off
2 cycles = 42 days of hormone pills, 7 days off,
3 cycles = 63 days of hormones, 7 days off
4 cycles = 84 days of hormones, 7 days off

The concept of taking the pill without a break to avoid the monthly period is not a new one; doctors have long adopted a process called tricycling (pronounced "tri-cycling") for women who suffer seriously from headaches or bad PMS during the pill-free week. In this process, three packets of pills are run together, avoiding bleeding for 62 days.

Pills may be prescribed in long cycles or continuously for girls with endometriosis, bad cramps, Polycystic Ovary Syndrome (PCOS), or other reasons. Continuously means that you will be taking one pill that contains the female hormones, estrogen and progesterone, every day. Taking the pill this way helps keep the lining of the uterus very thin. The goal is for you to have no periods. You will not take a week of placebo pills (sugar pills without hormones) and will not have a regular monthly menstrual period. You may have some irregular spotting or bleeding as your body gets adjusted to this new medication, especially in the first six months.

Vaginal Rings

Vaginal rings slowly release estrogen and progestin, or just progestin, into a woman's vagina. Vaginal rings come in only one size and a woman can put one in herself. They last from 1 month to 1 year. You can get pregnant as soon as you stop using a ring. the vaginal ring is worn for three weeks, and then stopped for a week for menstruation. Both methods are approximately 99% effective.

Vaginal ring

How do I take them?

How do I take them?

Take one pill at the same time every day. When you finish one pack of the hormone pills, begin another pack of pills the following day.

If you buy 21-day packs of pills, start a new pack the day after you finish all the pills in your current pack. If you buy 28-day packs of pills, take the three weeks of hormone pills but not the week of placebo pills (the last seven pills that are a different color). When you finish the hormone pills, throw the pack away and start a new pack the next day.

The Patch

The patch is a thin piece of plastic that sticks to the skin and releases both estrogen and progestin into the body. You must put on a new patch once a week for 3 weeks in a row, then no patch for 1 week. The patch can have the same side effects as combined pills.

The patch looks like a square Band-Aid and is worn on the skin. It contains hormone medicine similar to birth control pills but the dose absorbed through the skin is 60% higher than the birth control pills with 35ug of estrogen. This may increase the risks of side-effects such as blood clots and makes it particularly important that patch users not smoke. When used correctly, the patch is as effective as birth control pills in preventing pregnancy. Like birth control pills, your health care provider may also prescribe the patch for irregular periods, menstrual cramps, or endometriosis. Doctors and researchers found that the patch was 99% effective in preventing pregnancy.

Where on my body do I wear the patch?
The patch can be worn on the skin of your abdomen (stomach), buttocks, upper back or the outside part of your upper arm. Wherever you decide to put it, you must leave it there for 7 days.

If you forgot to restart your patch on time after your week off, apply it as soon as you remember. You MUST use another method of birth control such as condoms for at least 1 week. The first day that you apply your patch is considered Day 1 of your new patch cycle.

If your patch loosens, press down firmly along the edges of the patch with your finger for about 10 seconds. If your patch still doesn't stick, remove and apply a new patch.

The Birth Control Patch

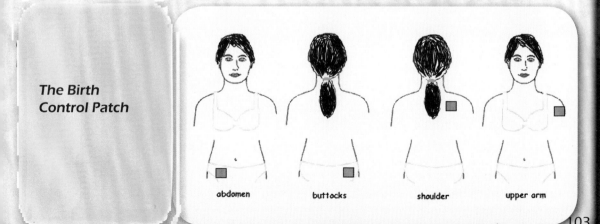

abdomen   buttocks   shoulder   upper arm

Birth Control Injections

In this family planning method, a woman is given injections of hormones every 1 to 3 months, usually at a health center or family planning clinic, by someone who knows how. The protection lasts until you need a new injection, and can be used without others knowing.

Progestin-only injections almost always cause changes in the monthly bleeding. You may have light bleeding every day or every once in a while. You will probably stop having monthly bleeding by the end of the first year. These changes are normal.

Progestin-only injections

Progestin-only injections, such as Depo Provera and Noristerat, contain only the hormone progestin. These are especially good for women who are breastfeeding and women who should not use estrogen. They are given **every 2 to 3 months**.

Women should not begin progestin-only injections if they have any of the conditions listed on page 97, if they are unable to get regular injections, or if they want to become pregnant within the next year.

The FDA now warns that prolonged use of projectin-only injections may cause decreased bone density.

Common side effects of progestin-only injections:

Because of the large doses of progestin given with each injection, women experience more changes in their monthly bleeding during the first few months than with other hormonal methods.

Other common side effects are:
• irregular bleeding or heavy spotting. If this is a problem, a health worker can give 2 cycles of a combined low-dose birth control pill to take along with the injections to stop the spotting. Most irregular bleeding will stop after a few months.
• no monthly bleeding.
• weight gain.

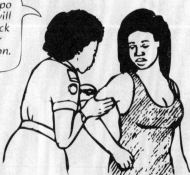

You are using Depo Provera, so you will need to come back in 3 months for your next injection.

How to use birth control injections:

It is best to get your first injection during your monthly bleeding. This way you know that you are not pregnant. You can start the injections anytime if you are breastfeeding and have not started your monthly bleeding.

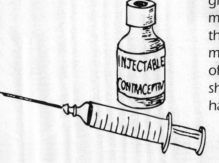

The injection protects you against pregnancy immediately if it is given within 5 days after your monthly bleeding begins. If the injection was given 6 or more days after the beginning of your monthly bleeding, you should use condoms or not have sex for the next 2 weeks.

You must have an injection every 3 months.

Try not to be late getting injections. The injection becomes less effective the longer you wait.

To stop using injections:

You can stop having birth control injections any time you want. But after you stop, it can take a year or more to become pregnant and for your monthly bleeding to return to normal. But it also may come back sooner. So if you do not want to become pregnant right away, you must use another family planning method during this time.

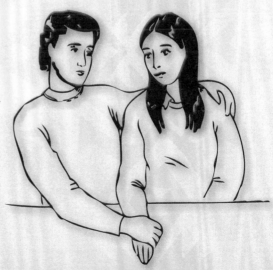

Intra- Uterine Devices (IUD)
(Devices that go into the womb)

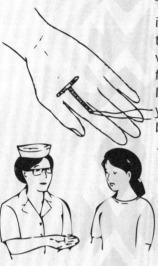

The IUD is a small object or device that is inserted into the womb by a specially trained health care provider. Once in the womb, the IUD prevents the man's sperm from fertilizing the woman's egg. The IUD can stay in the womb for up to 10 years (depending on the kind of IUD it is) before it must be removed and replaced. An IUD can be used without the man knowing you are using it (although sometimes a man can feel the strings). The most common IUDs are made of plastic, or plastic and copper.

IUDs do not protect against STIs, including HIV/AIDS. And if a woman has an STI, the IUD can lead to more serious complications, such as pelvic inflammatory disease (PID). PID can lead to infertility.

Mirena IUD
women who use Mirena often experience shorter and lighter periods. Some women's periods stop completely after a few months.
It works by delivering a very small amount of a progestin directly on the inner wall of the uterus. This dose is similar to taking two or three mini-pills a week.

Who should not use an IUD:
Do not use an IUD if you:
- are pregnant or might be pregnant.
- are in danger of getting an STI. (This includes any woman who has more than one partner, or whose partner may have other sex partners.)
- have ever had an infection in your tubes or womb, or an infection after giving birth or after having an abortion.
- have had a pregnancy in your tubes.
- have a lot of bleeding and pain during your monthly bleeding.

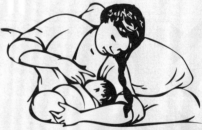

IUDs can be used safely by women who are breastfeeding.

Common side effects:
You may have some light bleeding during the first week after getting an IUD. Some women also have longer, heavier, and more painful monthly bleeding, but this usually stops after the first 3 months.

How to use the IUD:

An IUD must be inserted by a specially trained health care provider after doing a pelvic exam. The best time to have the IUD put in is during your monthly bleeding. After childbirth, it is best to wait 6 weeks for the womb to return to its normal size and shape before getting an IUD.

Occasionally an IUD will slip out of place. If this happens, it will not be effective in preventing pregnancy, so it is important to learn to check your IUD to make sure it is still in place. Most IUDs have 2 thread-like strings attached which hang down into the vagina. You should check the strings after each monthly bleeding to make sure the IUD is in place.

Warning signs for problems with an IUD:

Pelvic inflammatory disease is the most serious problem that can result from having an IUD. Most infections happen in the first 3 months, usually because the woman already had an infection when the IUD was put in. Or it may happen because the health worker did not put in the IUD under clean conditions.

If you have any of the following signs, you should see a health care provider trained to insert IUDs and to treat complications, or go to a hospital immediately:

- Your monthly bleeding is late.
- You have pain in your lower belly or pain during sex.
- You have a heavy or bad-smelling discharge from the vagina.
- You do not feel well, or have fever or chills.
- Your IUD string is missing, or is shorter or longer than usual.
- Your partner can feel the IUD (not just the strings) during sex.

To stop using an IUD:

When you want to stop using an IUD, it must be removed by a trained health care provider. Never try to remove an IUD yourself. You can become pregnant as soon as it has been removed.

Do not use an IUD if you are unable to get to a health center or clinic where you can have the IUD removed if necessary.

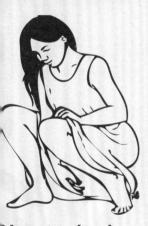

How to check the IUD strings:

1. Wash your hands.

2. Squat down and reach as far as you can into your vagina with your 2 fingers. Feel for the IUD strings, but do not pull them.

3. Take out your fingers and wash your hands again.

Natural Methods of Family Planning

There are also 3 methods to avoid pregnancy that do not require any devices or chemicals (as with barrier methods) or medicines (as with hormonal methods). The methods are:
- breastfeeding for the first 6 months
- the mucus method
- the rhythm method

Natural methods of family planning do not protect against STIs, including HIV/AIDS. If you use any of the natural methods listed in these pages, you still need to think about ways to protect yourself from these diseases.

Breastfeeding for the first 6 months
(lactational amenorrhea method, LAM)

Breastfeeding under certain conditions can prevent the ovaries from releasing an egg. This method does not cost anything, but it is most effective for only the first 6 months after childbirth.

Breastfeeding is an effective method of family planning only when these 3 conditions are true:

1. Your baby is less than 6 months old.

2. You have not had your monthly bleeding since giving birth.

3. You are giving your baby only breast milk, and feeding it whenever it is hungry—with no more than 6 hours between feedings—day and night. Your baby does not sleep through the night without feeding.

Use another method of family planning that is safe with breastfeeding as soon as any of the following things happen:

- Your baby is more than 6 months old, or
- Your monthly bleeding starts, or
- Your baby starts taking other kinds of milk or other foods, or starts sleeping for more than 6 hours during the night, or
- You must be away from the baby for more than 6 hours and cannot remove milk from your breasts during that time.

Traditional method that may work

Withdrawal or pulling out (coitus interruptus). With this method, a man pulls his penis out of the woman and away from her genitals before he ejaculates. This method is better than no method, but it does not always work. Sometimes a man is not able to pull out before he ejaculates. Even if the man pulls out in time, some liquid that contains sperm can leak out of his penis before ejaculation and cause pregnancy.

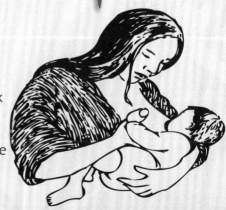

raditional
ethods that do
ot work or that
an be harmful

Washing out the
gina (douching)
ith herbs or powders
oes not prevent preg-
ancy. Sperm move
ry fast and some will
ach the inside of the
omb before they can
e washed out.

Urinating after sex
oes not prevent preg-
ancy. (But it can help
prevent infections of
e urine system.)

> All these methods
> require the man's
> cooperation or
> they will not be
> effective.

The Mucus Method and the Rhythm Method

To use either of these methods, you must understand when you are fertile during your monthly cycle. This is sometimes called 'fertility awareness'. Then, to avoid pregnancy, you and your partner must not have sex, or must use a barrier method of family planning, during your fertile days.

Because there are no costs or side effects, these methods can be used by women who cannot or do not want to use other methods, or when other methods are not available. To practice fertility awareness more effectively, both you and your partner should visit a specially trained health care provider to learn about your bodies and about fertility. It usually takes about 3 to 6 months of practice to learn how to use these methods.

The mucus & rhythm methods do not work as well if:

- you have little control over when you will have sex. During your fertile times, your partner must be willing to wait and not have sex or to use condoms or some other barrier method.
- your fertility signs change from month to month. You will not be able to know when you are fertile.
- you have just had a baby or miscarriage. It is hard to know when you are fertile at these times.

To make all natural family planning methods more effective:

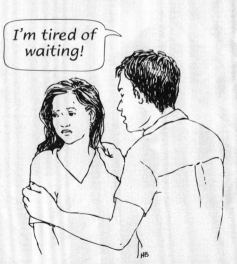

I'm tired of waiting!

- Have sex only on the days between the end of the fertile time and your next monthly bleeding.
- Use both the mucus method and the rhythm method at the same time.
- Use condoms whenever you are not sure if you are fertile, or do not have sex.

109

What you should know about a woman's cycle of fertility:

- A woman releases one egg each month.
- The egg is released from the ovary about 14 days before the next monthly bleeding.
- The egg lives for about 24 hours (1 day and 1 night) after it has been released from the ovary.
- The man's sperm (seed) can live up to 2 days inside the woman's body.

By itself, the mucus method is not as reliable as other methods of birth control and has an average failure rate of 20% per year.

Mucus Method (also called Ovulation method)

To use the mucus method, you must pay careful attention to the mucus (wetness) in your vagina. Your body produces wet mucus during your fertile time to help the sperm get into the womb. So if you check your mucus every day, you will know when you are becoming fertile. Then you can avoid sex during this time.

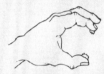

white, dry, sticky mucus = not fertile

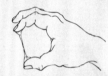

clear, wet, slippery mucus = fertile

How to tell when you are fertile:

1. Wipe the outside of your vagina with your finger or a piece of paper or cloth.
2. If there is mucus there, take some between your fingers. How does it feel? Wet and slippery? Dry and sticky?

How to use the mucus method:

- Do not have sex on any day you see or feel wetness or mucus. Or, if you want to have sex on those days, use a condom or a diaphragm without spermicide (these are the only methods that do not change the mucus).
- Do not have sex until 4 days after the last day of clear, slippery mucus.
- Do not have sex during your monthly bleeding. There is a small possibility you could be fertile and not be able to tell.
- Do not douche or wash out your vagina at any time.
- If you are having trouble knowing when you are fertile, or if you have a vaginal infection, you should use another method.

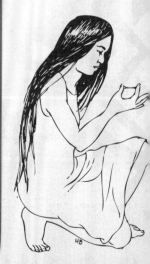

Rhythm Method

The rhythm method teaches you to find your fertile time by counting the days in your monthly cycle. You CANNOT rely on the rhythm method if:

- you are breastfeeding and your monthly bleeding has not returned.
- you have recently been pregnant and your monthly bleeding is not yet regular.
- you do not have regular periods.

How to use the rhythm method:

- Count the number of days in each of your monthly cycles for 6 months, from the first day of one monthly bleeding until the first day of the next.
- Pick out the longest and the shortest cycles.
- Take away or subtract 20 days from your shortest cycle and 10 days from your longest cycle. The time between these 2 days is your fertile time.
- Although you can have sex any time before or after your fertile time, the safest time is between the end of your fertile time and the beginning of your next monthly bleeding.

For example: Julia kept track of her monthly bleeding for 6 months. Her shortest cycle was 26 days and her longest cycle was 34 days:

To avoid pregnancy, Julia should not have sex, or she should use another family planning method, from day 6 after her monthly bleeding starts until day 24.

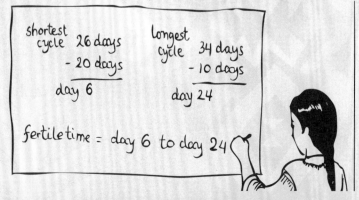

shortest cycle 26 days
− 20 days
day 6

longest cycle 34 days
− 10 days
day 24

fertile time = day 6 to day 24

Effectiveness
The rhythm method has an average failure rate of 13% to 20%. It is not recommended for women who have irregular cycles or who do not have menstrual cycles that are exactly the same number of days every month.

You must use another method of family planning while you are counting your 6 monthly cycles. But you should not use the pill, implants, or injections during the time you are counting, because these methods change the time when your monthly bleeding starts.

Emergency Contraception
(also called the "Morning After" pill or Plan B)

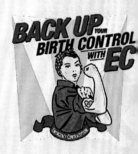

Is the Morning-After Pill Right for Me?
(from Planned Parenhood.org)

Accidents happen — that's why we have the morning-after pill (also known as emergency contraception). Did you have intercourse without using protection? Did you forget to use your birth control correctly? Did the condom break, leaving you worried about becoming pregnant? If so, emergency contraception might be a good choice for you.

Emergency methods are ways for women to avoid pregnancy after having unprotected sex. They are only effective if used soon after having sex. Emergency methods are safe and effective. But they are not as effective as consistent use of the other family

Emergency pills

The pills used for emergency family planning are often the same birth control pills that some women take each day. But in emergencies, you take a much higher dose for a short time. There are now also special emergency pills that have the high dose in 1 or 2 pills, sometimes called Plan B. For any of these, you must take the pills within 5 days of having unprotected sex, but they are most effective when taken within 72 hours after unprotected sex. The sooner you take the pills after unprotected sex, the more likely it is you will not get pregnant. **If you are already pregnant, taking emergency pills will not end the pregnancy or cause birth defects.**

Take as soon as possible and within 120 hours of unprotected intercourse. EC may be taken after 120 hours, but its effectiveness is much lower.

Some women experience nasea. If you vomit within a half hour, it might not work and you should take another dose. You might want to take it with food and some anti-nausea medication.

Emergency Contraception (EC) Pill, works by giving the body a short, high, burst of synthetic hormones. This disrupts hormone patterns needed for pregnancy. EC affects the ovaries and the development of the uterine lining, making pregnancy less likely. Depending upon where the woman is in her menstrual cycle, the hormones prevent pregnancy in different ways. It prevents ovulation (the egg leaving the ovary and moving into the fallopian tube). It blocks the hormones needed for the egg to be able to be fertilized. It may affect the lining of the uterus and alters sperm transport which prevents sperm from meeting the egg and fertilizing it.

How do I get the Morning After Pill?

Emergency Contraception is available from drugstores and health centers without a prescription for women and men 17 and older. If you are interested in getting emergency contraception and are 17 or older, you can either get it directly from a Planned Parenthood health center or from your local drugstore. If you are younger than 17, you'll need to go to a health center or private health care provider for a prescription.

You can also use a different dose of a number of brands of regular birth control pills. While these are not sold specifically as emergency contraceptive pills, they have been proven safe and effective for preventing pregnancy in the few days after sex. These daily birth control pills contain two hormones, progestin and estrogen.

If you are unable to obtain emergency contraception (Plan B) and would like to use your birth control pills, talk to your doctor or check out the following web sites for more information on EC:

www.plannedparenthood.org/ec

www.princeton.edu

ec.princeton.edu/questions/dose. html#dose

Until your next monthly bleeding, you should use a barrier method of family planning, like condoms, or not have sex. After your monthly bleeding, you can use any family planning method you choose. Your next monthly bleeding should begin in about 2 weeks. If it does not, you may have become pregnant despite the emergency family planning. You should continue to use a barrier method of family planning until you know for sure.

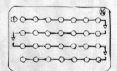

Choosing the Best Method

The best family planning method is the one you are most comfortable using. To choose the best method for you, it can be helpful to think about your day-to-day life, your relationships, concerns, needs, and desires. Whichever method you choose, it is important to understand and follow the instructions for how to use it effectively. Here are some ways to think about different methods based on your personal needs.

I want to keep having normal monthly bleeding

You might PREFER
    Barrier methods, IUD
You might AVOID
    Hormonal methods

I am breastfeeding my one year old baby

You might PREFER:
    Male or female condom, diaphragm, mini-pill, IUD

You might AVOID:
    Combined pill, implants, injections

My husband does not want to be involved in using a family planning method.

You might PREFER:
    Female condom, diaphragm, any hormonal method, IUD

You might AVOID:
    Male condom, natural family planning

I want to have a child within a year

You might PREFER:
    Any barrier method, combined pill, mini-pill, any natural method

You might AVOID:
    Implants, injections, IUD, sterilizati●

I think my partner has sex with others and may infect me with an STI.

You might PREFER:
    Male or female condom

You might AVOID:
    Any hormonal method, any natural method, IUD, sterilization

I do not want to put things in my vagina or my womb.

You might PREFER:
    Hormonal methods, male condom, natural methods

You might AVOID:
    Diaphragm, female condom, IUD

I do not want to have to do something every day

You might PREFER
    Implants, injections, IUD

You might AVOID
    Combined pill, mini pill, any natural method

I do not want any more children

You might PREFER:
    Sterilation, implants, injections, IUD

You might AVOID:
    Natural methods, barrier methods

My partner does not want me to use family planning

You might PREFER:
    Injections, implants, IUD

You might AVOID:
    Barrier methods, pills, natural methods

I want to be able to have sex anytime without interruption

You might PREFER:
    IUD, hormonal methods

You might AVOID:
    Barrier methods, natural methods

Dr C,

I remember clearly when I came to you, ten years ago, a single mom with three kids on housing assistance, food stamps, and living on student aid asking about a tubaligation. I thought I should get it done before I was removed from state-funded health coverage (as was happening to many adults then). Birth control was such a hassle, and besides, I thought, I will never find the right man to have more kids with...especially the right Indian man, at my age.

Your nurse went over the proper forms, consent, etc. I was told that sterilization was to be considered permanent, non-reversible. I was told all this, yes I know. I remember immediately after surgery I bled, a period. I looked down and regretted immediately what I had done. But, I told myself, "What does it matter? No man in your life anyway."

Eighteen months later I was in your office. I told you that I regretted the surgery. I cried. You said why? What could you have asked me that you didn't, you know, just so you would know the next time? I said, maybe you could have asked about my cultural beliefs. You looked at me like I had grown horns.

"Your cultural beliefs?" you said, "what does that have to do with it?"
"Well, I am Native American and having children is kind of an important thing in our culture." (I wasn't feeling very eloquent at the time).
"Oh" you said.

I asked you about tubal reversal surgery, which I had been researching because I had met an Indian man to whom I was engaged and we had discussed having children. You told me that reversal surgery was a waste of time and probably would not work. As I sobbed you suggested I try IVF, something you knew I could never afford – a cycle is, what 15,000, and has something like a 20% chance of success?

Luckily, you gave me Dr A's phone number (an IVF doctor). His partner Dr K did my surgery for the tubal reversal and the whole staff at the clinic was wonderful. Today I watch my two boys 4 and 6 run around and I often think that these two little people would not be alive today if I had listened to you. I am glad I did not listen to you, but I hope for the sake of some other Native woman that you listened to me.

P.S. I am no longer a single mom on housing, food stamps, etc. I have a Master's Degree, own my own home and my own business; and, partly motivated by my experiences, while I was in graduate school I published a peer review article on sterilization of Native American women and have given several lectures on the same subject.

Permanent Methods of Family Planning

Sterilization

(the operation for no more children)

There are operations that make it almost impossible for a man or a woman to have any children. Since these operations are permanent, they are only good for those women or men who are certain that they do not want any more children. To have one of these operations, you must go to a health center or hospital. The surgery is fast and safe, and does not cause side effects.

The operation for the woman (Tubal Ligation)

A tubal ligation is a slightly more difficult operation than a vasectomy, but it is still very safe. It takes about 30 minutes. A trained health care provider makes 1 or 2 small cuts in the woman's belly, and then cuts or ties the tubes that carry the eggs to the womb. It does not change a woman's ability to have sex or to have sexual pleasure.

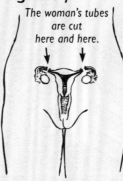

The woman's tubes are cut here and here.

The operation for the man (Vasectomy)

A vasectomy is a simple operation in which the tubes that carry the sperm from the testicles to the penis are cut. The man's testicles are not cut. This operation can be done in any health center where there is a trained care provider. It takes only a few minutes to do. The operation does not change a man's ability to have sex or to feel sexual pleasure. He still ejaculates semen but there are no sperm in the semen. The tubes may still have sperm in them for as long as 12 weeks after the operation, so you need to use another method of family planning during that time.

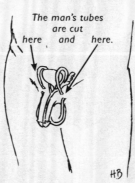

The man's tubes are cut here and here.

HB

Sterilization does not protect against STIs, including HIV/AIDS. So you will still need to think about ways to protect yourself from these infections.

Resource

**http://www.
plannedparenthood.
org/
1-800-230-PLAN**

Planned Parenthood

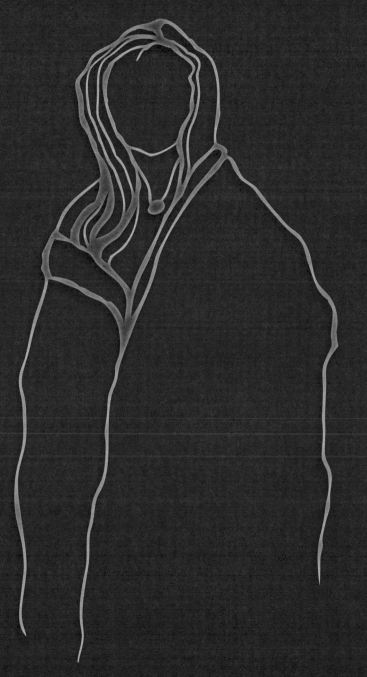

Section 2

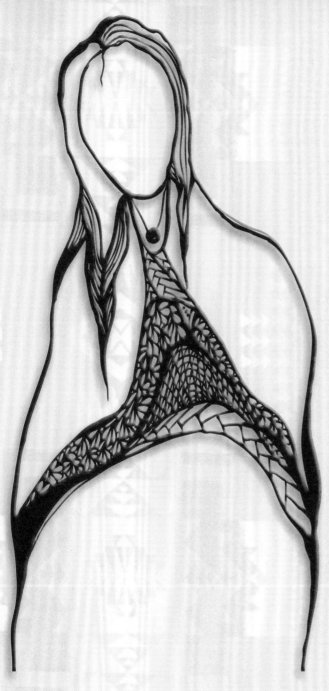

Sisters, you are
the best person to help
your daughter or your sisters with the dangers facing
them today. What do you do
if your daughter comes to you
or you hear she is ready for sex?
When discussing sex, don't just
talk about sex, talk about char-
acter, values and making good
choices. It is also extremely important that you be honest, for s
will hear sex stories from others,
some correct and some incorrect,
and it is best she is prepared the
right way. Further, it is important that you and your daught
understand many of today's
sexually transmitted infections
can be transmitted in a variety
of ways. If your child is old
enough to ask questions,
then gradually start dis-
cussing in a warm and loving environment.

STIs
(sexually transmitted infections)

Men and women can both get STIs. But a woman gets infected from a man more easily than a man gets infected from a woman. This is because a man enters some part of a woman's body during sex. Without a condom, the man's semen, which may carry infection, stays inside her body. This gives her a greater chance of getting an infection in the womb, tubes, and ovaries. When a woman has sores on her genitals or irritation from an infection in the vagina, she can also get HIV more easily.

Because most STIs are inside a woman's body, the signs of an STI in a woman are harder to see than in a man. So it is often hard to tell if a woman has an infection in her genitals— much less what kind of infection she has.

Please note, this chapter talks about sexually transmitted diseases and is not appropriate for young children.

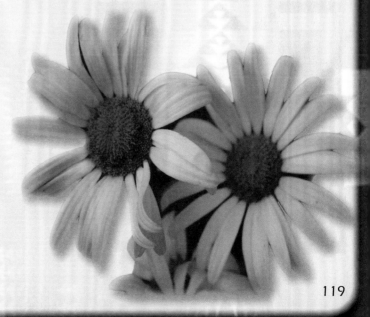

Sexually Transmitted Infections

Sexually transmitted infections, or STIs, are infections passed from one person to another during sex. Any type of sex can cause an STI. It can be penis to vagina sex, or penis to anus sex, or oral sex (mouth to penis, mouth to vagina). Sometimes STIs can happen from just rubbing an infected penis or vagina against another person's genitals. STIs can be passed from a pregnant woman to her baby before it is born, or during childbirth.

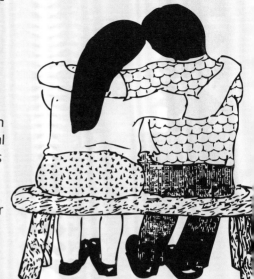

Unless they are treated early, STIs can cause:
- infertility in both men and women.
- babies born too early, too small, blind, sick, or dead.
- pregnancy in the tube (outside the womb).
- death from severe infection.
- lasting pain in the lower abdomen.
- cancer of the cervix.

Why so many women get STIs

It can be hard for a woman to protect herself from an STI. Often, she must have sex when her partner demands it. She may not know if her partner has sex with other partners, or if he is infected with an STI. If he has another partner who is infected, he may infect his wife. A woman may not be able to persuade her partner to use condoms. Latex condoms are the best way to protect both partners, but the man has to be willing to use them (see the "Family Planning" chapter for information on condom use.)

You may have an STI if you have one or more of these signs:
- an unusual or bad-smelling vaginal discharge
- itching genitals
- painful genitals
- sores or blisters on the genitals
- pain in your lower abdomen or pain during sex

How to know if you are at risk for an STI

Even if you do not have any signs, you may be at risk (more likely to have an STI) if:

• your partner has signs of an STI. He has probably passed the STI to you, even if you have no signs.

• you have more than one partner. The more partners you have, the greater the chance that one of them has passed an STI to you.

• you have had a new partner in the last 3 months. He may have had another partner just before you who had an STI.

• you think your partner might have other partners (for example, he lives away from home). This means he is more likely to become infected with an STI and infect you. In this chapter we recommend medicines that treat different STIs.

STIs: American Indians and Alaska Natives

The presence of a sexually transmitted disease can increase the chance of contracting or spreading HIV. High rates of Chlamydia trachomatis infection, gonorrhea, and syphilis among American Indians and Alaska Natives suggest that the same sexual behaviors that spread HIV are common among American Indians and Alaska Natives. According to 2005 surveillance data by race/ethnicity, American Indians and Alaska Natives had the 2nd highest rates of gonorrhea and Chlamydia trachomatis infection. American Indians and Alaska Natives had the 3rd highest rate of syphilis.

Treatment for STIs

If you have signs of an STI or think you are at risk for an STI, you should start treatment right away. Unfortunately, tests for STIs are not available in many places, may be expensive, and are not always accurate.

• Treat the infection right away. If you have signs described in this chapter, follow the treatments given.

• Do not wait until you are very ill. Treatment will protect you from more serious problems later on and will prevent the spread of STIs to others.

• Get tested if testing is available. You could be infected with another STI and have no signs.

• Help your partner get treated at the same time. If he does not get treated, he will infect you again if you have sex.

• Practice safer sex. You may get another STI or HIV/AIDS if you do not protect yourself (see "Family Planning" chapter).

• Try to get tested for HIV. STIs and HIV infection often occur together.

• Buy and take all the medicine as recommended. Even if your signs go away, you will not be cured until all the medicine has time to work. If the signs do not go away after taking the medicines, see a health provider. Pain or discharge could also be caused by another problem like cancer.

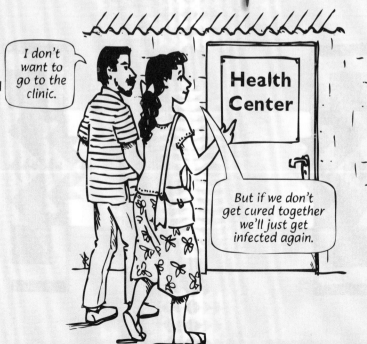

I don't want to go to the clinic.

Health Center

But if we don't get cured together we'll just get infected again.

What to do if you have signs of an STI or are at risk for an STI

STIs hurt men, too
Most women, and many men, who are infected with an STI do not have any signs.
When they are not treated, STIs can cause a man to:

• become infertile
• have lasting pain
• die of AIDS or other serious infections

Drug Resistance and STI Medicines

When using medicines for treating STIs, HIV/AIDS, and other diseases, it is very important to take all the medicine. If a person does not take enough of the right kind of medicine—or stops taking the medicine before the treatment is finished—the germs causing the infection are not all killed. The strongest germs survive and create stronger forms of the disease. Then a medicine that once worked against that disease is no longer able to cure it. This is called resistance.

For this reason, in many places gonorrhea has become resistant to the drugs usually used to treat it. Talk with a health provider to find out if there is drug resistance where you live, and what are the best medicines to treat STIs.

Be sure to take medicines correctly

Remember, when treating STIs, always:

• make sure your partner gets treated too.

• take all the medicine.

• stop having sex or use condoms during sex until your signs have gone away AND you and your partner have finished all the medicine.

• see a health provider if you do not get better by the end of your treatment.

• practice safer sex when you do have sex again.

Remember that most people have more than one STI or other infection of the genitals at the same time, so it is often necessary to take more than one medicine. Whichever medicines you choose, be sure to take them correctly.

You may also need to take a different medicine if:

• you are pregnant or breastfeeding and the medicine is not safe to take during those times.

• the STI you are trying to treat has become resistant to the medicine.

• you have an allergy to the medicine.

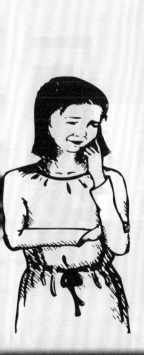

123

Abnormal Discharge

It is normal to have a small amount of discharge or wetness that comes from the vagina. This is the way the vagina cleans itself. The amount of discharge changes during the days of your monthly cycle. During your fertile time, your discharge is more wet and slippery, and clear in color. If you are pregnant, you may have more discharge.

A change in the amount, color, or smell of the discharge from your vagina sometimes means you have an infection, but it can be difficult to tell from your discharge what kind of infection you have.

Common Causes of Abnormal Discharge

Abnormal discharge can be a sign of a yeast infection or bacterial vaginosis, which are not sexually transmitted, or a sign of trichomonas, gonorrhea, and chlamydia, all of which are sexually transmitted. For other signs of these infections and how to treat them (see "Our Moon" chapter).

Yeast (candida, white discharge, thrush)

Yeast is not sexually transmitted. It does not cause complications, but it can be very uncomfortable. You are most likely to have a yeast infection when you are pregnant, taking antibiotics, or have some other illness like diabetes or HIV/AIDS.

Signs:
- white, lumpy discharge, like milk curd or yogurt
- bright red skin outside and inside your vagina that may bleed
- you feel very itchy inside or outside your vagina

Treatment:

Yeast is not dangerous, and it can often be cured using natural remedies. It is best to treat a pregnant woman before the birth, or the baby can get thrush.

One natural treatment is to mix 3 tablespoons of vinegar with 1 liter (quart) of boiled and cooled water. Soak a piece of clean cotton in the mixture and insert it into the vagina every night for 3 nights. Remove the cotton each morning.

Abnormal Discharge

Important: If you have discharge from the vagina with pain in the lower abdomen, you could have a serious pelvic infection. Get treatment immediately!

Prevention: Wearing loose clothing and underclothes made of cotton, rather than polyester or nylon, lets air around the genitals. This helps prevent yeast. Wash or change the underclothes often. Do not put soap in the vagina when bathing. Do not douche.

The bacteria that cause BV can sometimes infect the uterus (womb) and fallopian tubes. This type of infection is called pelvic inflammatory disease (PID). PID can cause infertility or damage the fallopian tubes enough to increase the future risk of ectopic pregnancy and infertility.

Bacterial vaginosis (BV)

The cause of BV is not fully understood. BV is associated with an imbalance in the bacteria that are normally found in a woman's vagina. The vagina normally contains mostly "good" bacteria, and fewer "harmful" bacteria. BV develops when there is an increase in harmful bacteria.

Not much is known about how women get BV. Any woman can get BV. However, some activities or behaviors can upset the normal balance of bacteria in the vagina and put women at increased risk including:

- Having a new sex partner or multiple sex partners,
- Douching, and
- Using an intrauterine device (IUD) for contraception.

Women do not get BV from toilet seats, bedding, swimming pools, or from touching objects around them. Women that have never had sexual intercourse are rarely affected. BV is treatable with antibiotics prescribed by a health care provider.

Itching of the genitals

Itching of the genitals can have many causes. Itching around the opening of the vagina could be yeast or trichomonas. Itching in the hair of the genitals or close to the genitals could be caused by scabies or lice. Scabies or lice can be easily treated with medicines found in most pharmacies. Some itching is caused by soaps or deodorants that have perfume in them. It can also be caused by plants and herbs that are used for douching or washing out the vagina. Wash with plain water to see if the itching goes away.

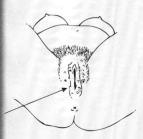

Genital herpes

Genital herpes is an STI caused by a virus. It produces sores on the genitals or in the mouth that come and go for months or years. There is no cure for herpes, but there is treatment to make you feel better. Not all herpes sores on the mouth are spread by sex. Children and adults often get sores on their mouths caused by a different herpes virus when they have a cold or fever.

125

Gonorrhea (clap, gono, VD) and Chlamydia

Gonorrhea and chlamydia are both serious STIs, but they are easy to cure if treated early. If not, they can cause severe infection and infertility in both women and men. In a man, the signs usually begin 2 to 5 days after he had sex with an infected person. But a man can have no signs and still be infected. In a woman, the signs may not begin for weeks or even months. Even if you do not have any signs, you can still pass gonorrhea and chlamydia to another person.

Signs in a woman:

- yellow or green discharge from the vagina or anus
- pain or burning when passing urine
- fever
- pain in the lower belly
- pain or bleeding during sex
- or no signs at all

Women with gonorrhea are at risk of developing serious complications from the infection, regardless of the presence or severity of symptoms.

Signs in a man:

- discharge from his penis
- pain or burning when he passes urine
- pain or swelling of the testicles
- or no signs at all

Chlamydia can be easily treated and cured with antibiotics. A single dose of azithromycin or a week of doxycycline (twice daily) are the most commonly used treatments. HIV-positive persons with chlamydia should receive the same treatment as those who are HIV negative.

Several antibiotics can successfully cure gonorrhea in adolescents and adults. However, drug-resistant strains of gonorrhea are increasing in many areas of the world, including the United States, and successful treatment of gonorrhea is becoming more difficult. It is important to take all of the medication prescribed to cure gonorrhea.

Preventing STIs can protect you and your partner from serious illness and infertility.

Gonorrhea and chlamydia have the same signs, so it is best, if possible, to get treated for both.

All sex partners should be evaluated, tested, and treated. Persons with chlamydia should abstain from sexual intercourse until they and their sex partners have completed treatment, otherwise re-infection is possible.

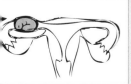

Complications of Chlamydia

In women, untreated infection can spread into the uterus or fallopian tubes and cause pelvic inflammatory disease (PID). This happens in up to 40 percent of women with untreated chlamydia.

PID can cause permanent damage to the fallopian tubes, uterus, and surrounding tissues. The damage can lead to chronic pelvic pain, infertility, and potentially fatal ectopic pregnancy (pregnancy outside the uterus). Women infected with chlamydia are up to five times more likely to become infected with HIV, if exposed.

To help prevent the serious consequences of chlamydia, screening at least annually for chlamydia is recommended for all sexually active women age 25 years and younger. An annual screening test also is recommended for older women with risk factors for chlamydia (a new sex partner or multiple sex partners). All pregnant women should have a screening test for chlamydia.

Complications among men are rare. Infection sometimes spreads to the epididymis (a tube that carries sperm from the testis), causing pain, fever, and, rarely, sterility.

Complications of Gonorrhea

In women, gonorrhea is a common cause of pelvic inflammatory disease (PID). About one million women each year in the United States develop PID. Women with PID do not necessarily have symptoms. When symptoms are present, they can be very severe and can include abdominal pain and fever. PID can lead to internal abscesses (pus-filled "pockets" that are hard to cure) and long-lasting, chronic pelvic pain.

PID can damage the fallopian tubes enough to cause infertility or increase the risk of ectopic pregnancy. Ectopic pregnancy is a life-threatening condition in which a fertilized egg grows outside the uterus, usually in a fallopian tube.

In men, gonorrhea can cause epididymitis, a painful condition of the testicles that can lead to infertility if left untreated.

Pelvic Inflammatory Disease (PID)

Pelvic Inflammatory Disease or PID is the name for an infection of any of the reproductive parts in a woman's lower abdomen. It is often called a 'pelvic infection'. Pelvic infection can happen if you have had an STI that was not cured, especially gonorrhea or chlamydia. It can also happen if you recently gave birth, had a miscarriage or abortion, or had an IUD inserted.

The germs that cause pelvic infection travel up from the vagina through the cervix and then into the womb, tubes, and ovaries. If the infection is not treated in time, it can cause chronic pain, serious illness, or death. An infection in the tubes can leave scars that make you infertile or at risk for a pregnancy outside the womb (tubal or ectopic pregnancy).

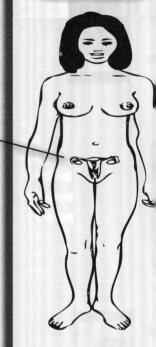

abcess

womb

tube

bacteria

vagina

Signs (you may have one or more of these):

- pain in the lower belly
- high fever
- you feel very ill and weak
- green or yellow bad-smelling discharge from the vagina
- pain or bleeding during sex

> **PID does not always cause pain.**

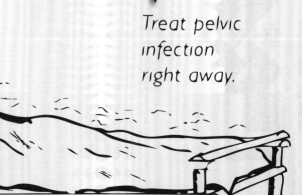

Treat pelvic infection right away.

128

How to prevent STIs

• Practice safer sex (see the chapter on "Family Planning").

• Use condoms every time you have sex. To learn how to encourage your partner to use condoms, see the "Family Planning" chapter.

Hepatitis B (yellow eyes)

Hepatitis B is a dangerous infection caused by a virus that harms the liver. Hepatitis B is spread when the blood, saliva (spit), fluid from the vagina, or semen of someone already infected with the virus gets into the body of another person. It spreads very easily from one person to another, especially during sex.

Signs:
- • fever
- • no appetite
- • tired and weak feeling
- • yellow eyes and/or skin (jaundice)

Treatment:

There is no medicine that will help. In fact, taking medicine can hurt your liver even more. Most people get better from hepatitis B. A small number of people may have liver problems that never go away, including cancer. Rest as much as you can, and eat foods that are easy to digest. Do not drink any alcohol for at least 6 months.
- • pain in the belly
- • dark urine and

Hepatitis C (HCV)

HCV occurs when blood from an infected person enters the body of a person who is not infected. HCV can be spread by sex, but this is rare. If you are having sex with more than one steady sex partner, use latex condoms* correctly and every time to prevent the spread of sexually transmitted diseases. HCV can be spread through sharing needles, through needlesticks or sharps exposures on the job, or from an infected mother to her baby during birth. Symptoms may include jaundice, fatigue, dark urine, abdominal pain or loss of appitite, though 80% of persons have no symptoms.

AVOID HEPATITIS!
HAVE SAFER SEX
AND
GET IMMUNIZED!

Cancer of the liver can be caused by hepatitis B and C

Long term effects may include chronic liver disease or even liver cancer. Drinking alcohol can make liver disease worse. There are treatment options for HCV, talk to your health care provider.

Trichomonas

Trichomonas is a very uncomfortable and itchy STI. Men usually do not have any signs, but they can carry it in the penis and pass it to a woman during sex. Trichomoniasis is caused by the single-celled protozoan parasite. The vagina is the most common site of infection in women.

Signs:

- gray or yellow, bubbly discharge
- bad-smelling discharge
- red and itchy genital area and vagina
- pain or burning when you pass urine

The infection also may cause discomfort during intercourse and urination, as well as irritation and itching of the female genital area. In rare cases, lower abdominal pain can occur. Symptoms usually appear in women within 5 to 28 days of exposure.

Trichomoniasis can usually be cured with the prescription drug, metronidazole, given by mouth in a single dose. Both partners should be treated at the same time to eliminate the parasite. Persons being treated for trichomoniasis should avoid sex until they and their sex partners complete treatment and have no symptoms.

Chancroid

Chancroid is an STI caused by bacteria. It can be cured with medicine if it is treated early.

Signs:

- one or more soft, painful sores on the genitals or anus that bleed easily
- enlarged, painful glands (lymph nodes, bubos) may develop in the groin
- slight fever

chancroid

If your partner will not use a condom, a diaphragm might give you a little protection against STIs.

- Wash the outside of your genitals after sex.
- Pass urine after having sex.
- Do not douche, or use herbs or powders to dry out the vagina. Douching (and washing out the vagina with soap) works against the natural wetness the vagina makes to stay healthy. When the vagina is dry, it can become irritated during sex, making it more likely to be infected with HIV and other STIs.
- You and your partner can have oral sex or other sexual touch instead of intercourse.

Most sores or ulcers on the genitals are sexually transmitted. It can be difficult to know which disease is causing the sores because the ones caused by both syphilis and chancroid often look alike. For this reason, it is best to give medicines that cure both of these STIs when treating genital sores.

Common Causes of Sores on the Genitals
(Genital Ulcers)

www.cdc.gov/std

Syphilis

Syphilis is a serious STI that has effects throughout the body and can last for many years. It is caused by bacteria and can be cured with medicine if treated early.

Signs:

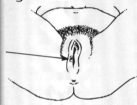

- The first sign is a small, painless sore that can look like a pimple, a flat, wet wart, or an open sore. The sore lasts for only a few days or weeks and then goes away by itself. But the disease continues to spread throughout the body.

- Weeks or months later, you may have a sore throat, fever, rash (especially on the palms of the hands and soles of the feet), mouth sores, or swollen joints.

All of these signs go away by themselves, but the disease continues. Even if you have no signs, you can still pass syphilis to others. Without treatment, syphilis can cause heart disease, paralysis, mental illness, and even death.

Pregnancy and Syphilis

A pregnant woman can pass syphilis to her unborn baby, which can cause it to be born too early, deformed, or worse. You can prevent this by getting a blood test and treatment during pregnancy.

If you are pregnant, try to get a blood test for syphilis.

HPV (Human Papillomavirus)

Genital HPV infection is a sexually transmitted infection (STI) that is caused by human papillomavirus (HPV). Human papillomavirus is the name of a group of viruses that includes more than 100 different strains or types. More than 30 of these viruses are sexually transmitted, and they can infect the genital area of men and women including the skin of the penis, vulva (area outside the vagina), or anus, and the linings of the vagina, cervix, or rectum. Most people who become infected with HPV will not have any symptoms and will clear the infection on their own.

Some of these viruses are called "high-risk" types, and may cause abnormal Pap tests. They may also lead to cancer of the cervix, vulva, vagina, anus, or penis. Others are called "low-risk" types, and they may cause mild Pap test abnormalities or genital warts. Genital warts are single or multiple growths or bumps that appear in the genital area, and sometimes are cauliflower shaped.

There is no "cure" for HPV infection, although in most women the infection goes away on its own. The treatments provided are directed to the changes in the skin or mucous membrane caused by HPV infection, such as warts and pre-cancerous changes in the cervix.

Most people who have a genital HPV infection do not know they are infected. The virus lives in the skin or mucous membranes and usually causes no symptoms. Some people get visible genital warts, or have pre-cancerous changes in the cervix, vulva, anus, or penis.

HPV is the main risk for Cervical Cancer!

HPV and Cervical Cancer

HPV can cause an infection in the cervix. The infection usually doesn't last very long because your body is able to fight the infection. If the HPV doesn't go away, the virus may cause cervix cells to change and become precancer cells.

Precancer cells are not cancer. Most cells with early precancer changes return to normal on their own. Sometimes, the precancer cells may turn into cancer if they are not found and treated. Very few HPV infections lead to cervix cancer.

Because HPV is so common, any woman who has ever had sex can get cervix cancer. However, most women who get HPV do not get cervix cancer. Women who have their Pap tests as often as they should are least likely to get cervical cancer. Some women have a greater chance of getting cervix cancer if they:
- have the HPV that can cause cervix cancer and it doesn't go away
- have HIV or AIDS
- smoke.

Women who do not have Pap tests at all or who do not have them as often as they should have the greatest chance of getting cervix cancer.

HPV and Genital Warts

Important
Large, flat, wet growths that look like warts may be a sign of syphilis (see the next page). Try to get a test for syphilis.

Warts are caused by some strains of the HPV virus. Warts on the genitals look like warts on other parts of the body. They can be raised or flat, single or multiple, small or large, and sometimes cauliflower shaped. It is possible to have genital warts and not know it, especially when they are inside the vagina or inside the tip of the penis.

The types of HPV that are found in the genital areas are usually passed on during sexual contact (sexually transmitted). HPV types that cause warts on the hands or feet do not cause genital warts or cervical cell changes. After sexual contact with an infected person, warts may appear within weeks or months, or not at all. Warts may go away without treatment, but it can take a long time. Usually they continue to get worse and should be treated.

Signs:
- itching
- small, painless, soft whitish or brownish bumps that have a rough surface. In women, these bumps usually grow on the folds of the vulva, inside the vagina, and around the anus. In men, they usually grow on the penis, (or just inside it) and on the scrotum, or the anus.

Warts grow faster during pregnancy. If you have a lot of them, this can cause problems with childbirth. Talk with your health care provider about this.

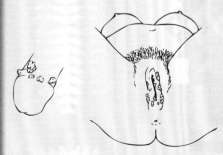

Visible genital warts can be removed by medications the patient applies, or by treatments performed by a health care provider. Some individuals choose to not have treatment to see if the warts will disappear on their own.

HPV Myths

Myths are stories that are not really true, but may get circulated between people to the point that some may believe they are true.

Here are some common myths about HPV. Myths are always false, so take a moment to read these pages to inform yourself about the truth about HPV.

1. Myth: I'm the only person I know with HPV.

Among those ages 15-49, only one in four Americans has not had a genital HPV infection. An HPV infection usually has no signs, so a person who has been infected may never know about it.   At any given time, only about 1% of all sexually active Americans have visible genital warts. Many more women have abnormal Pap smears because of an HPV infection, but in many cases health care providers may not have explained the link between HPV and cervical infection.

2. Myth: Only people who have casual sex get STDs.

Even with up to 12 million Americans contracting an STD each year. STDs can be passed along as readily in a loving, long-term relationship as in a one-night stand. And HPV is the virus to prove it. At least one study of middle-class, middle-aged women, most of them married with children, found that 21% were infected with cervical HPV.

3. Myth: In a monogamous relationship, an HPV diagnosis means someone has cheated.

This myth has been responsible for a great deal of anger, confusion, and heartache. The virus can remain in the body for weeks, years, or even a lifetime, giving no sign of its presence. Or a genital HPV infection may produce warts, lesions, or cervical abnormalities after a latent period of months or even years.

4. Myth: Genital warts lead to cervical cancer.

There are more than 70 types of human papillomavirus. Those most strongly associated with cancer are HPV types 16, 18, 31, 45. Genital warts are caused by HPV types that are virtually never found in cancer." These are the "low-risk" types, 6, 11, 42, 43, and 44.

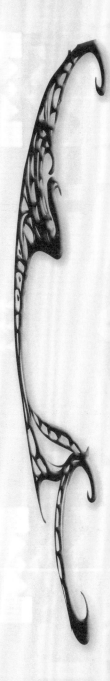

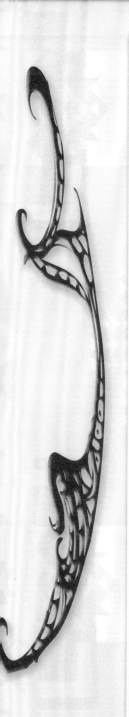

5. Myth: An abnormal Pap smear means a woman is at high risk for cervical cancer.

When a Pap test comes back as "abnormal," it means just that: Under the microscope the Pap test sample looks differnent from healthy, intact cervical cells. The difference could be due to local irritation, a non-HPV infection, or even a mistake in the preparation of the cell sample. A woman with an abnormal Pap smear is often asked to come back to the doctor's office and have the test repeated. Many reasons for an abnormal result last only a short time, and so repeating the Pap test after a few months usually weeds these out. Having an annual Pap test is key to finding abnormal cells at pre-cancer stages. According to the National Cancer Institute, about half of women with newly diagnosed cervical cancer have never had a Pap smear, and another 10% have not had a smear in the past five years.

6. Myth: Older women don't need Pap smears.

The myth can be deadly: ***One in four cases of cervical cancer, and 41% of deaths, occur in women age 65 and older.*** Continued Paps may be recommended because the HPV virus may be dormant for a number of years. Also, it may take 10-15 years for abnormal cell changes to develop into cervical cancer. What's best for you? Speak with your health care provider to see what is recommended, given your own medical history

7. Myth: Lesbians don't need regular Pap smears.

HPV can be passed through other forms of skin-to-skin contact. A regularly scheduled Pap smear is a smart health measure for gay and straight women alike.

8. Myth: If I've always used condoms, I'm not at risk for HPV.

Used correctly, condoms are very effective against STDs such as gonorrhea and HIV that are spread through bodily fluids. However, they are likely to be less protective against STDs that spread through skin-to-skin contact, such as HPV and herpes. That is not to say condoms are useless. In fact, studies have shown condom use can lower the risk of acquiring HPV infection and reduce the risk of HPV-related diseases, as well as help prevent other STDs and unintended pregnancy.

HIV/AIDS (Acquired Immune Deficiency Syndrome)

HIV/AIDS is a disease transmitted during sex by a virus called HIV. It is spread when blood, fluid from the vagina, or semen of someone already infected with the HIV virus gets into the body of another person.

Women can get HIV more easily than men during sex. You can get HIV from someone who looks completely healthy.

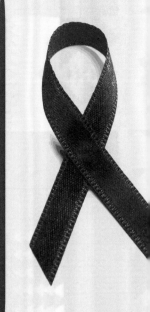

There is no treatment that can cure HIV, but treatment can lengthen and improve the life of someone with HIV. Practice safer sex to protect yourself and others from spreading HIV. If you think you have had unsafe sex with someone who might have HIV, see the next chapter.

Snapshot: HIV/AIDS in 2005 in Indian Country

In 2005 HIV/AIDS was diagnosed for an estimated 195 American Indians and Alaska Natives

In 2005 AIDS was diagnosed for an estimated 182 American Indians and Alaska Natives.

In 2005 an estimated 1,581 American Indians and Alaska Natives were living with AIDS.

In 2005 An estimated 81 American Indians and Alaska Natives with AIDS died.

http://www.cdc.gov/hiv/resources/factsheets/aian.htm

Resources:

www.cdc.gov/nchstp/dstd/disease_info.htm
www.cdc.gov/std/

www.nlm.nih.gov/medlineplus/sexuallytransmit-
teddiseases.html

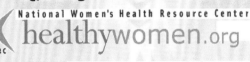
National Institutes of Health
The Nation's Medical Research Agency

www.4women.gov/FAQ/stdsgen.htm

1-800-994-9662 or
1-888-220-5446 for
the hearing im-
paired.

National Women's Health Resource Center
NWHRC
healthywomen.org

womenshealth.gov
The Federal Government Source for Women's Health Information

www.iwannaknow.org/
ASHA's STI Resource Center
1-800-227-8922
This line plays recordings about STI information 24 hours a day
and has health communication specialists available to answer
questions between 9am and 6pm, ET, Monday through Friday.

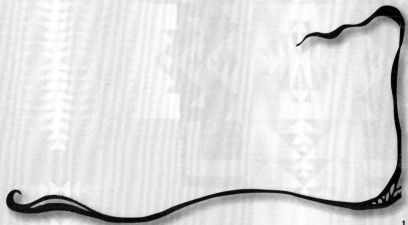

asha American Social Health Association

www.iwannaknow.org^{SM}

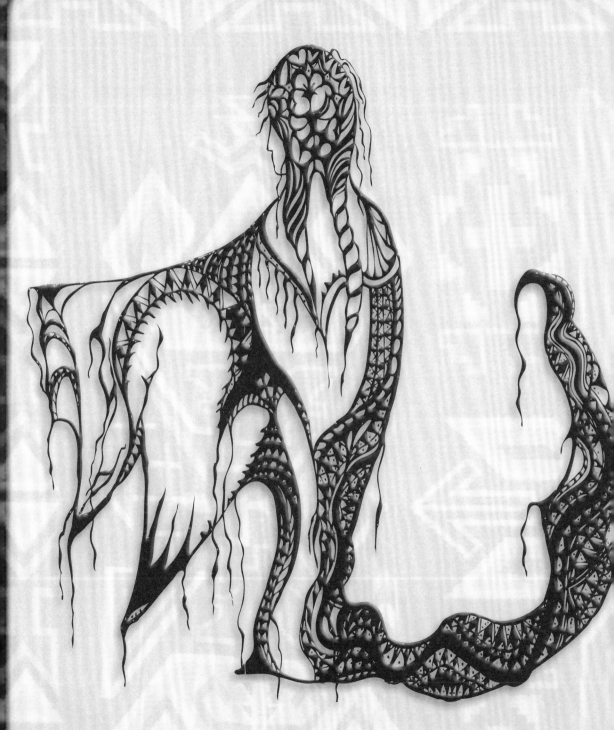

HIV/AIDS

(Human Immunodeficiency Virus/ Aquired Immune Deficiency Syndrome)

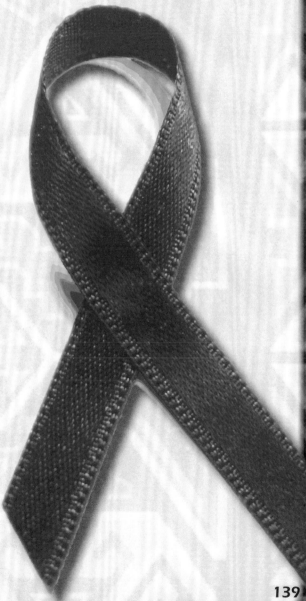

"AIDS is a disease that shines in hush and thrives on secrecy. It was prospering because people were choosing not to talk about it... I wanted to talk about AIDS so that at least my children, and yours, would be spared. They would know and have the information about AIDS before they became sexually active, and be able to talk about it."

—Noerine Kaleeba, Uganda

Millions of people are infected with HIV, the virus that causes AIDS worldwide. More and more of them are women. There is no cure for HIV or AIDS. But treatments are now available that can help people with HIV/AIDS live longer and healthier lives. To provide care for those who need it and to protect ourselves and each other from HIV and AIDS, we must be willing to talk about HIV with our families and friends.

Any woman may have to face HIV/AIDS. Most women do not think they are at risk of getting AIDS. They may think that only women who have many sex partners, or only women who use drugs, have any chance of becoming infected with HIV. This is not true. In some communities, it is married women who have the greatest risk of getting HIV.

What Are HIV and AIDS?

HIV (Human Immunodeficiency Virus) is a very small germ, called a virus, that you cannot see. AIDS (Acquired Immune Deficiency Syndrome) is a disease that develops later, after a person has been infected with HIV, the AIDS virus.

HIV

When a person becomes infected with HIV, the virus attacks the immune system, the part of your body that fights off infection.

HIV slowly kills the cells of the immune system until the body can no longer defend itself against other infections. Most people who are infected do not get sick from their HIV for 5 to 10 years. But eventually the immune system will no longer fight off common infections. Because HIV takes many years to make someone sick, most people with HIV feel healthy and do not know they have it.

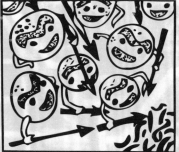

white blood cells

germs

The body has millions of white blood cells that attack germs and fight off infection.

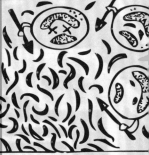

HIV kills the white blood cells until the are not enough cel left to attack the germs. This is whe the person has AID

AIDS

A person has AIDS when the immune system gets so weak that it can no longer fight off common infections and illnesses. The signs of AIDS are different in different people, and they can be different for women than for men. Often the signs are getting sick with other common illnesses.

How HIV/AIDS is spread

HIV lives in certain body fluids—blood, semen, and the fluids in the vagina—of people infected with HIV. The virus is spread when these fluids get into the body of another person. This means that HIV/AIDS can be spread by:

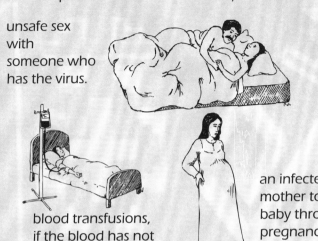

unsafe sex with someone who has the virus.

unclean needles or syringes, or any tool that pierces or cuts the skin **including unclean needles used for tatoos or piercings.**

blood transfusions, if the blood has not been tested to be sure it is free from HIV (rare in the US).

an infected mother to her baby through pregnancy, birth or breastfeeding.

infected blood that gets into cuts or an open wound of another person.

How HIV/AIDS is NOT spread

HIV does not live outside the human body for more than a few minutes. It cannot live on its own in the air or in water. This means you cannot give or get HIV in these ways:

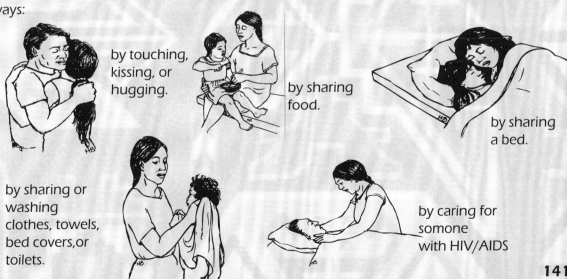

by touching, kissing, or hugging.

by sharing food.

by sharing a bed.

by sharing or washing clothes, towels, bed covers,or toilets.

by caring for somone with HIV/AIDS

141

HIV and AIDS are Different for Women because:

- women get infected with HIV more easily than men do. A man's semen stays in the woman's vagina for a long time. If there is HIV in semen it can pass easily into a woman's body through her vagina or cervix, especially if there are any cuts, sores, or STIs.

- women are often infected at a younger age than men. This is because young women and girls are less able to refuse unwanted or unsafe sex and are often married young to older men who are infected.

- women often live with untreated STIs, making it easier to become infected with HIV.

- women get more blood transfusions than men because of problems during childbirth.

- poor nutrition and childbearing may make women less able to fight disease.

- women may be blamed unfairly for the spread of AIDS, even though many men are unwilling to wear condoms or limit their number of sex partners.

- a pregnant woman infected with HIV can pass it to her baby.

- women are usually the caretakers for family members who are sick with AIDS, even if they are sick themselves.

Snapshot: HIV/AIDS in 2005 in Indian Country

In 2005 HIV/AIDS was diagnosed for an estimated 195 American Indians and Alaska Natives

In 2005 AIDS was diagnosed for an estimated 182 American Indians and Alaska Natives.

In 2005 an estimated 1,581 American Indians and Alaska Natives were living with AIDS.

In 2005 An estimated 81 American Indians and Alaska Natives with AIDS died.

Meth Use Increases the Risk of HIV in Indian Country

Native Americans are 4.2 times more likely to use crystal meth than Whites (2005 National Survey on Drug Use and Health). Methamphetamine users are at heightened risk for HIV and hepatitis from sharing syringes or drug works including water with infected users. Methamphetamine users are also at heightened risk for HIV and other STDs from prolonged unprotected sex with an infected partner.

aring or reusing wn" needle are some the behaviors that t women who use eth at increased risk r HIV.

Trends of Methamphetamine use in Indian Country:

- 12% of female American Indian 11th graders (Monitoring the Future 2005)
- 2.2% of American Indians and Alaska Natives treated for meth use in 2005 (SAMHSA Treatment Episode Data Set)
- Mexican drug distribution organizations target reservations. (Casper Star Tribune August 2005)

High Risk Injection Behaviors

- Reuse "own" syringe multiple times
- Sharing rinse water not seen as risky
- Women may be injected by others
- Days of bingeing and sleeplessness lead to inconsistent injection hygiene or direct sharing

Sexual Risks for Women

These behaviors put women at greater risk for HIV and STIs while using methamphetamines:

- "Do things I would never think of doing otherwise"
- Trade sex for meth
- Users may be focused on the drug - not condoms

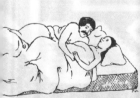

th users may be too used on the drug and "high", engaging ther risky behaviors h as needle sharing unprotected sex.

The healthcare system can help identify young users, screen for risk behaviors, provide confidential testing for HIV, hepatitis, and other STDS. If you or someone you know is using meth, your clinic or health care provider can help.

Source: Susan Dreisbach, Ph.D., Rural Center for AIDS/STD Prevention, University of Colorado Denver

Preventing HIV/AIDS

You can prevent AIDS in these ways:

- If possible, have sex with only one partner who has sex only with you.

- Practice safer sex—sex that prevents semen, blood and vaginal fluids from getting into your vagina, anus, or mouth. Use condoms regularly.

- Get tested for STIs and make sure partners do too.

- Avoid piercing or cutting the skin with needles or other tools that have not been disinfected between uses.

- Avoid blood transfusions except in emergencies.

- Do not share razors.

- Do not touch someone else's blood or wound without protection.

The HIV Test

When HIV enters the body, the body starts to make antibodies right away to fight the virus. These antibodies usually show in the blood 2 to 4 weeks later. The HIV test looks for these antibodies in the blood. It is the only way to know if a person has been infected with HIV. It is not a test for AIDS. A positive HIV test means that you are infected with the virus and your body has made antibodies to HIV. Even if you feel completely well, you can spread the virus to others.

A negative HIV test means 1 of 2 things:

- you are not infected with HIV, or

- you were recently infected but your body has not yet made enough antibodies to HIV to test positive. It can take up to 3 months after exposure to develop antibodies, and in very rare cases, up to 6 months.

Rapid Tests:

A rapid test is a screening test that produces very quick results, in about 20 minutes. Rapid tests use blood from a vein or from a finger stick, or a sample of saliva from your mouth to look for the presence of antibodies to HIV. As is true for all screening tests, a reactive rapid HIV test result must be confirmed with a follow-up confirmatory test before a final diagnosis of HIV infection can be made.

If you have tested negative for HIV but think you might be infected, you should take the test again in about 6 weeks. Sometimes a positive test also needs to be repeated. A health care provider can help you decide.

Rapid HIV testing is available in many health centers and hospitals at low or no cost. You can usually get test results the same day.

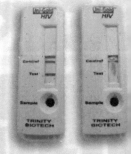

Resource:
http://www.hivtest.or

144

The HIV test should always be done:
• with your permission.
• with counseling before and after the test.
• with privacy. No one should know the results except you and those you want to know.

...sky Beliefs

...ese "myths" or un-
...ths in Indian County
...ay be leading to a
...ngerous epidemic of
...V in Indian Country.

...HIV does not exist in
...ral areas
...NTRUE! the HIV
...idemic is hitting the
...ral areas through
...ky behaviors such
... shared needles and
...protected sex.

...HIV/STD testing can-
...t be confidential
...NTRUE! Health care
...ovider teams un-
...rgo training and
...rtification to ensure
... patient information
...ept confidential.

When should you have the HIV test?

It may be more important to change unsafe behavior than to have an HIV test. But you and your partner may want to be tested if:

• you want to get married (or start a faithful sexual relationship with one person) or have children.
• you are pregnant and worried that you may be positive.
• you, your partner, or your baby have signs of AIDS.
• you or your partner have been having unsafe sex.

The advantages of knowing the test results

If your test is negative, you can learn how to protect yourself so that you stay negative and never get HIV/AIDS. If your test is positive, you can:

• prevent the spread of HIV to your partner or baby.
• get treatment early for health problems.
• make changes in how you live so you can stay healthy longer.
• get support from other HIV-infected people in your community.
• plan for yourself and your family's future.

HIV Testing Issues

Access to HIV testing and issues concerning confidentiality are important for many American Indians and Alaska Natives. For example, at the time of AIDS diagnosis, more American Indians and Alaska Natives, compared with persons of other races/ethnicities, resided in rural areas. Those who live in rural areas may be less likely to be tested for HIV because of limited access to testing. Also, American Indians and Alaska Natives may be less likely to seek testing because of concerns about confidentiality in close-knit communities, where someone who seeks testing is likely to encounter a friend, a relative, or an acquaintance at the local health care facility.

During 1997–2000, 50.5% of American Indians and Alaska Natives who responded to the Behavioral Risk Factor Surveillance System survey reported that they had never been tested for HIV. This percentage was higher in the southwestern United States, where 58.1% of the American Indians and Alaska Natives reported never having been tested.

http://www.cdc.gov/hiv/resources/factsheets/aian.htm

Living Positively with HIV and AIDS

No one—neither modern medicine nor traditional healers— has a cure for AIDS. But most people with HIV can be healthy for many years, especially with the right care and treatment.

During this time it can help to:
 • make the best of every moment of your life.
• spend time with friends and family.
• try to keep active by doing your daily work.
• be sexual if you want to. Enjoying sexual touch can help you stay healthier longer.

A negative test only means that you do not have HIV when the test is taken. If you do not protect yourself, you can still get infected.

Important
Practice safer sex.
Use condoms.

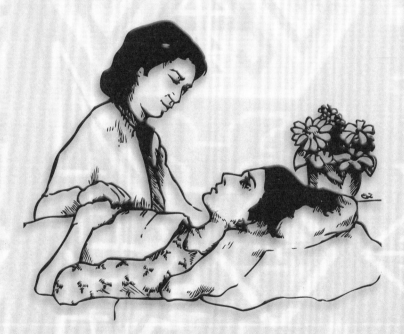

If your partner is HIV infected

Although it is risky, if you practice safer sex, the infected person can avoid passing HIV to his or her partner. Condoms are the best way to prevent HIV. Cover open skin wounds and get treated promptly for STIs. And remember, there are other ways to be sexual besides sexual intercourse.

Medication can prevent the transmission of HIV from mother to baby during childbirth - a great reason to get tested!

When a person has AIDS, the body's immune system is no longer able to fight off common infections and illnesses. The immune system gets weaker with each illness, making it even less able to fight infection the next time. This continues until the person's body is too weak to survive.

Preventing infections and illness is the best way to slow down the weakening of the immune system. It is also important to treat any infections to keep them from spreading or getting worse. This way a person with AIDS can stay healthy for as long as possible.

Medicines that treat AIDS

There is still no cure for AIDS, but antiretroviral medicines are now being used successfully to treat people who are sick with AIDS. Anti means against, and the virus that causes AIDS is called a retrovirus. If used correctly, antiretrovirals (called ARVs) fight against and kill much of the HIV. The immune system becomes stronger and the person with HIV is able to fight off infections and become healthier. But HIV is not cured. Small amounts of the virus always remain hidden in the body.

AntiRetroviral Therapy (ART) can help most people with HIV stay healthy for many years.

Taking antiretroviral medicines is known as ART. Clinics or health facilities and other programs may offer ART at low or no cost.

ART (Anti Retroviral Therapy**) works when used carefully.** ART means taking a combination of 3 antiretroviral medicines at least 2 times a day. Once a person with AIDS begins ART, the medicines must be taken faithfully every day. A woman on ART will gain weight, and look and feel healthier. But if she stops ART, misses doses of medicine, or takes them at the wrong times, her HIV can become stronger and make her sick again.

The Ryan White HIV/AIDS Treatment Modernization Act of 2006 is one of the primary ways the U.S. Government provides health care for people with HIV disease.

http://hab.hrsa.gov

ART and drug resistance: When people do not take ART at the right times every day, their HIV can become resistant, which means it changes so the medicine will not work as well against it. If drug resistant HIV spreads among many people, then ART medicines will no longer work very well. Taking ART correctly helps preserve its effectiveness for everyone.

How you can help prevent AIDS in the community

Education is one of the main ways a community can work to keep AIDS from spreading. Here are some ideas:

• Train girls and women to work as peer educators. They can talk with others alone or in groups to help girls and women understand their bodies and sexuality, and gain the selfconfidence and skills to demand safer sex.

• Use theater and media to help women feel it is OK to know about and to prevent AIDS. For example, use a play or comic book to show that 'good' girls or women can discuss AIDS with their partners, or can buy condoms and ask their husbands or boyfriends to use them.

At the same time, you can show different ideas about what it means to be a man or a woman. Help people question the idea that men should have many sex partners and that women should be passive about sex. Show how these ideas are dangerous to both men's and women's health.

• Talk openly about the dangers of shared needles or unsafe piercing or tatoo tools in the spread of HIV.

• Train men as outreach workers. They can go to the places where men gather and talk to them about AIDS.

• Help parents, teachers, and other adult role models become more comfortable talking about sex and AIDS with young people.

• Make sure that all people have access to information and sexual health services, including condoms, to keep AIDS from spreading in the community.

• Bring education about AIDS to community meeting places—like health fairs, sports events and pow wows.

RESOURCES:

www.cdc.gov/hiv/

National AIDS Hotlines at (800) 342-AIDS

The National Native American AIDS Prevention Center (NNAAPC) helps organizations that serve Native communities to plan, develop and manage HIV/AIDS prevention, intervention, care and treatment programs

www.nnaapc.org/

www.ihs.gov/MedicalPrograms/AIDS/index.asp
602-263-1502

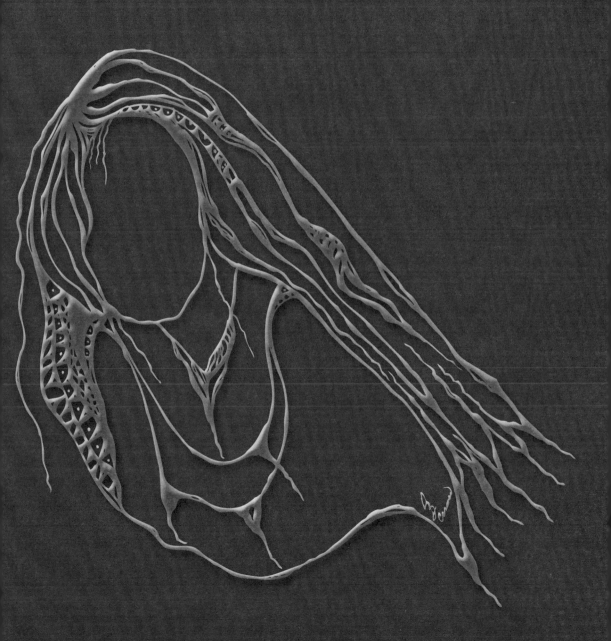

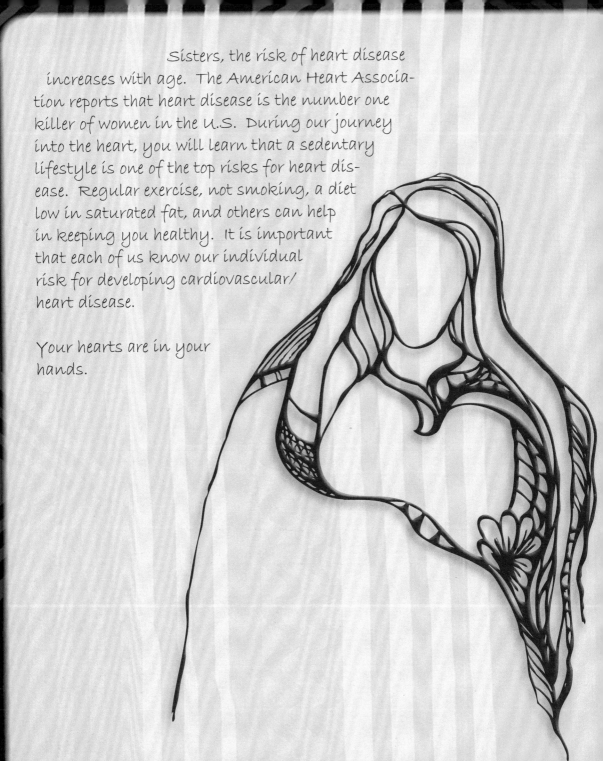

Sisters, the risk of heart disease increases with age. The American Heart Association reports that heart disease is the number one killer of women in the U.S. During our journey into the heart, you will learn that a sedentary lifestyle is one of the top risks for heart disease. Regular exercise, not smoking, a diet low in saturated fat, and others can help in keeping you healthy. It is important that each of us know our individual risk for developing cardiovascular/ heart disease.

Your hearts are in your hands.

Heart Health

Heart disease is the leading cause of death for American Indians and Alaska Natives.

Heart disease is a group of diseases of the heart and the blood vessel system in the heart. Coronary heart disease, the most common type, affects the blood vessels of the heart. It can cause angina or a heart attack. Angina is a pain in the chest that happens when the heart does not get enough blood. It may feel like a pressing or squeezing pain, often in the chest, but sometimes in the shoulders, arms, neck, jaw, or back. Having angina means you're more likely to have a heart attack. A heart attack happens when a blood vessel is blocked for more than 20 minutes.

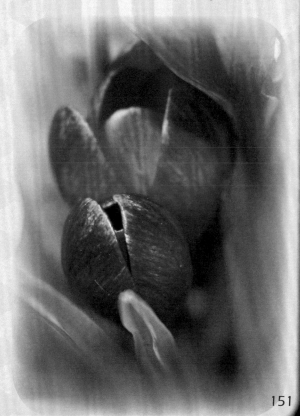

What is Heart and Vascular Disease?

Heart disease, sometimes called cardio vascular disease (CVD), is a term that includes several more specific heart conditions. The most common heart disease in the US is coronary artery disease (CAD). CAD occurs when the arteries that supply blood to the heart muscle become hardened and narrowed due to the buildup of plaque. The narrowing and buildup of plaques is called atherosclerosis. Plaques are a mixture of fatty and other substances including cholesterol and other lipids. Blood flow to the heart is reduced, which reduces oxygen to the heart muscle. This can lead to heart attack. Other heart conditions include angina, heart failure, and arrhythmias.

> Heart disease is more frequent in older people, especially in those who are overweight, who smoke, or who have high blood pressure or diabetes.

Coronary Heart Disease

The slow process of coronary heart disease begins during childhood when the arteries that carry blood from the heart become narrowed by a gradual build-up of fatty material within their walls. This condition is more commonly known as 'atherosclerosis".

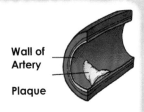

Wall of Artery

Plaque

Buildup of plaque

Partially blocked artery

Over time the artery may become so narrow that it cannot deliver enough oxygen-containing blood to the heart muscle when needed, such as during physical activity. This can lead to a severe pain called 'Angina'. This pain is similar to a cramp-like feeling and is due to the heart muscles becoming starved of oxygen rich blood.

Coronary heart disease can become more serious if a narrowed artery becomes blocked by a blood clot. This can result in a heart attack.

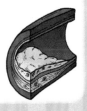

Heart Attack Explained

If the blood supply to the heart muscle is cut off, a heart attack can result. Cells in the heart muscle do not receive enough oxygen and begin to die. The more time that passes without treatment to restore blood flow, the greater the damage to the heart. Having high blood pressure or high blood cholesterol, smoking, and having had a previous heart attack, stroke, or diabetes can increase a person's chances of having a heart attack.

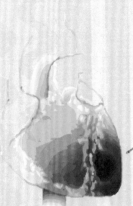
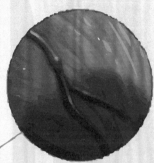

Death of heart tissue due to blocked coronary artery

Stroke
(Apoplexy, Cerebro-Vascular Accident, CVA)

In older people stroke or cerebro-vascular accident (CVA) commonly results from a blood clot or from bleeding inside the brain. The word stroke is used because this condition often strikes without warning. The person may suddenly fall down, unconscious. Her face is often reddish, her breathing hoarse and noisy, her pulse strong and slow. She may remain in a coma (unconscious) for hours or days. If she lives, she may have trouble speaking, seeing, or thinking, or one side of her face and body may be paralyzed. In minor strokes, some of these same problems may result without loss of consciousness. The difficulties caused by stroke sometimes get better with time.

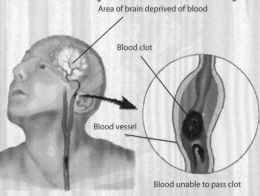

Area of brain deprived of blood

Blood clot

Blood vessel

Blood unable to pass clot

153

Signs of Heart Disease

- Anxiety and difficulty in breathing after exercise; asthma-like attacks that get worse when the person lies down (cardiac asthma).
- A rapid, weak, or irregular pulse.
- Swelling of the feet— worse in the afternoons.
- Shortness of breath without exercise, unexplained tiredness, weakness, dizziness.
- Sudden, painful attacks in the chest, left shoulder, or arm that occur when exercising and go away after resting for a few minutes (angina pectoris).
- A sharp pain like a great weight crushing the chest; does not go away with rest (heart attack).
- In women: nausea, clamminess, jaw pain.

What are symptoms of a heart attack?

The National Heart Attack Alert Program notes these major symptoms of a heart attack:

Chest discomfort. Most heart attacks involve discomfort in the center of the chest that lasts for more than a few minutes, or goes away and comes back. The discomfort can feel like uncomfortable pressure, squeezing, fullness, or pain.

Discomfort in other areas of the upper body. This can include pain or discomfort in one or both arms, the back, neck, jaw, or stomach.

Shortness of breath. This often comes along with chest discomfort. But it also can occur before chest discomfort.

Other symptoms women may have include:
- unusual tiredness
- trouble sleeping
- problems breathing
- indigestion (upset stomach)
- anxiety (feeling uneasy or worried)
- breaking out in a cold sweat
- experiencing nausea or light-headedness

> **IMPORTANT**
> Signs of dangerously high blood pressure:
> - frequent headaches
> - dizziness
> - ringing sound in the ears
>
> All these signs can also be caused by other diseases. For more information, see your health care provider.

> If you have any of these symptoms, call 911.

Different heart diseases may require different specific medicines, which must be used with great care. If you think a person has heart trouble, seek medical help. It is important that she have the right medicine when she needs it.

Living with Heart Disease

- People with heart trouble should not work so hard that they get chest pain or have trouble breathing. However, regular exercise helps prevent a heart attack.

- Persons with heart problems should not eat greasy food and should lose weight if they are overweight. Also, they should not smoke or drink alcohol.

- If an older person begins having attacks of difficult breathing or swelling of the feet, she should not use salt or eat food that contains salt. For the rest of her life she should eat little or no salt.

- Also, taking one aspirin tablet a day may help prevent a heart attack or a stroke.

Preventing and Treating High Blood Pressure

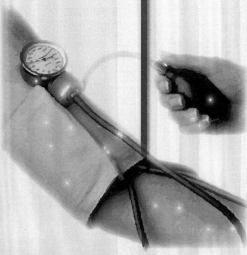

High blood pressure and hardening of the arteries (arteriosclerosis), which are the main causes of heart disease and stroke, can usually be prevented—or reduced—by doing the things recommended above. The lowering of high blood pressure is important in the prevention of heart disease and stroke. Persons who have high blood pressure should have it checked from time to time and take measures to lower it. For those who are not successful in lowering their blood pressure by eating less (if they are overweight), giving up smoking, getting more exercise, and learning to relax, taking medicines to lower blood pressure (antihypertensives) may help.

By the Numbers

Knowing your numbers is an important part of keeping your heart healthy. These numbers can help you and your doctor determine your risks and mark the progress you're making toward a healthier heart.

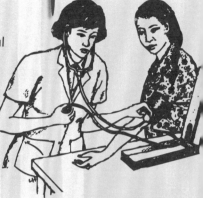

Target Blood Pressure:

less than 120/80

- **Total Cholesterol** Less than **200** mg/dL
- **LDL** ("Bad") Cholesterol LDL cholesterol goals vary.
    - Less than **100** mg/dL   Optimal
    - 100 to 129 mg/dL   Near Optimal/Above Optimal
    - 130 to 159 mg/dL   Borderline High
    - 160 to 189 mg/dL   High
    - 190 mg/dL & above Very High

- **HDL** ("Good") Cholesterol   **50** mg/dL or higher
- **Triglycerides**   less than **150** mg/dL
- **Blood Pressure**   less than **120/80** mmHg
- **Fasting Glucose**   less than **100** mg/dL
- **Body Mass Index (BMI)**   less than **25** Kg/m²
- **Waist Circumference**   less than **35** inches

- **Exercise** a Minimum of **30** minutes most days, if not all days of the week

If you are visiting a clinic for any reason, try to have your blood pressure checked at the same time.

Women can reduce their risk of heart disease by making the following lifestyle changes:

- Quitting Smoking
- Exercising Regularly
- Eating a Healthful, Low-Fat Diet
- Controlling High Blood Pressue
- Controlling Cholesterol Levels
- Controlling or Preventing Diabetes

If your blood pressure is very high, you may also need to take medicine.

Take the Heart Health Quiz!

True or False: Heart disease develops gradually over many years and can easily go undetected.

Heart disease takes years to develop and for women, it takes almost a decade longer to show up than it does for men. By then, most women are concerned with other potential health problems such as breast cancer, arthritis, or osteoporosis. (True)

True or False: Women are more likely to get heart disease after menopause.

Before menopause, women are relatively protected from heart disease because their bodies produce estrogen. But as women approach menopause, at about age 55, their hormone status changes. Studies show that the loss of natural estrogen as women age may contribute to a higher risk of heart disease after menopause. (True)

True or False: When a woman has a heart attack, she is more likely to survive it than a man.

A woman has a lower chance of surviving a heart attack compared to a man. According to the American Heart Association, 38 percent of women compared with 25 percent of men will die within one year after a heart attack. (False)

True or False: When women experience the symptoms of a heart attack, they may come on gradually rather than suddenly.

Many women experience the symptoms of a heart attack gradually. In fact, symptoms may even come and go. That's why it's so important for women to know and pay attention to the signs and symptoms. (True)

True or False: Women who smoke are twice as likely to have a heart attack over women who don't smoke.

Smoking is one of the most significant risk factors for women. According to the American Heart Association, smokers are 2 times more likely than non-smokers to suffer from a heart attack. (True)

True or False: Women with diabetes are three times more likely to develop heart disease.

According to the American Heart Association, compared to women of the same age without diabetes, women with diabetes have from three to seven times the risk of heart disease and heart attack. And diabetes doubles the risk of a second heart attack in women but not in men. (True)

American Indian / Alaska Native Heart Disease and Stroke Facts

• Heart Disease is the first and stroke the sixth leading cause of death Among American Indians and Alaska Natives.

• The heart disease death rate was 20 percent greater among American Indians and Alaska Natives than among all U.S. races when records were reveiwed from 1996-98.

• American Indians and Alaska Natives die from heart diseases at younger ages than other racial and ethnic groups in the United States. Thirty–six percent of those who die of heart disease die before age 65.

• Women who smo[...] risk having a hear[...] attack 19 years ear[...]er than non-smokir[...] women.
• Women with diab[...]tes are two to thre[...] times more likely t[...] have heart attacks[...]
• High blood pres[...]sure is more comm[...] in women taking oral contraceptives[...] especially in obes[...] women.

Preventing Heart Disease and Stroke
Among American Indians and Alaska Natives

Prevent and Control High Blood Cholesterol: High blood cholesterol is a major risk factor for heart disease. Preventing and treating high blood cholesterol includes eating a di[...] low in saturated fat and cholesterol and high in fiber, keeping a healthy weight, and gettin[...] regular exercise. All adults should have their cholesterol levels checked once every five year[...] If yours is high, your doctor may prescribe medicines to help lower it.

Prevent and Control High Blood Pressure: Lifestyle actions such as healthy diet, regu[...]lar physical activity, not smoking, and healthy weight will help you to keep normal blood pressure levels. A high blood pressure can usually be controlled with lifestyle changes and with medicines when needed.

Prevent and Control Diabetes: Diabetes has been shown to be a very important risk facto[...] for heart disease among American Indians and Alaska Natives. People with diabetes have a[...] increased risk for heart disease but can reduce their risk. Also, people can take steps to redu[...] their risk for diabetes in the first place, through weight loss and regular physical activity. For[...] more information about diabetes, see CDC's diabetes program Web site.

No Tobacco: Chewing, dipping, and cigarette smoking are non-traditional uses of tobacco[...] among American Indians and Alaska Natives. Smoking increases the risk of high blood pres[...]sure, heart disease, and stroke.

Moderate Alcohol Use: Excessive alcohol use increases the risk of high blood pressure, he[...] attack, and stroke. People who drink should do so only in moderation and always responsib[...] More information on alcohol can be found at CDC's alcohol and public health Web site.

Regular Physical Activity: Adults should engage in moderate level physical activities for a[...] least 30 minutes on most days of the week.

Words to Our Sisters and Daughters Who Want to Stay Healthy When They Are Older

Many of the health problems of middle and old age, including high blood pressure, hardening of the arteries, heart disease, and stroke, result from the way a person has lived and what she ate, drank, and smoked when younger. Your chances for living and staying healthy longer are greater if you:

1. Eat well—enough nutritious foods, but not too much rich, greasy, or salty food.

Avoid getting overweight. Use vegetable oil rather than animal fat for cooking.

2. Do not drink a lot of alcoholic drinks.

3. Do not smoke.

4. Keep physically and mentally active.

5. Try to get enough rest and sleep.

6. Learn how to relax and deal positively with things that worry or upset you.

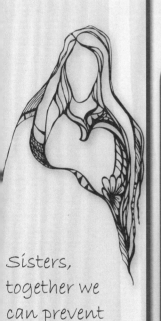

Sisters, together we can prevent heart disease.

Compared with Men:

According to the American Heart Associaion,

• 38% of women and 25% of men will die within one year of a first recognized heart attack.

• 35% of women and 18% of men heart attack survivors will have another heart attack within six years.

• 46% of women and 22% of men heart attack survivors will be disabled with heart failure within six years.

• Women are almost twice as likely as men to die after bypass surgery.

• Women are less likely than men to receive beta-blockers, ACE inhibitors or even aspirin after a heart attack.

• More women than men die of heart disease each year, yet women receive only:

> • 33% of angioplasties, stents and bypass surgeries
> • 28% of inplantable defibrillators and
> • 36% of open-heart surgeries

• Women comprise only 25% of participants in all heart-related research studies.

Eating for a Healthy Heart

Heart disease is the leading cause of death for American Indians and Alaska Natives today. We can do something to prevent heart disease. Healthy eating is one way to keep a healthy heart.

Native foods and traditional ways can help us stay healthy. Native foods can still be found in many places today.

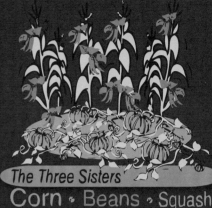

The Three Sisters
Corn • Beans • Squash

• Grow traditional plants such as beans, corn, chile, pumpkin, squash, and melons.
• Choose berries, nuts, plants, fish, caribou, deer, rabbit, duck, and other native foods more often.

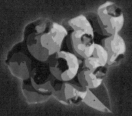

• Use traditional ways of preparing food like drying, baking, stewing, and boiling.

Today, many American Indian families choose foods that are higher in fat, saturated fat (animal fat), cholesterol, calories, salt, and sodium. We also eat more than we used to. These habits can lead to heart disease.

Here are tips for making heart healthy choices:

• Choose fish, fowl, deer, and caribou.
• Eat lean cuts of beef, pork, and mutton.
• Cut the fat from meat and throw it away. Take off the skin from chicken and turkey.
• Remove fat from canned meat.
• Eat rice, corn, oats, and beans.
• Eat salads and sandwiches with little or no dressing.
• Eat fruits and vegetables.
• Drink fat-free or low-fat milk and choose fat-free and low-fat cheese.
• Bake, boil, broil, steam, or roast! Fry foods less often. Use small amounts of vegetable oil instead of lard or shortening.
• Drain the liquid from canned vegetables and the syrup from canned fruits.

from: http://hp2010.nhlbihin.net/FactSheets/treat.htm
(National Heart Lung and Blood Institute & Indian Health Service)

Resources:

WomenHeart
the National Coalition for Women
with Heart Disease
www.womenheart.org/

American Heart Association
www.goredforwomen.org

http://www.cdc.gov/wisewoman/

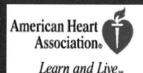

**http://www.nhlbi.nih.gov/health/
hearttruth/**

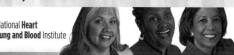

Go Red For Women is the American Heart Association's nationwide movement that celebrates the energy, passion and power we have as women to band together and wipe out heart disease. Thanks to the participation of millions of people across the country, the color red and the red dress have become linked with the ability all women have to improve their heart health and live stronger, longer lives.

Taking care of your heart is more important than you might know. Too few people realize that heart disease is the No. 1 killer of American women — and of men. But the good news is that heart disease can largely be prevented. Go Red For Women empowers women with knowledge and tools so they can take positive action to reduce their risks of heart disease and stroke and protect their health.

The movement gives women tips and information on healthy eating, exercise and risk factor reduction, such as smoking cessation, weight maintenance, blood pressure control, and blood cholesterol management.

www.goredforwomen.org

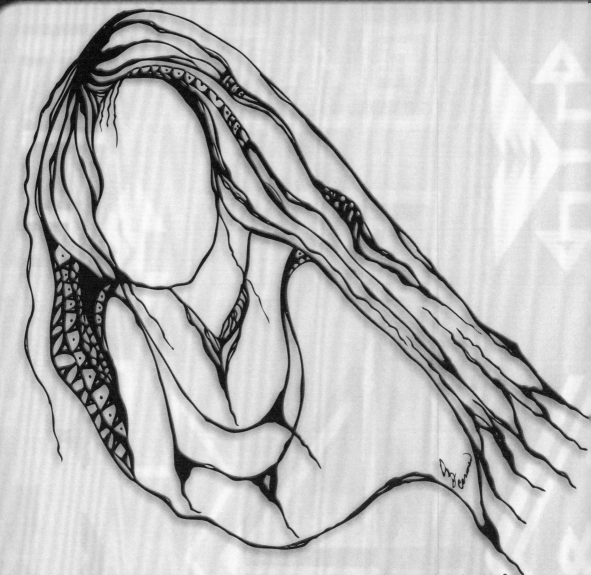

Sisters, like Cancer, Diabetes is a silent disease, it kind of creeps up on you. Diabetes occurs when your body no longer makes insulin or not enough. As you will learn in this section, there are two types of Diabetes; Type 1, which requires insulin shots and Type 2, which sometimes require a pill and sometimes requires insulin. Both insulin shots and pills assist your Pancreas and make insulin. Native peoples suffer from higher Diabetes rates than any other ethnic group/race. The why's are not exactly known, but we are no longer hunters or gatherers of food. Our lifestyle's have changed and so has our ability to keep diseases away.

Diabetes

Diabetes has something to do with having too much or too little sugar in the blood. But what does that mean? Everybody has some amount of sugar, or glucose, in their blood. Glucose comes from the food we eat and gives us energy. Nearly everything we eat gets broken down into glucose. It helps cells to grow and get the power they need to do their job.

Most people's bodies do an amazingly good job of controlling the amount of glucose in their blood. One of the body's organs, the pancreas, makes insulin. Insulin does most of the work in moving glucose out of the blood to where it's needed in the rest of the body's cells. The insulin works to move the glucose from the blood stream into the cells so it can be used. In a person who doesn't have diabetes, the pancreas produces just the right amount of insulin needed by the body.

But when someone has diabetes, their body has trouble controlling the level of glucose in its blood. Either the person's pancreas can't make insulin (Type 1 diabetes), or can't make enough insulin, or their body has a problem using the insulin it does make (Type 2 diabetes).

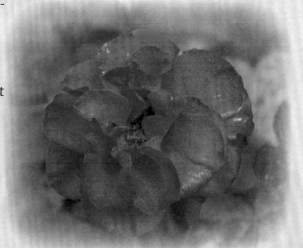

Types of Diabetes

Type 2 Diabetes

Type 2 Diabetes is the most common form of diabetes. In this type of diabetes, the pancreas still produces insulin, but, either the body does not produce enough insulin or the cells ignore the insulin.

Type 2 diabetes usually develops in adults over 35 years old, and especially in those who are overweight. But recently type 2 diabetes has begun to appear more in children and teenagers, as more and more of them are becoming overweight.

Type 2 diabetes is generally connected with older age, obesity (being overweight), a history of diabetes in the family, having had gestational diabetes (diabetes only while you are pregnant), and lack of physical exercise. It also seems to be tied to race or ethnicity. People who are African American, Hispanic or Latino American, Native American, and members of some groups of Asian Americans and Pacific Islanders have a greater chance of developing type 2 diabetes.

About 90 to 95 percent of people diagnosed with diabetes have type 2. The symptoms can include extreme tiredness, being unusually hungry or thirsty, losing weight suddenly, urinating more often than normal, blurry vision, and sores or infections that take a long time to heal. These symptoms can come on gradually, or there may not be any symptoms at all. Usually, type 2 diabetes can be controlled by losing weight, improving nutrition and increasing exercise. But many people may need to take medication by mouth or inject or pump insulin (or sometimes both) to control the disease.

When glucose buil[d] up in the blood in-stead of going into cells, it can cause tv problems:

1. Right away, you cells may be starve[d] for energy.

2. Over time, high blood glucose leve[l] in the blood may h[e] your eyes, kidneys, nerves or heart.

Some people diagnosed with diabetes have n[o] symptoms. Find out more at you[r] clinic.

Type 2 Diabetes

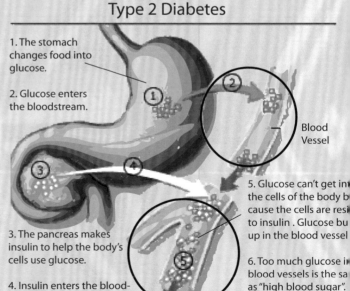

1. The stomach changes food into glucose.

2. Glucose enters the bloodstream.

3. The pancreas makes insulin to help the body's cells use glucose.

4. Insulin enters the blood-stream to help the glucose get into the cells to be used for energy.

Blood Vessel

5. Glucose can't get in[to] the cells of the body b[e] cause the cells are resi[stant] to insulin . Glucose bu[ilds] up in the blood vessel

6. Too much glucose i[n] blood vessels is the sa[me] as "high blood sugar".

7. High blood sugar causes damage to the body over time.

Gestational Diabetes

For women who do not currently have diabetes, pregnancy brings the risk of gestational diabetes. Gestational diabetes develops in 2% to 5% of all pregnancies but disappears when a pregnancy is over. Women who have had gestational diabetes or have given birth to a baby weighting more than 9 pounds are at an increased risk for developing type 2 diabetes later in life.

Diabetes is more likely to develop during pregnancy than at other times. If you are pregnant and are always thirsty or are losing weight, see a health worker to test your blood sugar.

Type 1 Diabetes

Type 1 diabetes is usually diagnosed in children and young adults, and was previously known as juvenile diabetes. In type 1 diabetes, the body does not produce insulin. Insulin is a hormone that is needed to convert sugar (glucose), starches and other food into energy needed for daily life.

Good News!
Type 2 diabetes can be prevented!

Before people develop type 2 diabetes, they almost always have "**pre-diabetes**" – blood glucose levels that are higher than normal but not yet high enough to be diagnosed as diabetes. Recent research has shown that some long-term damage to the body, especially the heart and circulatory system, may already be occurring during pre-diabetes. Research has also shown that if you take action to manage your blood glucose when you have pre-diabetes, you can delay or prevent type 2 diabetes from ever developing.

If you have pre-diabetes, you can and should do something about it. People with pre-diabetes can prevent or delay the development of type 2 diabetes through changes to their lifestyle that include modest weight loss and regular exercise. It is recommended that those with pre-diabetes reduce their weight by 5-10 percent and participate in some type of modest physical activity for 30 minutes daily. For some people with pre-diabetes, intervening early can actually turn back the clock and return elevated blood glucose levels to the normal range.

Eating Healthy

People with diabetes must pay close attention to their dietary intake, portion sizes, and meal frequency. What you eat, or more specifically the carbohydrates (or carbs) in the food you eat, are the body's main source of glucose. Foods that contain carbohydrates include sugar, starchy foods like potatoes and pasta, and grain-based foods like breads and cereals. Carbohydrates can also be found in dairy products and fruits and vegetables, as well as many beverages.

If you have diabetes or pre-diabetes talk to a registered dietician to plan healthy meals and snacks.

Fats and Sweets:

Limit the amount of fats and sweets you eat. Fats and sweets are not as nutritious as other foods. Fats have a lot of calories. Sweets can be high in carbohydrate and fat. Some contain saturated fats, trans fats, and cholesterol that increase your risk of heart disease. Limiting these foods will help you lose weight and keep your blood glucose and blood fats under control.

Fruits:

Eat fruits raw or cooked, as juice with no sugar added, canned in their own juice, or dried.

Buy smaller pieces of fruit.

Choose pieces of fruit more often than fruit juice. Whole fruit is more filling and has more fiber.

Save high-sugar and high-fat fruit desserts such as peach cobbler or cherry pie for special occasions.

Starches:

Buy whole grain breads and cereals.

Eat fewer fried and high-fat starches such as regular tortilla chips and potato chips, french fries, pastries, or biscuits. Try pretzels, fat-free popcorn, baked tortilla chips or potato chips, baked potatoes, or low-fat muffins.

Use low-fat or fat-free plain yogurt or fat-free sour cream instead of regular sour cream on a baked potato.

Use low-fat or fat-free substitutes such as low-fat mayonnaise or light margarine on bread, rolls, or toast.

Eat cereal with fat-free (skim) or low-fat (1%) milk.

Alcoholic Drinks

Alcoholic drinks have calories but no nutrients. If you have alcoholic drinks on an empty stomach, they can make your blood glucose level go too low. Alcoholic drinks also can raise your blood sugar and blood fats. If you want to have alcoholic drinks, talk with your doctor or diabetes educator about how much to have.

Staying Active

Should I Stop Exercising When I Reach My Ideal Weight?

Exercise is a lifetime commitment. Regardless of your weight, you should exercise at least three to four times per week for 20 to 40 minutes each session. Ideally, you should exercise every day to help manage your type 2 diabetes long-term.

A Little Exercise Goes a Long Way

You don't have to spend hours exercising to look and feel better! Just 30 minutes a day will do. You can even split it up into 2 or 3 parts. Try a 10-minute walk after every meal. Or think of ways to

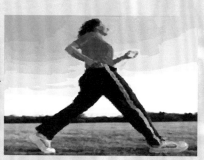

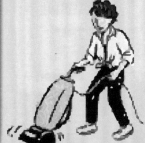

build extra activity into your day. You don't have to go to a gym. Just walk, wash the car, weed the garden, or clean the house. The goal is to find the balance between eating and exercise - making sure you burn up the calories you eat!

General Exercise Guidelines

• Check with your health care provider before you begin a diabetes exercise program. Tell your doctor what kind of exercise you want to do so adjustments can be made to your medicine schedule or meal plan, if necessary.

• Start slowly and gradually increase your endurance.

• Choose an activity that you enjoy. You'll be more likely to stick with a program if you enjoy the activity. **Make exercise a lifetime commitment.** Consider walking, riding a stationary bicycle, swimming or muscle stretching.

• Exercise at least three to four times per week for 20 to 40 minutes each session. Ideally, you should exercise every day. A good exercise program should include a 5- to 10-minute warm-up and at least 15 to 30 minutes of continuous aerobic exercise (such as walking or biking) or muscle stretching exercises, followed by a 5-minute cool down.

• Wear good shoes and practice proper foot care.

• Drink water before, during and after exercise to prevent dehydration.

• Do not ignore pain -- discontinue any exercise that causes unexpected pain. If you continue to perform the activity while you are in pain, you may cause unnecessary stress or damage to your joints.

Women with Diabetes
Complications and Related Conditions

Heart Disease and Stroke
People with diabetes have extra reason to be mindful of heart and blood vessel disease. Diabetes carries an increased risk for heart attack, stroke, and complications related to poor circulation.

Kidney Disease
Diabetes can damage the kidneys, which not only can cause them to fail, but can also make them lose their ability to filter out waste products.

Eye Complications
Diabetes can cause eye problems and may lead to blindness. People with diabetes do have a higher risk of blindness than people without diabetes. Early detection and treatment of eye problems can save your sight.

Diabetic Neuropathy and Nerve Damage
One of the most common complications of diabetes is diabetic neuropathy. Neuropathy means damage to the nerves that run throughout the body, connecting the spinal cord to muscles, skin, blood vessels, and other organs.

Foot Complications
People with diabetes can develop many different foot problems. Foot problems most often happen when there is nerve damage in the feet or when blood flow is poor. Learn how to protect your feet by following some basic guidelines.

Skin Complications
As many as one-third of people with diabetes will have a skin disorder caused or affected by diabetes at some time in their lives. In fact, such problems are sometimes the first sign that a person has diabetes. Luckily, most skin conditions can be prevented or easily treated if caught early.

Having diabetes increases your risk for many serious complications. Some complications of diabetes include: heart disease (cardiovascular disease), blindness (retinopathy), nerve damage (neuropathy), and kidney damage (nephropathy). Your clinic and health care provider are valuable resources for helping identify and reduce complications from diabetes.

People with diabetes ideally should get a checkup every three months. Talk to your health care provider about routine diabetes checkups.

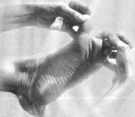

Foot Checks look for:
- corns and calluses
- blisters
- ingrown toenails
- bunions
- hammertoes
- planter's warts
- dry and cracked skin
- athlete's foot

Some complications may happen more often in women with diabetes. Here are some examples:

Depression

The rate of depression in people with diabetes is much higher than in the general population. Women experience depression about twice as often as men. The risk of depression increases in women with diabetes. Many hormonal factors may contribute to the increased rate of depression in women – particularly such factors as menstrual cycle changes, pregnancy, miscarriage, postpartum period, pre-menopause, and menopause. Many women also face additional stresses such as responsibilities both at work and home, single parenthood, and caring for children and for aging parents.

Polycystic Ovarian Syndrome

Polycystic Ovarian Syndrome (PCOS) is the most common cause of female infertility. Many women with PCOS also have diabetes. In women with PCOS, eggs from the ovaries may not make it to the womb to be fertilized. As a result, women with PCOS often don't have menstrual periods, or they have periods only on occasion.

No one knows the exact cause of PCOS, but studies are looking at whether it is caused by genetics. Studies are examining the relationship between PCOS and the body's ability to produce insulin.

Other symptoms include acne, obesity, high blood cholesterol, high blood pressure, excessive hair growth, and baldness in a similar pattern as seen in men or thinning hair.

Eating Disorders

Research suggests that eating disorders are probably more common among women with diabetes than women who do not have diabetes. Bulimia is the most common eating disorder in women with type 1 diabetes. Among women with type 2 diabetes, binge eating is more common.

Eating disorders are illnesses with a biological basis influenced by emotional and cultural factors. The stigma associated with eating disorders has kept some women suffering in silence. If you have questions about eating disorders, trust your health care provider to help find answers.

169

Frequently Asked Questions about Women and Diabetes

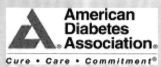

American Diabetes Association.
Cure • Care • Commitment®

Why are women with diabetes predisposed to developing recurrent yeast infections?
The glucose (sugar) in your body is the perfect trigger to encourage and grow yeast within your body.

What are the complications of using birth control pills while having diabetes?
Birth control pills may raise your Blood Glucose(BG) levels. Using them for longer than a year or 2 may also increase your risk of complications. For instance, if you develop high blood pressure while on the pill, you increase the chance that eye or kidney disease will worsen.

Will menopause affect my diabetes?
Yes. The changes in hormonal levels and balance, may lead to Blood Glucose levels that are out of control. Women with diabetes are also at risk of developing premature menopause and consequent increased risks of cardiovascular disease.

Are there any diabetes medications that have a higher incidence of side effects amongst women who use them?
Yes, the oral medications classified as thiazolidinediones (TZDs) may cause women who are not ovulating and haven't gone through menopause to begin ovulating again, enabling them to conceive. Also, oral contraceptives may be less effective when taking this medication.

Is their a time frame that women with diabetes should follow for check-ups such as gynecological exams?
Check-ups should be performed on a regular, consistent basis to ensure that the diabetes is not negatively affecting the reproductive organs. Your health care provider will determine how often you should visit with him/her depending on your overall health.

I had diabetes before I was pregnant. Now that I am pregnant, how often should I monitor my BG levels?

Most health care professionals recommend that a woman with pre-existing diabetes (both type 1 & type 2) who becomes pregnant monitor her BG levels up to 8 times daily. In terms of your day-to-day routine, you should probably monitor: before each meal, 1 or 2 hours after each meal, at bedtime, occasionally at 2-3 a.m.

I had gestational diabetes. How soon after having the baby should I get my blood glucose rechecked?

About 6-8 weeks after delivery. Like 90% of the women with gestational diabetes, your BG levels will probably return to normal right after your baby is born. However, you still run the risk of developing type 2 diabetes. In fact, 5% of women with gestational diabetes will have type 2 diabetes and 15% will have pre-diabetes by the time of this first screening.

What are the risks of hormone replacement therapy?

The risks are increased incidence of breast cancer and uterine cancer while using estrogen. However, when estrogen and progesterone are administered together and in the correct doses, the risk of cancer of the uterus or endometrium is reduced.

Will my children inherit diabetes from me?

It all depends on risk factors that include:

- no diabetes in the family – 11% chance of type 2 diabetes by age 70 and 1% chance of type 1 diabetes by age 50.
- One parent with type 2 diabetes (diagnosed before the age of 50) – 14% chance of type 2 diabetes.
- Both parents with type 2 diabetes (overall risk) – 45% chance of type 2 diabetes.

However, even for those at higher risk because diabetes runs in a family, type 2 diabetes can be prevented or significantly delayed. Ask your health care provider to screen for diabetes and pre-diabetes. Healthy habits such as maintianing a healthy weight and getting routine exercise can help someone at risk to prevent diabetes. Setting healthy eating and exercise habits for your children are probably the most important thing you can do to help prevent diabetes in future generations.

Living Healthy with Diabetes

If you or a loved one has been diagnosed with diabetes, your doctor may have talked to you about "managing your diabetes". Successful management of diabetes often happens with moderate changes in lifestyle and with the help of a team of others. Your diabetes team might include your primary care provider, your dentist, a dietician, your clinic Diabetes Coordinator, Community Health Representatives, your family, your friends and ultimately, your community.

Besides eating a healthy (low carbohydrate and fat) diet and getting routine exercise, a person with diabetes will need to monitor their own blood glucose, possibly take medications and get checkups at your clinic every three months.

The Indian Health Service recommends the following clinical care for someone with diabetes. Talk with your doctor to make sure you are receiving the right care at the right time intervals. By getting routine checkups, your health care provider can adjust medication and can find and treat complications of diabetes before they become a problem.

Diabetes checkups may include:
- height and weight
- blood pressure
- HbA1c test
- Cholesterol, HDL, LDL check
- review of medicines
- help with self monitoring your blood sugar
- depression screen
- foot check
- eye check
- kidney and liver function test
- Immunizations
- nutrition, exercise and other education
- help with quitting tobacco use
- a chance for you to ask questions about diabetes

> Check your feet once a day to see if you have any sores or signs of infection.

Resources

Special Diabetes Programs for Indians (SDPI) at your IHS, Tribal or Urban Indian Health Clinic

Indian Health Service Division of Diabetes Treatment and Prevention

http://www.ihs.gov/ MedicalPrograms/Diabetes/index.asp

 NARA's Diabetes Prevention and Treatment Program
503-230-9875

Diabetes in American Indians and Alaska Natives

from Indian Health Service Diabetes FactSheet 2007

16.3% = Percent of American Indian and Alaska Native adults have diagnosed diabetes (compared with 8.7% of non-Hispanic whites)

1,758 = Number of American Indian and Alaska Native youth under the age of 19 who have diagnosed diabetes (2005)

68% = Percent increase in diabetes from 1994 to 2004 in American Indian and Alaska Native youth aged 15-19 years

95% = Percent of American Indians and Alaska Natives with diabetes who have type 2 diabetes (as opposed to type 1 diabetes)

30% = Estimated percent of American Indians and Alaska Natives who have pre-diabetes

2.2 = Times higher Likelihood of American Indians and Alaska Natives to have diabetes compared with non-Hispanic whites

58% = Increase in diabetes prevalence among American Indians and Alaska Natives aged 20–29 from 1990 to 1998, as compared with 9.1% in the U.S. general population

3 = Times higher Death rate due to diabetes for American Indians and Alaska Natives compared with the general U.S. population (2004)

Additional Resources

American Diabetes Association

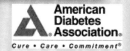

www.diabetes.org

1-800-DIABETES (1-800-342-2383). Monday - Friday, 8:30 AM - 8 PM EST

National Diabetes Education Program

www.ndep.nih.gov/

The National Institute of Diabetes and Digestive and Kidney Diseases

www2.niddk.nih.gov/

Centers for Disease Control and Prevention

http://www.cdc.gov/diabetes/

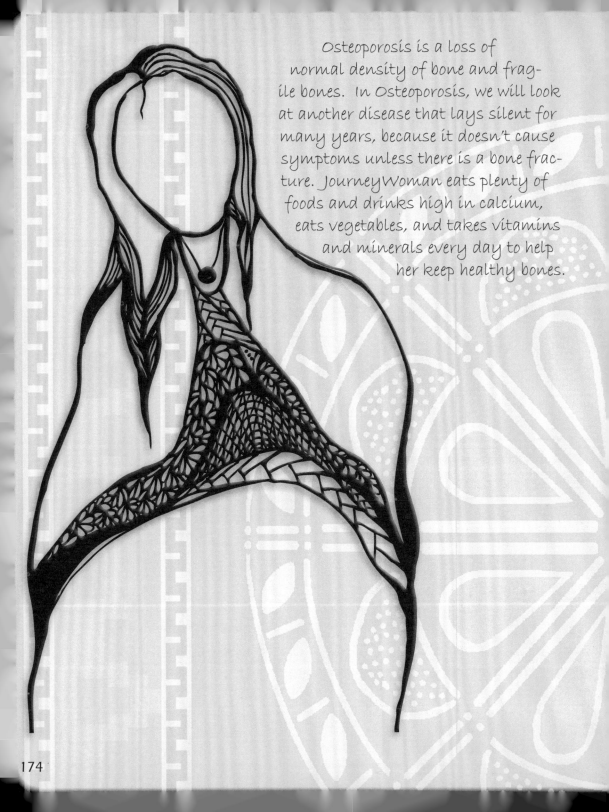

Osteoporosis is a loss of normal density of bone and fragile bones. In Osteoporosis, we will look at another disease that lays silent for many years, because it doesn't cause symptoms unless there is a bone fracture. JourneyWoman eats plenty of foods and drinks high in calcium, eats vegetables, and takes vitamins and minerals every day to help her keep healthy bones.

Healthy Bones

Osteoporosis (oss-tee-oh-puh-ro-sis) is a condition that means your bones are weak, and you're more likely to break a bone. Since there are no symptoms, you might not know your bones are getting weaker until you break a bone! A broken bone can really affect a woman's life. It can cause disability, pain, or loss of independence. It can make it harder to do daily activities without help, such as walking. This can make it hard to participate in social activities. It can also cause severe back pain and deformity.

A generation ago, most people considered osteoporosis and broken bones to be a part of normal aging. We now know a lot about how you can protect your bones throughout your life with nutrition and exercise. And although it's never too late to start protecting your bones, the best time to begin is while you're young.

If you already have osteoporosis or are at risk for it, the good news is that in the last 15 years, effective treatments for osteoporosis have been found. They're not a cure, but they can help, especially when you exercise and eat right.

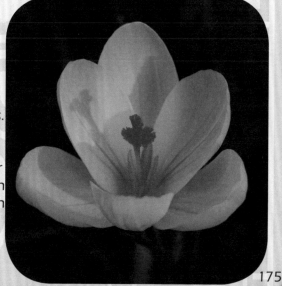

The U.S. Surgeon General reports that half of all women older than 50 will break a bone because of osteoporosis. One in four men will, too. And breaking a bone when you're older is serious. It leads to pain and immobility, which in turn can lead to isolation, depression, and other health problems.

The word osteoporosis means porous bone. If you looked at healthy bone under a microscope, you would see that parts of it look like a honeycomb. If you have osteoporosis, however, the holes and spaces in the honeycomb are much bigger than they are in healthy bone. And as your bones become less dense, they get weaker and easier to break. Fractures from osteoporosis can occur in almost any bone, but you are most likely to break bones in your wrist, spine, and hip.

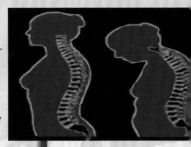

Osteoporosis is often called a "silent disease" because bone loss occurs without symptoms. People may not know that they have osteoporosis until their bones become so weak that a sudden strain, bump or fall causes a fracture or a vertebra in the back-bone to collapse. Collapsed vertebrae may initially be felt or seen in the form of severe back pain, loss of height, or stooped posture.

What bones does osteoporosis affect?

Osteoporosis can happen to any of your bones, but is most common in the hip, wrist, and in your spine, also called your vertebrae (ver-tuh-bray). Vertebrae are important because these bones support your body to stand and sit upright. See the picture below.

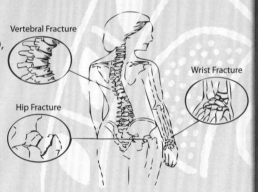

Vertebral Fracture

Wrist Fracture

Hip Fracture

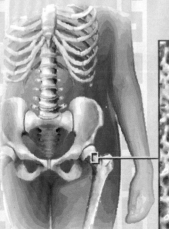

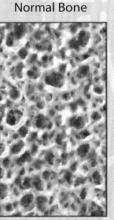

Normal Bone

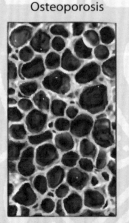

Osteoporosis

Any bone can be-come weak, but of special concern are fractures of the hip and spine. A hip fra ture almost always requires hospital-ization and major surgery. It can hurt a person's ability to walk unassisted and may cause disability or even death. Weak nesses and cracks in the spine can also lead to serious harm, includ ing loss of height, severe back pain, and deformity (hunched back).

Bone changes over a lifetime

Throughout life, your skeleton loses old bone and forms new bone. Children and teenagers form new bone faster than they lose the old bone. In fact, even after they stop growing taller, young people continue to make more bone than they lose. This means their bones get denser and denser until they reach what experts call peak bone mass. This is the point when you have the greatest amount of bone you will ever have. It usually occurs between the ages of 18 and 25.

After you achieve peak bone mass, the balance between bone loss and bone formation might start to shift. In other words, you may slowly start to lose more bone than you form. In midlife, bone loss usually speeds up in both men and women. For most women, the pace really picks up after menopause, when estrogen levels drop sharply. The more bone you have at the time of peak bone mass, before bone loss starts, the better protected you will be against weak bones.

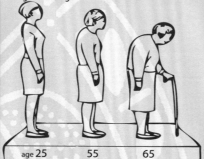

age 25   55   65

Prevention

By about age 20, the average woman has acquired 98 percent of her skeletal mass. Building strong bones during childhood and adolescence can be the best defense against developing osteoporosis later. There are four steps, which together can optimize bone health and help prevent osteoporosis. They are:

1) A balanced diet rich in calcium and vitamin D.

2) Weight-bearing and resistance-training exercises.

3) A healthy lifestyle with no smoking or excessive alcohol intake.

4) Talking to one's healthcare professional about bone health. Bone density testing & medication when appropriate.

177

Calcium Prevents Bone Loss

The bones of the human skeleton contain 99.5% of the total calcium in the body. The calcium within bones is available to the body should the body need it for other purposes. Since we all lose bone mass as we age, if you've built up bone mass early in life, the loss is less likely to cause devastating problems. That's why dietitians stress the importance of calcium for children and teens.

But even if you're past the teenage years, you can still benefit from calcium. According to the U.S. Institute of Medicine, the average healthy adult needs between 1,000 and 1,300 milligrams of calcium per day. An 8 ounce glass of milk has 300 mg. Calcium-rich foods include dairy products, dark-green leafy vegetables, broccoli, tofu & fortified breads & cereals. If you don't like these foods or if you're lactose intolerant, talk with your doctor about supplements.

Keep in mind that while supplements and fortified foods can be useful in getting enough calcium, it's important not to overdo it. According to the National Institutes of Health, getting 2,000 mg/day or more of calcium can produce adverse health effects. Use of supplements should always be discussed with a doctor first.

Recommended Calcium

Age	Daily Needs
1-3 years	500 mg
4-8 years	800 mg
9-18 years	1,300 mg
19-49 years	1,000 mg
50+ years	1,200 mg

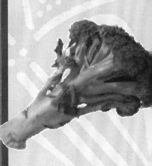

Calcium and Lactose in Common Foods

Vegetables	Calcium Content	Lactose
Soymilk, fortified, 1 cup	200–300 mg	0
Sardines, w/edible bones, 3 oz.	270 mg	0
Salmon, canned, w/bones, 3 oz.	205 mg	0
Broccoli, raw, 1 cup	90 mg	0
Orange, 1 medium	50 mg	0
Pinto beans, 1/2 cup	40 mg	0
Tuna, canned, 3 oz.	10 mg	0
Lettuce greens, 1/2 cup	10 mg	0
Dairy Products		
Yogurt, plain, low-fat, 1 cup	415 mg	5 g
Milk, reduced fat, 1 cup	295 mg	11 g
Swiss cheese, 1 oz.	270 mg	1 g
Ice cream, 1/2 cup	85 mg	6 g
Cottage cheese, 1/2 cup	75 mg	2–3 g

"I don't like milk and milk doesn't like me. The doctor says I'm "Lactose Intolerant", how can I still get enough calcium in my diet?"

You need vitamin D to absorb calcium

Your body needs vitamin D to absorb calcium. Your skin makes vitamin D when it is exposed to the sun. In fact, sunlight is the main source of vitamin D for many people, but we know that getting sun is a risk factor for skin cancer. Vitamin D is usually added to the milk you buy at the grocery store (but not to other milk-based products, like cheese, yogurt, and butter). Liver, fatty fish, and egg yolks also contain vitamin D. If you don't get enough of the nutrient from food, consider taking a multivitamin or a vitamin D supplement. (Many calcium supplements also contain vitamin D.)

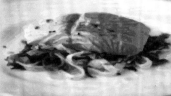

Salmon is an excellent source of calcium and Vitamin D

Weight bearing exercise makes bones stronger

You know that your muscles get bigger and stronger when you use them. Well, bones are similar: they get stronger and denser when you make them work. And "work," for bones, means handling impact and weight.

You can work your bones by doing activities that make you move against gravity, such as fast walking, running, dancing, and playing soccer. Biking and swimming are not weight-bearing exercises, so if you like these activities, try to add in other activities that do work your bones. You can also work your bones by lifting weights or doing resistance exercises. Resistance exercises include certain muscle strengthening exercises, using elastic fitness bands, and using weight machines.

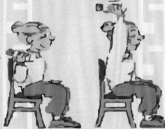

Magnesium

The American Dietetic Association (ADA) says magnesium is also important for maintaining healthy bones and a healthy heart. The recommended amount, according to ADA is 400 milligrams of magnesium a day. Food sources include whole grain breads and cereals, as well as nuts, seeds, and fresh fruits and vegetables.

What Can I Do For My Bones?

The recipe for bone health is simple:

- get enough calcium and vitamin D, and eat a well-balanced diet
- do weight-bearing and resistance exercises
- don't smoke
- drink alcohol only in moderation
- talk to your doctor or health care provider about your bone health

Of course, there are risk factors for osteoporosis that you cannot control. These include your family history, your age, your sex, having a small frame, and your race. (Keep in mind that people of any race can get osteoporosis.) But concentrating on the factors that you do control can have a big impact on your bones. Even so, on average, Americans are not getting enough calcium, vitamin D, and exercise to keep their bones healthy.

If you think you are at risk for osteoporosis, don't be shy about asking your doctor or health care provider if you need a Bone Mineral Density (BMD) test. Some good reasons to have one include:

- being a woman older than 65
- being a man older than 70
- being a middle-aged woman or man who also
    - _has broken a bone as an adult
    - _has a family history of osteoporosis or broken bones
    - _currently smokes cigarettes
    - _weighs very little (less than 127 pounds)
- having a medical condition known to cause osteoporosis, such as low testosterone levels in men, rheumatoid arthritis, intestinal disorders, or certain cancers
- taking medications known to cause osteoporosis, such as glucocorticoids (steroids), thyroid medications in excess, antiseizure medications, and certain breast cancer medications
- breaking bones in accidents that seem minor
- losing height or becoming hunched over

Most Bone Mineral Density (BMD) tests measure the amount of bone in the hip, spine or sometimes other bones. The test is quick, painless, and not invasive. BMD-testing equipment uses radiation, but it's a very low dosage.

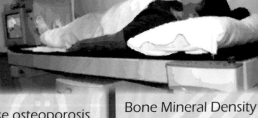

Bone Mineral Density (BMD) test

Heavy drinking weakens bones

Heavy drinking reduces bone formation. It might also affect your body's calcium supply. Drinking alcohol can also make you more likely to fall, which is how many people break bones.

Smoking weakens bones

Smoking is bad for your bones for many reasons. First, the nicotine and other chemicals in cigarettes are toxic to your bone cells. Smoking also might make it harder for you to absorb calcium. Plus, smoking lowers estrogen levels in women, which is a problem because estrogen helps protect bones. Finally, smoking can make exercise harder. It's no surprise, then, that researchers say smokers are more likely than nonsmokers to break bones.

Resources:

The National Osteoporosis Foundation
Phone: (202) 223-2226

www.nof.org

Toll free: 1 (800) 223-9994

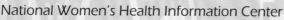
National Osteoporosis Foundation
NOF.ORG

National Women's Health Information Center
800-994-9662 or
888-220-5446 (TDD)
Monday through Friday
(9:00 to 6:00 pm, eastern time)

http://www.4women.gov/FAQ/osteopor.htm

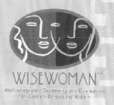
womenshealth**.gov**
The Federal Government Source for Women's Health Information

http://www.cdc.gov/wisewoman/
1–800–CDC–INFO
(1–800–232–4636)

WISEWOMAN™
Well-integrated Screening and Evaluation
for Women Across the Nation

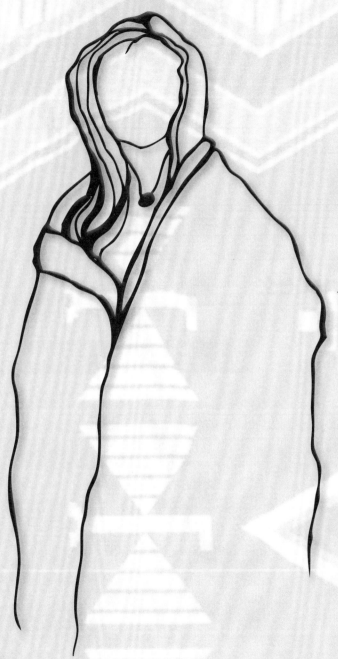

Your urinary system filters waste and extra fluid from your blood. In Problems of the Urine System, we will travel through the urinary system and look at problems caused by aging, illness, or injury. As we age, changes in our kidneys cause them to lose ability to remove waste from our blood, as well as loss of muscle coordination.

Our Urinary System

Many women can tolerate amazing amouts of pain and discomfort. A urinary tract infection is a pain or discomfort that is best to be taken care of as soon as you feel the symptoms. A bladder infection can be very easy to treat, sometimes even with home remedies. However, if left untreated an infection in the bladder can lead to an infection in the kidneys.

There are 2 main kinds of urine system infections. A bladder infection is the most common and the easiest to treat. A kidney infection is very serious. It can lead to permanent damage to the kidney or worse.

What causes bladder and kidney infections?
Infections of the urine system are caused by germs (bacteria). They get into the body from the outside through the urinary opening near the vagina. Infection is more common in women than in men because a woman's lower urine tube is much shorter. This means germs can more easily climb up the short urine tube into the bladder.

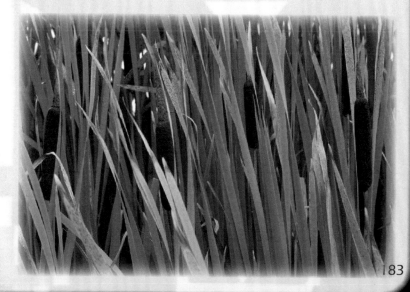

Infections in the Urine System

Germs often enter a woman's urine system or start to multiply when she:

- has sex. During sex, germs from the vagina and anus can be pushed up through the urinary opening into the lower urine tube. This is one of the most common causes of a bladder infection in women. To prevent infection, pass urine after having sex. This washes out the urine tube (but does not prevent pregnancy).

- goes for a long time without drinking, especially if she works outside in hot weather and sweats a lot. Germs will start to multiply in the empty bladder. Try to drink at least 8 glasses or cups of liquid a day. When working in the hot sun, drink even more.

- goes for a long time without urinating (for example, when traveling). Germs that stay in the urine system for a long time can cause an infection. Try to pass urine every 3 to 4 hours.

- not keeping genitals clean. Germs from the genitals—and especially the anus—can get into the urinary opening and cause infection. Try to wash the genitals every day, and always wipe from front to back after passing stool. Wiping forward can spread germs from the anus into the urinary opening. Also, try to wash your genitals before having sex.

Bladder infection signs:
- need to pass urine very often. (It may also feel as though some urine is still left inside.)
- pain or a burning feeling while passing urine
- pain in the lower belly just after passing urine
- urine smells bad, or looks cloudy, or has blood or pus in it. (Dark urine can also be a sign of hepatitis)

Kidney infection signs:
- any bladder infection signs
- fever and chills
- lower back pain, often severe, that can go from the front, around the sides, and into the back
- nausea and vomiting
- feeling very ill and weak

A girl or woman of any age—even a small baby—can get an infection of her urine system.

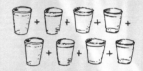

When a woman has a kidney infection, she may be in great pain and feel very ill. This can be very frightening. If this happens to you, try to get a family member or a friend to help you get to a health clinic. health clinic.

If you have signs of both a bladder and a kidney infection, you probably have a kidney infection.

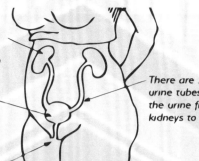

There are 2 kidneys They make urine by cleaning waste from the blood

There are 2 upper urine tubes They carry the urine from the kidneys to the bladder

The bladder is a bag It stretches and gets bigger as it fills with urine and gets small after you pass urine

When you pass urine the urine goes down the lower urine tube and comes out a small hole in front of your vagina

Bladder infections can often be treated with home remedies. Start treatment as soon as you notice the signs. A bladder infection can sometimes travel quickly up the urine tubes into the kidneys. It is important to go to your clinic if the bladder infection does not go away within a day or two.

Prevention and Treatment of a Bladder Infection:

A bladder infection is a bacteria infection that may need to be treated by antibiotics. Talk to you doctor for more information. If you feel you may be getting a bladder infection, here are some suggestions to keep it from getting worse:

- **Drink a lot of water.** Try to drink at least one cup of clean water every 30 minutes. This will make you pass urine often. Sometimes the germs will wash out of your urine system before the infection gets worse.
- **Stop having sex for a few days,** or until the signs have gone away.
- **Make a tea** from flowers, seeds, and leaves that are known to help cure urine infections. Ask the Elders in your community which plants will help.
- **Drinking cranberry juice**, at least 3 glasses a day, will change the pH (acidity) of your urine which makes urine less hospitable to common bacteria that cause UTI.

Treatment for a Kidney Infection:

- If you have signs of a kidney infection, home remedies are not enough. **Go your your health clinic immediately.** Start taking prescribed medicines right away. Return to your clinic if you do not start to feel better after 2 days.

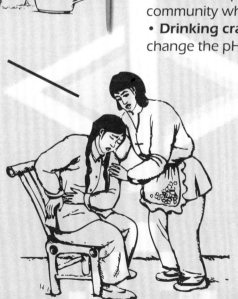

on't orry, ary, will ke you the alth nic."

Blood in Urine

Kidney or bladder stones

These are small hard stones that start to grow in the kidney, and then move through the urine system.

Signs:

- Sudden, very bad pain:

  in the back where the kidneys are,

  or in the side near the kidneys,

  or lower down in the urine tubes or bladder.

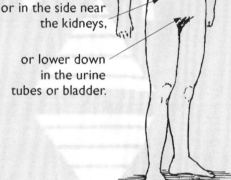
B Carter

Other signs or Kidney stones are:

- Blood in the urine. This can happen if the stones scratch the inside of the urine system.

- Difficulty passing urine. This can happen if a stone blocks the tubes.

Blood in the urine

If your urine has blood in it, and if there are no other signs of a **bladder or kidney infection**, you may have bladder or kidney stones.

Though less common, tuberculosis (TB) can damage the bladder and kidneys and cause blood in the urine.

Treatment:

- Drink large amounts of liquid (at least 1 or 2 cups every 30 minutes). This will help wash the stone out of the kidney and down the urine tube.

- Take a pain medicine such as tylenol or aspirin. If the pain is very bad, get medical help. Sometimes the blocked urine tubes become infected. Treat this problem the same way you would treat a kidney infection.

- **See your doctor if you have any questions or concerns. Your doctor can discuss other treatment options.**

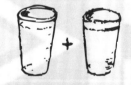

Drink 1 to 2 cups every 30 minutes to help wash the stone out of the kidney.

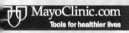

Kidney and Urologic Home

National Kidney and Urologic Disease Information Clearing House (NKUDIC)
http://kidney. niddk.nih.gov

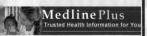

MayoClinic.com
Tools for healthier lives

http://www. mayoclinic.com/ health/urinary- tract-infection/ DS00286

Medline Plus
Trusted Health Information for You

http://www. nlm.nih.gov/ medlineplus/ kidneysanduri- narysystem.html

This may happen because:
- the muscles around your bladder and womb have become weak. The 'squeez-ing exercise' (see below) may help strengthen these muscles.
- a growth (like a fibroid) in your abdomen is pushing against the bladder so it cannot hold much urine.
- you have a bladder infection.
- you have diabetes.

Poor control of urine (incontinence)
This can be caused by weak or damaged muscles around the bladder. It happens mainly to older women or to women after childbirth. The urine leaks out when a woman puts pressure on the weak muscles in her lower belly during sex, or by laughing, coughing, sneezing, or lifting. The 'squeezing exercise' may help.

Need to pass urine often

The squeezing exercise
This exercise can help strengthen weak muscles that cause you to pass urine often or to leak urine. First practice while you are passing urine. As the urine comes out, stop it by tightly squeezing the muscles in your vagina. Count to 10, then relax the muscles to let the urine come out. Repeat this several times Some women may need surgery to help control leaking urine. If your urine leaks a lot and this exercise does not help, get advice from a health worker trained in women's health. The squeezing exercise is good for all women to do every day. It helps keep muscles strong and can prevent problems later in life. Once you know how, practice the squeezing exercise at other times during the day. No one will know. Try to practice at least 4 times a day, squeezing your muscles 5 to 10 times each time.

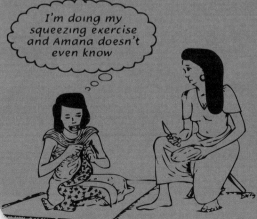

I'm doing my squeezing exercise and Amana doesn't even know

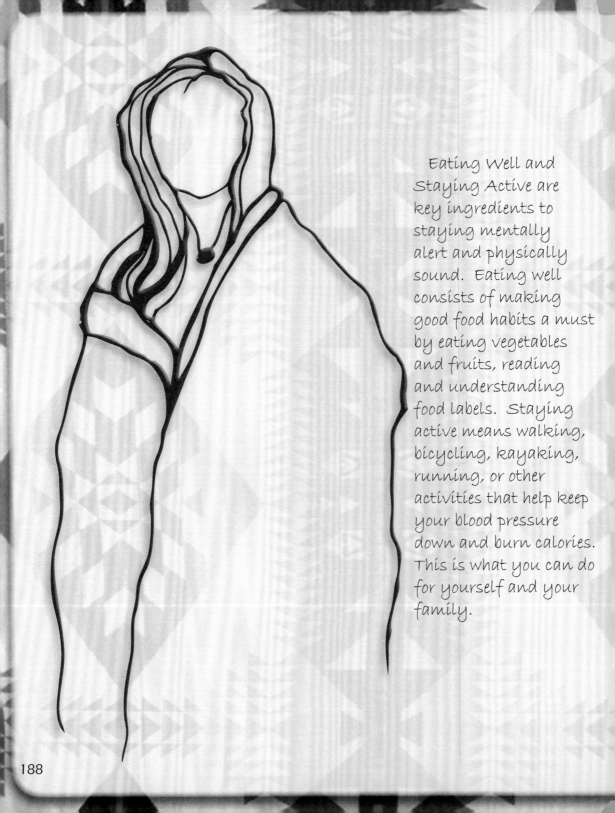

Eating Well and Staying Active are key ingredients to staying mentally alert and physically sound. Eating well consists of making good food habits a must by eating vegetables and fruits, reading and understanding food labels. Staying active means walking, bicycling, kayaking, running, or other activities that help keep your blood pressure down and burn calories. This is what you can do for yourself and your family.

Nutrition

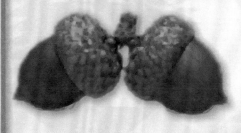

A woman needs good food to do her daily work, to prevent illness, and to have safe and healthy births. And yet, women in Indian Country often suffer from poor nutrition. This can cause exhaustion, weakness, disability, and general poor health.

There are many reasons for poor nutrition and not eating well. One main reason is lack of access to nutrional food. Another is not making it a priority to take the time to prepare and eat nutrional meals. Modern life makes us think it is easier to "just go through the drive through" for dinner than to take the time to prepare a well balanced meal. Recipes from our grandmothers may have worked well for them, but in today's time, when we may not get as much exercise, we need to cut down on the fat content of our meals and make sure we get the right balance of nutrition in the food we eat. As women, we set the example for our families and our children for how to eat healthy. We, as Native Women, have challenges to face in our generation including diabetes, cancer and heart disease. Serving and eating a nutritious meal will help not only us and this generation, but will influence following generations.

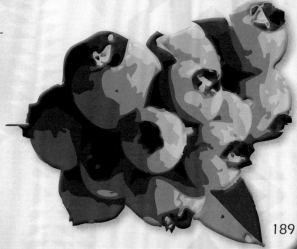

189

Eating Healthy

In much of Indian Country people eat one main low-cost food with almost every meal. Depending on the region, this may be rice, potatoes or bread (including buns, pasta or pizza crust). This main food usually provides most of the body's daily food needs. By itself, however, the main food is not enough to keep a person healthy. Other 'helper' foods are needed to provide protein (which helps build the body), vitamins and minerals (which help protect and repair the body), and fats and sugar (which give energy). The healthiest diets have a variety of foods, including some foods with protein, and fruits and vegetables rich in vitamins and minerals. You need only a small amount of fat and sugar to be healthy.

Other health problems that can be caused or made worse by poor nutrition:

• constipation
• diabetes
• osteopororis (weak bones)
• heart disease
• cancer
• fatigue
• weakened immune system
• acid indigestion, and heartburn
• high blood pressure

New Food Pyramid
www.Stanford.edu

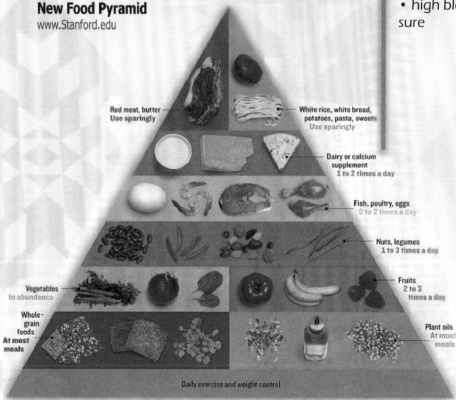

Red meat, butter
Use sparingly

White rice, white bread, potatoes, pasta, sweets
Use sparingly

Dairy or calcium supplement
1 to 2 times a day

Fish, poultry, eggs
0 to 2 times a day

Nuts, legumes
1 to 3 times a day

Vegetables
In abundance

Fruits
2 to 3 times a day

Whole-grain foods
At most meals

Plant oils
At most meals

Daily exercise and weight control

Good nutrition means eating enough food and the right kind of food for the body to grow, be healthy, and fight off disease.

You can buy more nutritious food than packaged food for the same amount of money.

Low sugar and sodium frozen, canned and dried fruits and vegetables are a good source of nutrition.

When money is limited, it is important to use it wisely. Here are some suggestions for getting more vitamins, minerals, and proteins at low cost:

1. **Protein foods.** Beans, peas, lentils, and other similar foods (called legumes) are a good, cheap source of protein. Eggs are one of the cheapest sources of animal protein. Liver and fish are often cheaper than other meats and are just as nutritious.

2. **Grains.** Rice, wheat, and other grains are more nutritious. Whole grains, such as whole wheat bread or flour or brown rice are more nutritious and add fiber.

3. **Fruits and vegetables.** The sooner you eat fruits and vegetables after harvesting, the more nutrition they have. When you store them, put them in a cool, dark place to preserve vitamins. Cook vegetables in as small an amount of water as possible, because vitamins from the vegetables go into the water during cooking. Then use the water in soups. Many wild fruits and berries are rich in vitamin C and natural sugars, and can provide extra vitamins, fiber, antioxidants and energy.

4. **Milk and milk products.** They are rich in body-building proteins and in bone building calcium.

5. **Avoid spending money on packaged foods.** If parents took the money they often use for sweets or sodas and spent it on nutritious foods, their children would be healthier for the same amount of money.

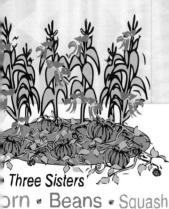

Three Sisters
orn • Beans • Squash

The Three Sisters of Native American agriculture: corn, beans and squash, were used by various tribes in North America. The three plants are companions; they help each other by maximizing growing conditions for one another. The corn, tall and firm, grows in the center of a circular bed and serves as a support for climbing pole beans. The beans fix nitrogen in the soil, important for nitrogen loving, heavy feeding corn. The squash surrounds the corn and beans and covers the ground, serving to hold moisture in the soil, and – as Native American lore explains – the prickles on squash stems act as repellant to pests such as hungry raccoons.

Important Vitamins and Minerals

There are 3 important vitamins and minerals that women need, especially women who are pregnant or breastfeeding. The 3 are: iron, folic acid (folate), calcium.

Iron

Iron is needed to make blood healthy and to help prevent weak blood (anemia). A woman needs to get a lot of iron throughout her life, especially during the years she has monthly bleeding and during pregnancy.

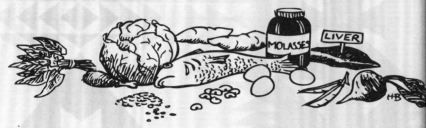

It is best to eat iron foods along with citrus fruits or tomatoes. These contain vitamin C, which helps your body use more of the iron in the food.

These foods have a lot of iron:
• meat
• chicken
• sardines
• beans
• oyster
• dried fruit (prunes and raisons)

These foods also have some iron:
• yams
• broccoli
• dried fruit
• sunflower, sesame, pumpkin seeds
• strawberries
• dark green leafy vegetables
• cabbage with dark-colored leaves
• potatoes
• cauliflower
• lentils, peas
• brussels sprouts
• eggs
• fish

Good sources of folic acid are:
• dark green leafy vegetables
• whole grains
• mushrooms
• liver
• meats
• fish
• nuts
• peas and beans
• eggs

Folic acid (folate)

The body needs folic acid to make healthy red blood cells. Lack of folic acid can lead to anemia in women and severe problems in newborn babies. So getting enough folic acid is especially important during pregnancy.

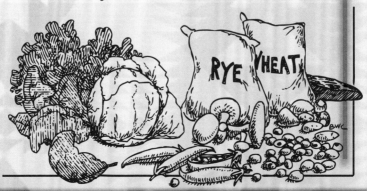

Dark yellow, orange and green leafy vegetables, and some orange fruits, are rich in vitamin A.

These foods contain calcium:
• milk, yogurt
• cheese
• ground sesame
• bone meal
• cooked green leafy vegetables
• almonds
• beans, especially soy, white beans
• shellfish
• salmon canned with bones

Sunshine will help you use calcium better. Try to be in the sun at least 15 minutes every day. Remember that it is not enough to just be outdoors. The sun's rays must touch the skin.

Everyone needs calcium to make their bones and teeth strong. In addition, girls and women need extra calcium:
• during childhood. Calcium helps a girl's bones grow strong so she can skip, hop and play.
• during pregnancy. A pregnant woman needs enough calcium to help the baby's bones grow, and to keep her own bones and teeth strong.
• during breastfeeding. Calcium is necessary for making breast milk.
• during mid-life and old age. Calcium is needed to prevent weak bones (osteoporosis).

Problems from eating too much food or the wrong kinds of food

Women who do not have healthy foods to eat, especially if they are very overweight and their diets have too much fat or sugar, are more likely to have high blood pressure, heart disease, a stroke, gallstones, diabetes, and some cancers. Being very overweight can also cause arthritis in the legs and feet.

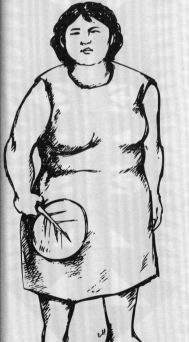

Make sure you get enough exercise and eat more fruits and vegetables. Here are some suggestions for cutting down the amount of fat in the diet:

• Cook with broth or water instead of using butter, lard, or oil.

• Remove fat from meat before cooking. Do not eat the skin of chicken or turkey.

• Avoid processed snack foods that are high in fat, like chips and muffins from the store.

Resources

National Agricultural Library
Food and Nutrion Information Center
www.nal.usda.gov

Nutrtion.gov
www.nutriton.gov

Native Web Food Resource database
www.nativeweb.org/resources/food/

NativeTech: Indigenous Food and Traditional Recipes
www.nativetech.org/recipe

A Pueblo hot dog story

During the 1950's many young Indian people were sent to faraway places to learn a skill and a job, on a program called "relocation".

Two young men were sent to San Francisco, from the reservation. The first day they were there, they walked the streets looking up at the tall buildings and busy people moving like ants.

Walking made them hungry so they started looking for a place to eat, coming from the reservation the BIA Relocation Program didn't allow much, so they wanted to eat something that wasn't too costly.

So they seen a vendor with a sign "Hot Dogs", and a hot dog was only 25 cents each. So they thought that was cheap enough and ordered two. The vendor put each hot dog in a brown sack and they walked away. It was their first experience eating a hot dog.

One opened up his sack and looked, and then he nudged his friend and asked, "What part did you get"?

A typical hot dog with bun has 377 calories .

(55 grams of carbohydrates and 16 grams of fat)!

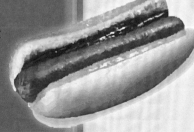

Section 4

Everyday is a battle to
begin to be healthy or maintain a healthy
balance; to keep depression from secretly
creeping into our emotions and body; to
be strong against the temptations of
quick fixes that hook us for life, and
then feed upon our bodies, pulling
out all of the needed vitamins
and minerals only to be replaced
with life-threatening illnesses.
Well-Being is a journey
into the dark side of life,
for in life, there is the
good and bad. We will
talk about depression,
alcohol and drugs,
and understand
that choices that
we make will
influence our
lifetime.

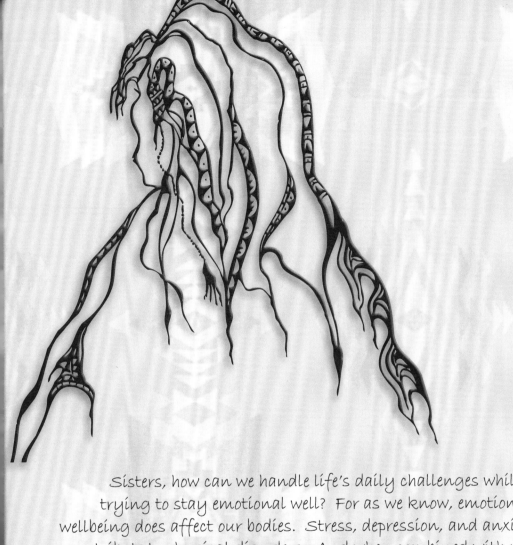

Sisters, how can we handle life's daily challenges while trying to stay emotional well? For as we know, emotional wellbeing does affect our bodies. Stress, depression, and anxiety can contribute to physical disorders. And when combined with mental health issues, can become a two-pronged problem; how to treat the mental and emotional health issues while caring for the physical body? Emotional Well-Being discusses some of the above challenges and others. Please use this chapter as a guide to understanding that we are human and every day is not sunny, but you can make your own sunshine. And, if you suffer from depression, stress, or not sure of what, please seek help.

Emotional Wellbeing

Life events like having a baby or losing a loved one can effect our mind and spirit. If the difficulty continues and keeps a woman from carrying out her daily activities—for example, if she becomes so tense and nervous that she may find it difficult to care for her family -her emotional wellbeing may be out of balance. These inbalances are harder to identify than problems in the body, which we can often see or touch. Yet challenges to one's emotional wellbeing needs attention and treatment, just as physical problems do.

Just as a woman's body can be healthy or unhealthy, so can her mind and spirit. When her mind and spirit are healthy, she has the emotional strength to take care of her physical needs and those of her family, to identify her challenges and attempt to solve them, to plan for the future, and to form satisfying relationships with others.

Mental and emotional challenges to our well-being are normal and natural and everyone experiences them from time to time. When people are sick, hungry, lonely or tired they may have problems thinking, concentrating, making decisions or remembering. A woman may benefit from help with her mental or emotional health problem. This chapter describes the most common emotional and mental challenges and their causes. It also offers suggestions for how a woman can help herself or others with these problems.

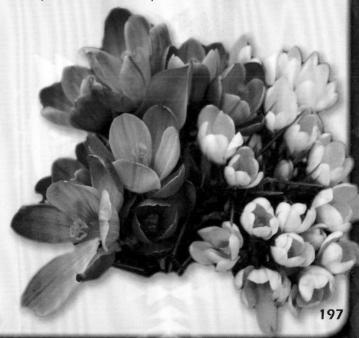

Challenges to Emotional Wellbeing

A woman usually experiences challenges to her emotional or mental health when these pressures are stronger than her ability to cope. Also, not all mental health problems have causes that can be identified. Sometimes we just do not know why someone experiences a mental health problem.

To have better mental health, women need to exercise more control and power over their lives.

Stress in daily life

Daily activities and events often put pressure on a woman, causing tension in her body and mind (stress). Stress can come from physical problems, like illness or overwork. Or it can come from emotional events, like conflict in the family or being blamed for problems that a woman has no control over. Even events that often bring pleasure—like a new baby or getting a job—can be stressful because they create changes in a woman's life.

When a woman faces a lot of stress every day and for a long time, she may begin to feel overwhelmed and unable to cope. The problem may be made worse if she has been taught to take care of others first and neglects her own needs. With little time to rest or to enjoy things that could help reduce her stress, she may ignore signs of illness or overwork. And as a woman, she may feel she has limited energy or power to change her situation.

Often a woman is made to feel that she is weak or ill. But the real problem may be something that is not fair or no right in life.

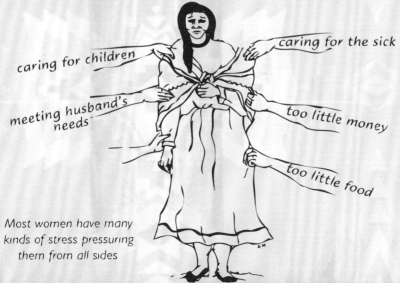

caring for children

caring for the sick

meeting husband's needs

too little money

too little food

Most women have many kinds of stress pressuring them from all sides

Self-esteem

When a woman feels she makes a valuable contribution to her family and community, she is said to have good self-esteem. A woman with good self-esteem knows that she is worthy of being treated with respect.

> It is easy not to notice the stress in daily life because it is always there. But it takes a lot of a woman's energy to cope with this kind of stress.

Self-esteem begins to develop in childhood. The amount of self-esteem a woman develops depends on how she is treated by the important people in her life—like her parents, brothers and sisters, neighbors, teachers, and spiritual guides. If these people treat her as someone who deserves their attention, if they praise her when she does something well, and if they encourage her to try things that are difficult, she will begin to feel she is valued. In some cases, girls have a hard time developing good self esteem. For example, if girls are criticized a lot or their hard work goes unnoticed, they are more likely to grow up feeling unworthy. Then, as women, they may not believe they deserve to be treated well by their husbands, spend money on herself or to have health care when they are sick, or to develop their skills. When women feel this way, they may even think that their lack of importance in the family and community is natural and right—when, in fact, it is unfair and unjust. Self-esteem is an important part of good mental health. When a woman enhances her self-esteem she will feel more able to cope with (manage) daily problems and better able to work for changes that can improve her life and her community.

Building self-esteem

Building self-esteem is not an easy task. This is because a woman cannot just decide to value herself more. Rather, she must change deeply held beliefs that she may not know she has. Often these changes must happen indirectly, through experiences that allow a woman to see herself in a new way. Change can come through building on strengths a woman already has, like her ability to form close, supportive relationships with others, or from learning new skills.

> A woman's self-esteem will influence the choices she makes about her health.

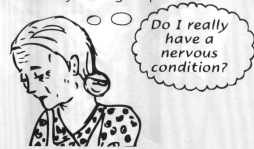

Do I really have a nervous condition?

Often a woman is made to feel that she is weak or ill. But the real problem may be something that is not fair or not right in life

199

Changes in a woman's life and community

In many parts of Indian Country and in Alaskan Villages, communities are finding strength in holding on to traditions, yet at the same time they are riding the wave of modern life. Many of these changes require families and communities to alter their entire way of life. For example:

Loss and death

When a woman loses someone or something important—a loved one, her work, her home, or a close friendship—she may feel overwhelmed with grief. This can also happen if she becomes ill or develops a disability.

Grieving is a natural response that helps a person adjust to loss and death. But if a woman faces many losses at once, or if she already has a lot of daily stress, she may begin to experience an imbalance in her mental or emotional well being. This can also happen if a woman is unable to grieve in traditional ways—for example, if she has moved to a new community where her traditions are not practiced and friends and family are far away.

Trauma

When something horrible has happened to a woman or to someone close to her, she has suffered a trauma. Some of the most common kinds of trauma are violence in the home, historical violence, rape, war, torture, forced relocation and natural disasters. Trauma threatens a person's physical or mental well-being. As a result, a person feels unsafe, insecure, helpless, and unable to trust the world or the people around her. It usually takes a long time for a woman to recover from trauma, especially if it was caused by another person, not by nature. Trauma suffered as a child, before she could understand what was happening or talk about it, can affect a woman for many years without her even knowing it.

When families and communities break apart, or when life changes so much that old ways of coping do not work, people may begin to have mental health problems.

Although there are many kinds of mental health problems, the most common ones are anxiety, depression and misuse of alcohol or drugs. In most communities, women suffer from these problems more than men do. But men are more likely than women to have problem misusing alcohol or drugs.

Physical problems

Some mental or emotional imbalances are caused by physical problems, such as:

- hormones and other changes in the body
- malnutrition.
- infections, such as HIV.
- environmental exposure including pesticides, herbicides, and industrial solvents.
- liver or kidney disease.
- too much medicine in the body, or the side effects of some medicines.
- drug and alcohol misuse.
- strokes, dementia, and head injuries.
- diabetes

Having your regular doctor screen for depression is a common practice, especially if you have diabetes.

Depression and other Diseases

Some imbalances to mental and emotional wellbeing are caused by a change in one's health status like being daignosed with diabetes, cancer, hepatisis C or HIV. One may think she has just received a death setence . It is normal to experience difficult thoughts and feelings about the diagnosis.

Talking with someone right away can help reduce the stress that can come from such news. Letting family and friends know that you are going through a difficult time can help reduce stress.

Seeking out more information about the illness and the treatments can help bring balance back into one's life. Talking with your health care provider or counselor can help.

Don't hesitate to talk to your doctor about your emotional well-being. Your doctor can help.

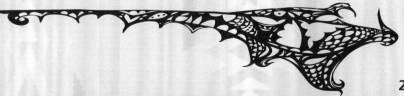

Common Mental Health Problems for Women

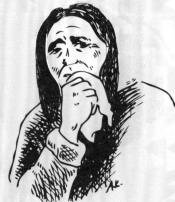

Depression (extreme sadness or feeling nothing at all)

It is natural for a person to feel depressed when she experiences a loss or death. But she may have problems with depression if the signs below last for a long time.

Signs:
- feeling sad most of the time
- difficulty sleeping or sleeping too much
- difficulty thinking clearly
- loss of interest in pleasurable activities, eating, or sex
- physical problems, such as headaches or intestinal problems, that are not caused by illness
- slow speech and movement
- lack of energy for daily activities
- thinking about death or suicide

Suicide

Serious depression can lead to hopeless thinking or suicide (killing oneself). Almost everyone has thoughts of suicide once in a while. But if these thoughts come more and more often or get very strong, a woman needs help right away.

A woman can talk with her health care provider or a trusted counselor about her thoughts, and they can develop a plan for safety. A woman can also ask a friend to join her in staying safe.

A woman can also ask a health care provider or counselor for more help if she does not think she can stay safe. Doctors, nurses, counselors, ministers and case managers can help promote safety.

Planning for Safety

Many Tribes and Urban Indian programs have health clinics and social service programs. Keep local phone numbers handy.

List telephone numbers and hot line numbers with other emergency services so they can be found easily. Do whatever it takes to stay safe even if it means calling 911.

Physical changes and disease caused by stress

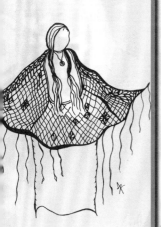

When a person experiences stress, the body gets ready to react quickly and fight off the stress. Some of the changes that occur are:

- The heart starts beating faster.
- The blood pressure goes up.
- A person breathes faster.
- Digestion slows down.

If the stress is sudden and severe, a woman may feel these changes in her body. Then, once the stress is gone, her body returns to normal. But if the stress is less severe or happens slowly, she may not notice how the stress is affecting her body, even though the signs are still there.

Stress that goes on for a long time can lead to the physical signs common in anxiety and depression, like headache, intestinal problems, and lack of energy. Over time, stress can also cause illness, like high blood pressure. In some places, emotional problems are not considered as important as physical problems. When this happens, people may be more likely to have physical signs of anxiety and depression than other signs. While it is important not to ignore physical signs, it is important to also be sensitive to the emotional causes of illness.

Dancing, singing, playing, reading, writing, laughing, painting, even hugging a tree can help reduce stress.

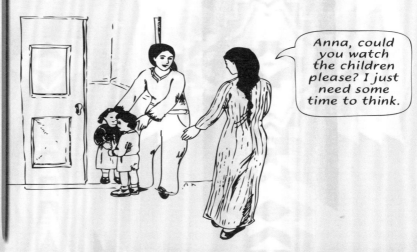

Anna, could you watch the children please? I just need some time to think.

203

Anxiety (feeling nervous or worried)

Everyone feels nervous or worried from time to time. When

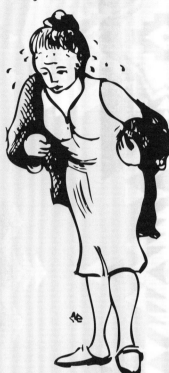

these feelings are caused by a specific situation, they usually go away soon afterwards. Sometimes the anxiety continues or becomes more severe, or if it comes without any reason, then she may have a problem with anxiety.

Signs:
- feeling tense and nervous without reason
- shaking hands
- sweating
- feeling the heart pound (when there is no heart disease)
- difficulty thinking clearly
- frequent physical complaints that are not caused by physical illness and that increase when a woman is upset

Panic attacks are a severe kind of anxiety. They happen suddenly and can last from several minutes to several hours. In addition to the signs above, a person feels terror or dread, and fears that she may lose consciousness (faint) or die. She may also have chest pain, difficulty breathing, and feel that something terrible is about to happen.

When a woman has severe chest pain or difficulty breathing, she should get medical help. These may be a sign of serious physical illness.

There are many healthy tools that help manage anxiety, reduce stress and promote peace of mind

1. Relaxation
2. Slow breathing
3. Visualization
4. Take breaks from worry
5. Talk with a friend or counselor

Post-traumatic stress disorder (PTSD) is an intense physical and emotional response to thoughts and reminders of the event that last for many weeks or months after the traumatic event. The symptoms of PTSD fall into three broad types: re-living, avoidance and increased arousal. Other symptoms linked with PTSD include: panic attacks, depression, suicidal thought and feelings, drug abuse, feelings of being estranged and isolated, and not being able to complete daily tasks.

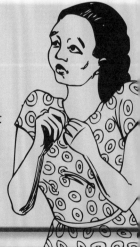

Reactions to Trauma

After a person has experienced trauma, she may have many different reactions, such as:

- Going over the trauma again and again in her mind. While she is awake, she may keep remembering the terrible things that happened. At night she may dream about them or be unable to fall asleep because she is thinking about them.

- Feeling numb or feeling emotions less strongly than before. She may avoid people or places that remind her of the trauma.

- Becoming very watchful. If she is constantly looking out for danger, she may have difficulty relaxing and sleeping. She may overreact when startled.

- Feeling very angry or full of shame about what happened. If a person has survived a trauma where others died or were seriously injured, she may feel guilty that others suffered more than she did.

- Feeling separate and distant from other people.

- Having outbursts of strange or violent behavior, in which she is confused about where she is.

For severe problems, medicines may be necessary. Try to talk to a health provider who knows about medicines for mental health problems.

Many of these signs are normal responses to a difficult situation. For example, it is normal to feel angry that a trauma has happened, or to be watchful if the situation is still dangerous. But if the signs are so severe that a person cannot carry out daily activities, or If the problems become worse or last longer than one month after the event, the person may be suffering from post-traumatic stress disorder (PTSD).

Coping with traumatic events.

- Understand that your symptoms may be normal, especially right after the trauma.
- Keep to your usual routine.
- Take the time to resolve day-to-day conflicts so they do not add to your stress.
- Do not shy away from situations, people & places that remind you of the trauma.
- Find ways to relax and be kind to yourself.
- Turn to family, friends, and spiritual leaders for support, and talk about your experiences and feelings with them.
- Participate in cultural and recreational activities.
- Recognize that you cannot control everything.

A person may be mentally ill if she has any of these signs:

- She hears voices or sees unusual things that others do not hear or see (hallucinations).
- She has strange beliefs that interfere with daily life (delusions)—for example, she thinks that loved ones are trying to rob her.
- She no longer cares for herself—for example, she does not get dressed, clean herself, or eat.
- She behaves in a strange way, like saying things that make no sense.

People who are not mentally ill sometimes act this way, particularly if these behaviors are part of their community's beliefs or traditions. For example, if a woman says that she received guidance in a dream, she may be drawing upon traditional sources of knowledge and guidance—not suffering from mental illness.

Getting care for mental illness

Although in most places family members play a role in caring for those with mental illness, it is best if the person can also be treated by a trained mental health worker. In some situations medicines are necessary, but they should never be the only treatment. Traditional healers can also play an important role in treating mental illness. If they come from the same community as the person with the problem, they may know and understand her. Some healers also have treatments or rituals that can help a woman overcome her problem. Ask these questions before deciding on a treatment:

- What is the purpose of each step in the treatment? What should be expected to happen?
- If the person is not a danger to herself or others, can she get mental health care while living at home, or living together with others in her community?
- Will the family be involved in the treatment?
- Is the person providing treatment respected in the community?
- Do any of the treatments cause physical harm or shame?

> No matter what treatment is given, a person with a mental illness should be treated with kindness, respect, and dignity.

> Similar signs can be caused by illness, poisoning, medicines, drug abuse, or damage to the brain.

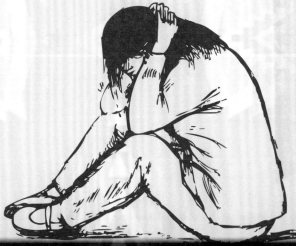

Helping relationships

In a helping relationship, two or more people make a commitment to get to know and understand each other. This can happen in any relationship—between friends, family members, or women who work together, or in a group that already meets for another purpose. Or a new group may form because the people share a common problem. These are often called 'support groups'.

Building a helping relationship

Even when two people know each other well, helping relationships develop slowly, because people usually hesitate to share their problems. It takes time to get over these worries and begin to trust one another. Here are some ways to build trust between people or members of a group:

- Try to be open to hearing everything another person says, without judging it.

- Discuss safety early on in forming relationships or women's groups. Share a list of local resources such as hot lines, local clinic, social services and emergency numbers so that everyone has them.

- Try to understand how the other person feels. If you have had a similar experience, think about how you felt. But avoid seeing someone else's experience as exactly like your own. If you do not understand her, do not pretend that you do.

- Do not tell another person what to do. You can help her understand how the pressures of her family, community, and work responsibilities affect her feelings, but she must make her own decisions.

- Never think of a woman as beyond help.

- Respect the woman's privacy. Never tell others what she has told you unless it is necessary to protect her life. Always tell her if you plan to speak with someone else for her protection.

Many people with mental illness regain balance in their lives and are active in their community as co-workers, life-time mates, and caregivers in their family. National organizations like NAMI and CAMI have a strong network to help families understand and cope with the mental challenges of a family member.

nami.org
1-800-950-NAMI
(6264)

Helping Yourself and Helping Others

A person suffering from mental health problems can begin to feel better with treatment. Many communities now have mental health services. Talk to your doctor or someone from your health clinic.

Personal coping skills

Women do not often take time out of their busy day to do something for themselves. But every woman needs to put her problems aside sometimes and do what she likes. Simple things that you may not do very often—like spending time alone, or shopping, gardening, or cooking with a friend—can all be helpful.

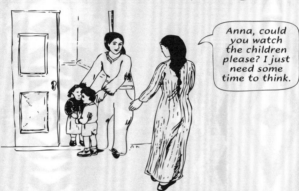

Anna, could you watch the children please? I just need some time to think.

Creating pleasing surroundings. Try to fix your living space so that it feels right to you. No matter how small it is, you will feel more order and control when it is arranged the way you like. Try to have as much light and fresh air as possible.

Try to have some beauty around you. This could mean putting some flowers in the room, playing music, or going where there is a nice view.

Practice traditions that build inner strength. Many communities have developed beliefs and traditions that help calm the body and mind, as well as build inner strength. For example: prayer, dance, song, meditation, and rituals.

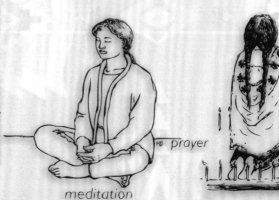

prayer

meditation

Activities to let your feelings out.

Making up poems, songs, and stories can be helpful when you have trouble saying things to others. Or you can draw your feelings without using words—you do not have to be an artist.

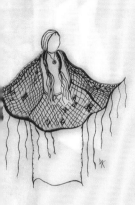

Our story is about how we learned to make Indian baskets as a group of Indian women. We were beginners at weaving with our fingers and with plant materials, we had not known about. Even though we watched our grandmothers and mothers weave cradleboards and baskets, we never learned for one reason or another and we were growing older each day. How would our children and grandchildren learn we asked ourselves?

The day Minerva Soucie announced that she had received a grant to teach basket weaving in the Burns Paiute community was a joyous day for many of us who have always wanted to learn, but never had the opportunity to. Now, we had a master weaver, who lived so close and was willing to teach us the basics of weaving.

Minerva had been exposed to weaving in her youth, observing the old ladies working on Paiute cradleboards, tanning bear and deer hides, and learning how to twine from her mother, Bernice Beers Teeman. It seemed that now the time was right for us to learn.

Our weaving group started out small, meeting on Monday cultural day at the social hall behind the Church of Living Waters, located on the Burns Paiute Reservation. Rev. Anne Scissions had invited her to work with the women's group and that was how it began.

We started out as a weaving group and a year later, we were weaving and supporting each other through; our illness', heartbreak, stress, pain, family duress, loss of friends, financial Issues and childhoods experiences. This year, we all went through issues that affected us or our families that were painful and stressful, but we all came out strong.

We had evolved into a support group that is full of; love, respect, caring, harmony, support, wisdom, spirituality, team work, encouragement and self esteem. We are blessed to find one another.

A weaver's story
Newe Mau Go-nee
Weaving Circle

is often easier to urn an existing roup into a upport group han to create new one. But e careful when hoosing helping relationships. orm relationships nly with people ho will respect ur feelings and ur privacy.

Meeting together with others can help a woman:

Helping Yourself and Helping Others

Starting a Women's group

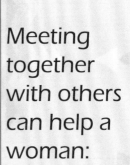

1. Find two or more women who want to start a group.
2. Plan when and where to meet. It helps to find a quiet place, such as a school, health clinic, Elder's center, or place of worship. Or you can plan to talk while doing a craft such as sewing, weaving or beading.
3. At the first meeting, discuss what you hope to accomplish. If you are in a group, decide how the group will be led and whether new members can join later.

Although the person who began the group will probably need to take the lead at the first meetings, she should not make decisions for the group. Her job is to make sure everyone has a chance to talk and to bring the discussion back to the main point if it wanders off. After the first few meetings, members may want to take turns leading the group. Having more than one leader can also help shy women lead.

Some women may feel more comfortable listening as they work with their hands—for example, as they weave or sew.

Women's groups can be made up of many women or just two to three women. Here are tips on how your group can help each other talk about uncomfortable issues and give each other support.

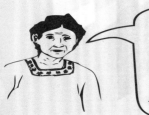

Sometimes we would arrive at the meeting in a bad way. We didn't have any wish to speak. We felt without energy. Then a hug from someone or the spirits of others would be catching. And all of us would feel more strength.

Meeting together with others can help a woman:

- Get support.
- Mental health problems often drain a woman's energy and make her discouraged.
- Meeting together can give a woman more energy, which then helps her cope with daily problems.

• recognize feelings. Sometimes women hide their feelings (or do not even realize they have them) because they think the feelings are bad, dangerous, or shameful. Hearing others talk about feelings can help a woman notice her own.

> Some of us had been sexually abused in the past, but we had never been able to share it with others. It was only in the group that we could talk about these terrible things.

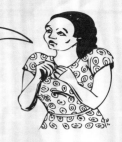

• put forth solutions. Solutions that are discussed in a group are often more easily accepted and used than those that a woman thinks of by herself.

> There are things from our past that we have never discussed with our partners. In the group we talked about how to deal better with these things. We get strength from each other.

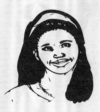

control impulsive reactions. Group members can help a woman think through a problem, so that she will not act on her first impulse, without thinking.

> The group helped me to see others' points of view and to not get carried away by my feelings. This has helped me understand why other people react the way they do.

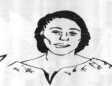

• understand underlying causes. By talking together, women begin to realize that many of them suffer from the same kinds of problems. This helps them identify root causes of the problem.

> I often think poorly of myself and feel as if I am to blame for my family's situation. But it is not our fault that we are poor. Talking about this with others has helped me to understand why we women suffer the way we do.

• develop collective power. Women acting together are more powerful than a woman acting alone.

> We all decided to have a ceremony and then accompany one of our members to get a death certificate for her partner and arrange the title for her land. If she had to do these things alone it would be very difficult.

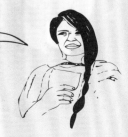

Exercises for learning how to help

Most members of a group need to understand what a helping relationship is and what makes it work before they can really help one another with a mental health problem.

These exercises can help:

1. Sharing experiences of support. To become more aware of what support is, the leader can ask members to tell a personal story in which they have received or given support. Then the leader asks questions like: What kind of help was it? How did it help? What are the similarities and differences between the stories? This can help the group come up with general ideas about what it means to support and help another person. Or the leader can pose a story of someone with a problem—for example, a woman whose husband drinks too much and beats her. She becomes withdrawn and pretends nothing is wrong, but no longer participates in the community. Then the group can discuss: How could we as a group help her? How can she help herself?

2. Practicing active listening. In this exercise the group divides into pairs. One partner talks about a topic for about 5 to 10 minutes, then the partners switch roles. When the partners are finished, they think about how well it worked. They ask each other questions like: Did you feel listened to? What difficulties did you have? Then the leader begins a general discussion among everyone about the attitudes that best show listening and concern. The leader can also emphasize that listening sometimes means talking: asking questions, sharing experiences, or saying something that makes the other person feel understood. It may also mean admitting that you have tried but still do not understand. The other partner listens, without interrupting or saying anything, except to encourage the speaker to say more. The listener shows that she is listening by her attitude and by the way she moves her body.

Then the partners switch roles. When the partners are finished, they think about how well it worked. They ask each other questions like: Did you feel listened to? What difficulties did you have?

Some women may feel more comfortable listening as they work with their hands—for example, as they weave or sew.

Once the group has learned how to help and support one another, they can be healers for one another. Here are some ways for the group to help healing begin:

Exercises for healing mental health

1. Share experiences and feelings in the group. People who have mental health problems often feel very alone. Just being able to talk about a problem can be helpful. After one person has told her story, the leader can ask for other similar experiences. When everyone has listened to these, the group can discuss what the stories have in common, whether the problem was partly caused by social conditions, and if so, what the group might do to change these conditions. A woman can also practice this exercise at home whenever she has difficulty sleeping, or feels tense and afraid. Breathing deeply helps calm nervous feelings.

If you start to feel uncomfortable or frightened at any time during a relaxation exercise, open your eyes and breathe deeply.

2. Learn to relax. This exercise is particularly helpful for people who are suffering from stress. In a quiet place where everyone can sit down, the leader asks the group to follow these instructions:
• Close your eyes and imagine a safe, peaceful place where you would like to be. This might be on a mountain, by a lake or ocean, or in a field.
• Keep thinking about this place as you breathe deeply in through your nose and then out through your mouth.
• If it helps, think of a positive thought, such as "I am at peace," or "I am safe."
• Keep breathing, focusing either on the safe place or the thought. Do this for about 20 minutes.

3. Creating a story, drama, or painting. The group can make up a story about a situation similar to those experienced by members of the group. The leader starts the story, and then another member continues to tell another part—and so on until everyone has contributed something and the story is complete. (The group can also act out the story as it is told or paint a picture of the story.)

Then the group analyzes the different ideas that have been developed.

These questions can help people begin to talk:
• What feelings or experiences are most important in this story?
• Why did these feelings occur?
• How is the person coping with these feelings?
• What can help her develop a new balance in her life?
• What can the community do to help?

Helping women with reactions to trauma

• The most important way to help someone suffering from trauma is to help her learn to trust others again. Let her control how fast the relationship between you develops. She needs to know you are willing to listen, but that she can wait until she feels ready to talk. Doing everyday activities together may be best at first.

• It may help a woman to talk about her life before the trauma as well as her current experiences. This may help her realize that although life has changed a lot, in many ways she is the same person as before. If it seems right, encourage her to do some of the same activities she enjoyed before or that were part of her daily routine.

• Some painful things may be too difficult to talk about, or may be 'buried' away where they cannot be remembered. Exercises like drawing or painting, or a physical activity like walking, can help a person express or relieve these painful feelings.

• If a woman dreams of the trauma, she can put an object from her new life next to her as she sleeps. This helps her remember, when she wakes from a bad dream, that she is safe now.

• If reminders of the trauma make a woman react in fearful ways, help her make a plan for those reminders that cannot be avoided. For example, a woman might tell herself: "His face is like the man who attacked me, but he is a different person and does not wish to hurt me".

• If a person was raped or beaten, remind her that she is not responsible for what she said or did while being hurt. All responsibility lies with those who hurt her. Help her understand that one aim of abuse is to make a person feel she can never feel whole again, but that this is not true.

Professional Help

Many communities, Tribes, Urban Indian programs and IHS facilities have mental health professionals that can help someone deal with trauma. Talk to your health care provider for more information.

If a woman has made a plan for killing herself, she needs help right away.

If there are mental health services in her community, find out if someone can talk with her regularly. Medicine for depression may also be helpful.

Helping someone who wants to end her life

Anyone who suffers from serious depression is at risk for suicide. A woman may not readily talk about thoughts of suicide, but she will often admit them if asked. If she does, then try to find out:

- Does she have a plan about how to kill herself?
- Does she have a way to carry out the plan?
- Has she ever tried suicide before?
- Is her judgment affected by alcohol or drugs?
- Is she isolated from family or friends?
- Has she lost the desire to live?
- Does she have a serious health problem?
- Is she young and going through a serious life problem?

If the answer to any of these questions is 'yes', she is at a greater risk for attempting suicide than other people. To help, first try talking with her. Some people may begin to feel better simply by telling you about their problems. If so, or if she still feels bad but is more in control of her feelings than before, ask her to promise that she will not hurt herself without talking to you first. If talking about her problems does not help, or if she cannot promise to talk to you, then she needs to be watched closely.

Always tell the person considering suicide that you plan to talk with others to help protect her. Talk to her family and friends, encouraging someone to be with her at all times. Ask them to remove dangerous objects from her surroundings.

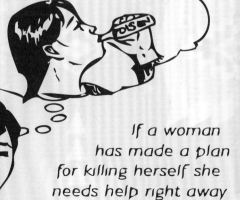

If a woman has made a plan for killing herself she needs help right away

Ways to Improve Your Community's Mental Health

Identify those at risk for mental health problems.
Women are at risk if they have:
- had mental health problems in the past.
- lost family members or are separated from their families.
- witnessed violence or have violent partners.
- little social support.

Look for other behaviors that may indicate mental health problems. If you suspect that someone has a mental health problem, get to know her better. Listen to what other people are saying about her behavior and the ways she has changed.

Build on a woman's strengths.
Every woman has developed ways of coping with everyday problems. Help a woman identify the positive ways she has dealt with problems in the past and how she might use these strengths in her present situation.

Remember that there are no quick solutions.
Beware of anyone who promises this. Work within a woman's traditions and culture. Every community has traditional ways of dealing with mental health problems, such as prayer and ritual. These practices are not always helpful, but they should always be considered and used as much as possible. Try to learn as much as you can about a woman's traditions and how they may be a source of strength for her. Anything that helps a woman recognize or give meaning to her experience can help her mental health.

Ask for help when you need it.
If you do not have experience with a mental health problem, try to talk to a trained mental health worker who does. Listening to other people's mental health problems can make you feel burdened, especially if you listen to a lot of people. Watch yourself to see if you are feeling pressured, if you are losing interest in helping others, or if you get irritable or angry easily. These are signs that you are making other people's problems your own. Ask for help, and try to get more rest and relaxation.

Resources:

www.tribalconnections.org/ehealthinfo/
mentalhealth.html

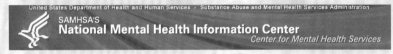
TRIBAL CONNECTIONS — eHEALTH INFORMATION RESOURCES

mentalhealth.samhsa.gov/

United States Department of Health and Human Services · Substance Abuse and Mental Health Services Administration

SAMHSA'S
National Mental Health Information Center
Center for Mental Health Services

www.nlm.nih.gov/medlineplus/mentalhealth.
html

Covenant House Hotline: 800-999-9999
Crisis line for youth, teens, and families. Gives callers locally based referrals throughout the United States. Provides help for youth and parents regarding drugs, abuse, homelessness, runaway children, and message relays. Operates 24 hours, seven days a week.

**National
Alliance on
Mental Illness**
nami.org
1-800-950-NAMI
(6264)

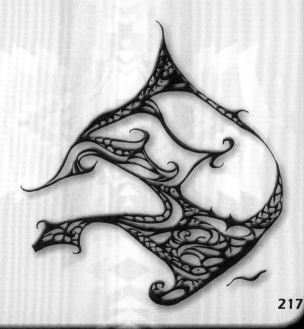

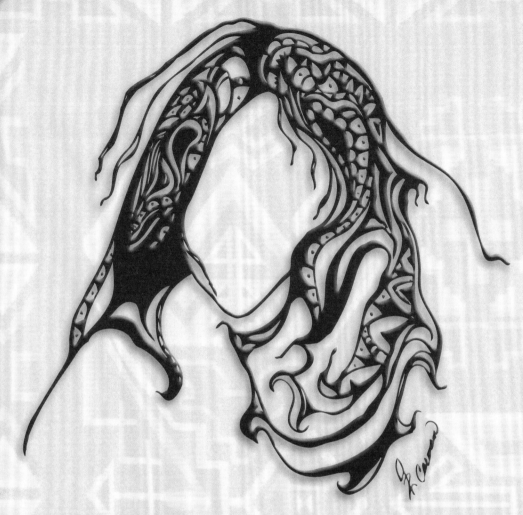

This is a hard topic for JourneyWoman to lead you through. Alcohol, drugs, and now meth are taking our young people on a different and violent path. JourneyWoman has not been spared; both grandparents were alcoholics as is her son, who, the only time she does not worry about, is when he is in jail. Unfortunately, in Indian County, this scenario is replayed every minute. A mother's tears do not stop.

Alcohol and Drug Abuse

Many kinds of drugs are used in everyday life. In some places, drugs or brewed drinks have a sacred role in traditions. In other places, alcoholic drinks like wine or beer are commonly served with meals or social events. And some drugs are used as medicines.

Why do people begin to use alcohol or drugs?

People often begin to use alcohol or drugs because of social pressure. Boys and men may face pressure to drink or use other common drugs to prove their manhood. A man may believe that the more he drinks, or the more drugs he uses, the more manly he is.

Many girls and women may also face social pressure to start drinking or using drugs. They may feel that they will appear more grown-up or more modern. Or they may think they will be accepted more easily by others.

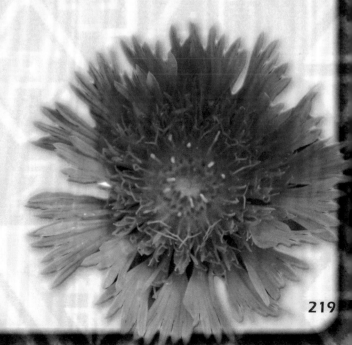

Use and Misuse of Alcohol and Drugs

When does use become misuse?

Whatever the reason for starting, alcohol and drugs can easily become misused. A person is misusing drugs or alcohol if she loses control over when she uses alcohol or drugs, over the amount she uses, or over the way she acts when using alcohol or drugs.

Here are some common signs that people are misusing drugs or alcohol.

- they feel they need a drink or a drug to get through the day or night. They may use it at unusual times or places, such as in the morning, or when they are alone.

- they lie about how much they or others use, or hide it.

- they have money problems because of how much they spend on buying drugs or alcohol. Some people commit crimes to get money for drugs or alcohol.

- they ruin celebrations because of how much they drink alcohol or use drugs.

- they are ashamed of their behavior while using drugs or alcohol.

- they are not working as well as before or are not going to work as often because of using alcohol or drugs.

- they have problems with violent behavior. Someone may become more violent towards their spouse, children, or friends.

CAGE Screening for Alcoholism

Cut down on drinking – have tried repeatedly without success

Annoyed by criticism about drinking habits

Guilty feelings about drinking

Eye opener drink needed in the morning

"One Drink" =
1 shot hard liquor (1.5 o
1 glass of wine (5 oz)
1 beer (12 oz)

How much is too much?

The American Medical Association's Maximum Drinking Limits for alcohol consumption:
- For healthy men up to age 65: no more than 4 drinks in a day AND no more than 14 drinks in a week.
- For healthy women (and healthy men over age 65): no more than 3 drinks in a day AND no more than 7 drinks in a week.
- Even lower limits or abstinence (not drinking any alchohol) is recommended for some as medically indicated: for example, for patients who take medications that interact with alco hol, have a health condition made worse by alcohol, or are pregnant (abstinence advised)

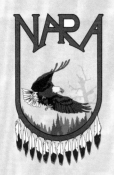

reatment Resource in
ortland, Oregon

NARA RESIDENTIAL
REATMENT CENTER
7645 NW St. Helens
Highway
Portland, Oregon
7231
03.621.1069

NARA OUTPATIENT
REATMENT CENTER
631 SW Columbia
Portland, Oregon
7201
03.231.2641

Why People Misuse Drugs and Alcohol

Many people end up misusing drugs and alcohol in order to escape from problems in their lives.

All types of people do this. But people whose parents misused alcohol or drugs are much more likely to try and solve their problems in the same way. This is because a 'weakness' to misuse drugs or alcohol may be passed from parents to children. And as children watch their parents use alcohol or drugs to escape problems, they learn this same behavior.

Alcohol and drug misuse is also common among people who do not feel any hope about changing the miserable conditions of their lives. People who are displaced from their homes or facing desperate problems—like losing their jobs or way of earning a living, losing family members, or being abandoned by a partner—are also more at risk for misusing drugs and alcohol.

Women often begin to misuse drugs or alcohol because they do not feel that they have any control over—or power to change—their lives. They may feel dependent upon, or at the mercy of, their partner or male family members. And if women have low status in the community, it may be hard for them to value themselves.

Unfortunately, drugs and alcohol usually make all these problems worse, and people feel even less able to improve their lives. Instead of looking for ways to improve their situations, most people who misuse drugs or alcohol spend their time, money, and health on trying to avoid and forget their problems.

eens and Alcohol:
Alcohol is the most frequently used drug by high school niors, and its use is increasing. Boys usually try alcohol for the first time at just 11 years old, ile the average age for American girls' first drink is 13. In short, our nation's youth are flirting with disaster. Underage drinking is a factor in nearly half of all teen automobile crashes, e leading cause of death among teenagers. Alcohol use contributes to youth suicides, micides and fatal injuries – the leading cause of death among youth after auto crashes. cohol abuse is linked to as many as two-thirds of all sexual assaults and date rapes of teens d college students. Alcohol is a major factor in unprotected sex among youth, increasing eir risk of contracting HIV or other transmitted diseases.

Dependence and addiction

When a person misuses drugs or alcohol, both the mind and the body can begin to feel an overpowering need for the drug. When the mind feels this need, it is called dependence. When a person's body feels such a strong need for the drug that she gets sick without it, it is called physical addiction.

Alcohol and some drugs can cause addiction. Once a person becomes addicted, she will need more and more alcohol or drugs to feel their effects.

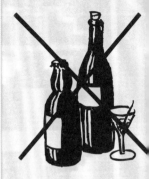

Any use of drugs and alcohol is dangerous if a person:
- is driving, using a machine, or dangerous tool.
- is pregnant or breastfeeding.
- is caring for small children.
- is taking medicine, especially medicines for pain, sleep, fits (seizures), or mental health problems.
- has liver or kidney disease.

Common health problems

People who use alcohol and drugs a lot get sick more often and more severely than others. They are more likely to have:
- poor nutrition, which causes more sickness.
- diabetes or complications from diabetes.
- cancer, and problems of the heart, liver, stomach, skin, lungs and urine system—including ones that cause permanent damage.
- brain damage or fits (seizures).
- memory loss—waking up not knowing what happened.
- mental health problems, such as seeing strange things or hearing voices (hallucinations), being suspicious of others, having flashbacks, or feeling severe depression or anxiety. death from using too much at one time (overdose).

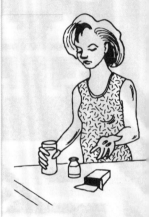

Misuse of drugs can include misuse of prescription drugs or taking prescription drugs from other people.

In addition, injuries or death from accidents happen more often to these people (and often to their families). This is because they make bad decisions or take unnecessary risks, or because they can lose control of their bodies while using alcohol or drugs. If they have unprotected sex, share needles used to inject drugs, or trade sex for drugs, they are at risk for hepatitis and sexually transmitted infections.

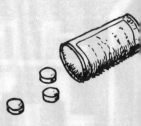

Drugs and Alcohol can be Worse for Women

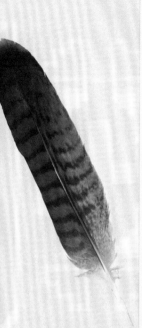

In addition to the problems that anyone who misuses drugs or alcohol may suffer, women face some special health problems.

- Women who drink large amounts of alcohol or use a lot of drugs are more likely to get liver disease than men.

- Many women and girls are pushed into sex they do not want when they drink alcohol or use drugs. This may result in unwanted pregnancy, STIs, and even HIV/AIDS.

- If used during pregnancy, drugs and alcohol can cause children to be born with birth defects and mental disabilities, such as:

    - problems of the heart, bones, genitals, head and face.
    - low birth weight.
    - slow growth.
    - learning difficulties.

A baby can be born dependent on drugs and suffer the same signs of withdrawal as an adult.

Women feel more shame

In most communities, women's behavior in public is more strictly controlled than men's behavior. Often it is considered normal for men to use alcohol or drugs, but not for women to do so. If a woman loses control of her behavior because of using too much alcohol or drugs, she is thought to be a 'loose woman', even if she is not having sex with others.

To avoid the shame that comes from making her drug or alcohol misuse public, a woman is more likely to drink steadily over a long period of time, rather than drinking a lot at one time. This kind of drinking makes it easier for her to control her behavior. She is also more likely to keep her misuse a secret and to put off getting treatment. All these behaviors increase the harm that comes from alcohol or drug misuse.

Overcoming Problems with Alcohol and Drugs

Misusing alcohol and drugs makes violent situations worse, especially in the home. Women who have partners who misuse drugs and alcohol often suffer injuries and even death.

Although it may seem difficult to overcome a dependence or addiction to alcohol and drugs, it can be done. There are 2 stages: quitting and then learning ways to stay free of drugs and alcohol.

Quitting

If you think you have a drinking or drug problem and want to quit:

1. Admit you have a problem.

2. Decide to do something TODAY.

3. Stop. Or use less and then stop. Many people can stop drinking or using drugs all at once. All it takes for them is the will to stop and the belief they can do it. Others need help from a group or treatment program like Alcoholics Anonymous (AA) that helps people with drinking or drug problems. There may also be other groups or treatment programs in your area. Most women feel more comfortable in a group with women only. If there are no groups in your area, try starting your own group with someone who has been successful in helping people to stop drinking or using drugs.

> It may be dangerous to stop alcohol use abruptly, you may need to find a "detox" program to safely withdrawal. from drinking.

4. If you start drinking or using drugs again, do not blame yourself. But try to stop again right away.

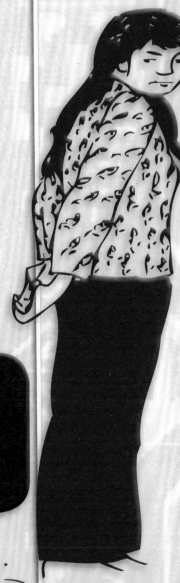

Living with Someone Who Has a Drinking or Drug Problem

Often women must care for someone, like a partner or a male relative, who has a drinking or drug problem. Living with someone with these problems is very difficult, especially if the person does not want to change. You can help yourself and your family if you:

- Do not blame yourself. It is not always possible to help another person control his or her drug or alcohol use.

- Try not to rely on the person's opinion of you to feel good about yourself.

- Try to find a support group for you and your family. Sometimes this is the only way a family can cope with the problem.

Some herbal teas can help the liver cleanse the body of poisonous effects of alcohol or drugs. A traditional healer may be able to suggest good local herbs.

How to help someone with a drinking or drug problem:

- Help him or her admit he or she has a problem. This may be all that is needed for them to use less or stop, unless they are addicted.

- Talk to them about stopping when they are not drunk or on drugs.

- Try not to blame him or her.

- Help her or him to avoid situations where he may feel pressured to drink or take drugs. This means not being with people with the same problem, even if they are friends.

- Help him or her to find other ways to cope with life's problems and to have better mental health.

- Help them make a plan for stopping and follow that plan.

When someone is addicted to alcohol, lack of alcohol in the body can cause seizures, and in extreme cases, death.

Physical Addiction and Withdrawal

When a person is physically addicted to alcohol or a drug and quits using it, she will go through a period of withdrawal. During this time her body must get used to being without the drug.

Alcohol addiction and withdrawal. After quitting drinking, it can take about 3 days for most signs of withdrawal to stop. Many people get through these days without problems. But since some people have very serious signs, it is important to have someone watch over the person and give

Learning to stay free of drugs and alcohol

Once a person has overcome physical addiction, it is important to learn how to stay free of drugs and alcohol to prevent the problem from developing again. The best way to do this is to learn better skills for coping with life. This is not easy to do and will take time.

A woman who has misused alcohol or drugs often feels powerless and full of shame. She needs to learn that she is able to make changes to improve her life. One way to begin is to make small changes that help prove to herself and to others that she can cope with problems. Here are some ideas that have helped women build coping skills:

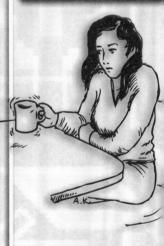

*   Develop a network of support among those close to you and ask for help when you need it. It is much easier to think about problems and begin to solve them when you can talk and work with others.
*   Try to solve one problem at a time. That way, problems will not seem so large that you cannot cope with them.
*   Try to tell a friend or someone you trust about things that worry or upset you, or that make you sad or angry. You may begin to understand why you feel the way you do and what you can do to feel better.
*   Work with other people on a project to improve your community. This proves to you and to others that you know how to work for change. You may also find that doing this helps you make personal changes, too.
*   Meet together regularly with other people who are working to stay free of alcohol or drugs.

Early signs of withdrawal:
*   slight shaking
*   nervous and irritable feelings
*   sweating
*   trouble eating and sleeping
*   aches all over the body
*   nausea, vomiting, stomach pain

If you are trying to stay free of drink or drugs, avoid places where you will feel pressure to use them.
Work with others to organize social vents where drugs and alcohol are not used.

esources:
ww.niaaa.nih.
ov/

AAA NATIONAL INSTITUTE ON
ALCOHOL ABUSE AND ALCOHOLISM
of the NATIONAL INSTITUTES OF HEALTH

ibstance Abuse
eatment Locator
tp://dasis3.sam-
a.gov/

SAMHSA
Substance Abuse & Mental Health
Services Administration
U.S. Department of Health
and Human Services

Preventing Drug and Alcohol Misuse

To prevent drug and alcohol misuse successfully, you must consider the social forces that contribute to drug use. How did the problem start? What makes people use more? Are there new pressures on men or women that make it harder for them to control their use of alcohol and drugs? How can the drugs or alcohol be made less important in your community?

Once you understand the reasons for the problem, your can identify causes including social pressures to drink or use drugs. This puts you more in control and able to prevent drug and alcohol misuse,

Helping young people resist alcohol and drugs

Many people who have drug and alcohol problems as adults began using them when they were young. Drugs or alcohol can seem like an easy way to have fun or escape from problems, especially if others are using them. Young people often feel confused and powerless about the many changes they must cope with—their growing bodies and new responsibilities. Young people are also influenced by many pressures, especially their friends, older people they admire, and advertising.

One way to reduce drug and alcohol misuse is to help young people learn to resist harmful pressures. Here are some ideas that have worked in many communities:

- Encourage the schools in your community to teach young people about the problems of using drugs and alcohol.
- Make it harder for people to sell drugs to young people.
- Organize to remove advertisements that make cigarettes and alcohol look glamorous and modern.
- Become a good role model. If you drink a lot or use drugs, chances are your children will too.
- Teach your own children about the problems drug and alcohol use can cause. They can then influence their friends.
- Help young people have fun without drugs and alcohol.
- Help your children develop skills and self-esteem to resist the social pressure to use drugs and alcohol.

227

Violence against women, including domestic violence, is not new to Indian Country; it has just been well hidden. No longer can we bury our head in the sand and pretend it does not exist, no longer can we keep it a private matter, for when domestic violence happens, it happens to everyone in the village or community. It may start with a slap to the face by a partner or someone else and trickle down to children and continue the downward spiral to mothers, fathers, friends, cousins, aunties, teachers, and on and on.

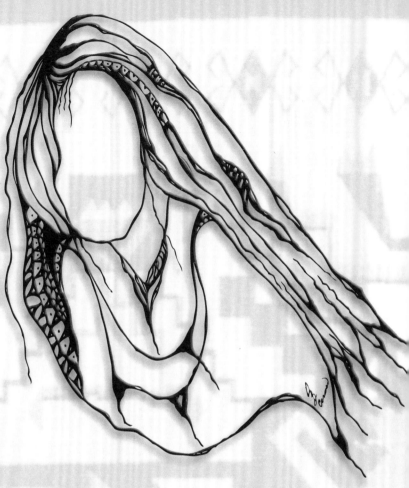

JourneyWoman is a domestic violence survivor. In the 1970s, there were no resources available to help women, men, or children, such as me. For many years, I was ashamed and did not talk about a time when I was beaten, verbally abused and thought of as "nothing." But, I became a fighter for my children and myself and eventually became a strong woman. If Journey Woman can do it, so can you.

I hope this chapter on domestic violence will empower, teach, and enlighten you about different types of violence, some of the reasons behind violence, and what you can do you are in a relationship where you are being physically hurt, mentally brow-beaten verbally told you are nothing, remember, you are something; a two-legged human be who deserves the very best in life, for you and your family. Don't be afraid, seek hel

Violence Against Women

Every day, women are slapped, kicked, beaten, humiliated, threatened, sexually abused, and even murdered by their partners. But often we do not hear about this violence, because the women who are abused may feel ashamed, alone, and afraid to speak out. Many doctors, nurses, and health workers do not recognize violence as the serious health problem it is.

This chapter is about different types of violence that occur to women and girls. It can help you understand why violence happens, what you can do about it, and how you can work for change in your community.

Although this chapter talks about violence between a woman and a man, violence can happen in any close relationship: for example, between a mother in- law and her son's new wife, between parents and their children, between an older and younger child, between family members and an older person living in the home, and between partners of the same sex.

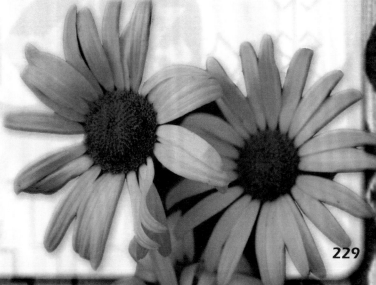

Why Does a Man Hurt a Woman?

A man may offer many excuses for hurting a woman—that he was drunk, that he lost control, or that she 'deserved it'. But a man chooses to use violence because it is a way he can get what he needs or what he feels is rightfully his as a man. When a man does not feel that he has power over his own life, he may use violence to try and control another person's life. It is natural for someone to want to control his or her own life in normal ways, but it is wrong to try and control someone else's life, especially with violence. Here are some of the reasons why some men hurt women:

1. Violence works.
   - It offers the man a quick end to a disagreement without having to talk about the real problem or find a real solution.
   - A man may find the fight exciting, and have lots of energy afterward. He may want to have these feelings again.
   - If a man uses violence, he 'wins' and gets his way. The victim is likely to give him his way again the next time to avoid being hurt. This gives the man even more power.

2. The man has a wrong idea about what it means to be a man.
   - If a man believes that to be a man, he must control what a woman does, he may feel it is OK to hurt her.
   - Some men think that they have a 'right' to certain things—to a 'good' wife, to sons, to making all the decisions in the family—just because they are men.

3. The man feels that the woman belongs to him, or that he needs her.
   - If the woman is 'strong', the man may feel afraid that he will lose her, or that she does not need him. He will take steps to make her more dependent on him.

4. He does not know any other way to be.
   - If a man has seen his father or other people in his life react with violence when life is difficult and stressful, then he may have never learned any other way to behave.

Violent or abusive relationships often happen when one person has more power over the other. These reasons may explain why a man abuses his wife, but they **do not** give him permission to do so.

One form of abuse often turns into another.
In many cases, verbal abuse becomes physical abuse after a while. It may not seem like it at first, but the man may slowly begin to 'accidentally' push or bump the woman, or begin to sit down in the place the woman usually sits, so that she has to move. If this behavior works for him, it may get worse until he becomes violent. Not all women who suffer other forms of abuse are beaten, but all women who have been beaten have suffered from other forms of abuse.

There are many different ways that a man tries to gain power over a woman. Beating is only one of them. But all of them can hurt a woman.

Kinds of Violence

Imagine that the circle below is a wheel. Power and control are at the center of the wheel because they are the reasons behind all of the actions. Each section of the wheel is a behavior that a violent man may use to control a woman. Violence is the rim of the wheel—what holds it together and gives it strength.

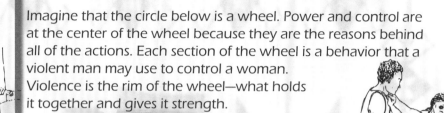

VIOLENCE

Emotional Abuse

The man insults the woman, puts her down, or makes her think she is going crazy.

Sexual Abuse

The man makes the woman do sexual things against her will, or physically attacks the sexual parts of her body. He treats her like an object.

Isolation

The man controls everything the woman does—who she sees and talks to, and where she goes.

Controlling Money

The man tries to keep the woman from getting a job or making her own money. He makes her ask him for any money she needs. Or he may force her to work and then take the money she earns.

Power and Control

Making Threats

The man uses a look, action, tone of voice, or makes threats, that make the woman feel afraid that he will hurt her.

Because he is a 'Man'

The man uses the fact that he is a man as an excuse to treat the woman like a servant. He makes all the decisions and tells her that, as a woman, she has no right to object.

Using Children

The man uses the children to make the woman feel guilty, or to hurt her.

Blaming Her

The man says that the abuse did not really happen, that it was not serious, or that it was the woman's fault.

VIOLENCE

231

The Story of
Jalene and Darren

Darren was 12 years older than Jalene and was already a successful car mechanic and wood carver when they met. He sold his art to the store where Jalene worked as a clerk. Darren was charming and would talk about the kind of life they could have together. He told Jalene he would buy her anything she wanted and take her anywhere she wanted to go. He often bought her new clothes that he liked to admire her in, telling her how pretty she would be if she stopped dressing the way she did.

He eventually began to see her every day, and soon asked her to quit her job and marry him. After they married, Jalene expected Darren to keep his promises. Instead, things began to change. He would not allow her to go out, because she "looked so ugly." In fact, he took all the beautiful clothes he had bought her and burned them, saying, "That stupid, ugly woman didn't deserve such clothes."

One day Darren came home in the middle of the day and punched a hole in the wall, accusing Jalene of sleeping with his friend. When she said that she had just gone to visit her mother, Darren called her a lying whore and hit her. He said she would not go to visit her family—they did not want her either. He never said anything more about it, but when he came home later that night, he brought her a present and told her how much he loved her and wanted to take care of her.

When Jalene got pregnant, she thought Darren would start treating her better. But it seemed to give him more excuses to hurt her. When he got angry, he started hitting and kicking her in the stomach. She was terrified she would lose the baby, but she had no place to go. She believed Darren when he said her family did not want her, and besides, she had no money of her own. There were times when Darren would go several weeks without losing control, and Jalene would convince herself that everything was OK. He really did love her, after all. If only she could learn how to avoid setting him off. She would try even harder than before, but nothing helped.

Through the years, Darren drank too much, threw her against walls, and would force her to have sex even when her body ached from his beatings. Jalene awoke one night to find him holding a knife to her throat. The next day, he told her she was imagining things, that she was crazy. He always said that if she told anyone "lies" about him he would kill her. She didn't tell anyone and she went out as little as possible. She hated the thought of anyone seeing her bruises and knowing what he did to her.

Jalene often thought about leaving, but she did not know where to go. After 12 years of being his wife, not only was Jalene afraid of what he would do to her, but without him she would have no home, no money, no father for her children. Darren had said bad things about her to the people at the store where she used to work, and she knew that, because of her children she would have a hard time finding work and childcare. Jalene felt so alone.

Jalene's father was dead now and her mother lived with her brother's family at another tribe in another state. They did not have room for her and her children. Her sister was deeply religious and told Jalene it was her duty to stay with her husband, no matter what. "That is the way it is meant to be, we all have to make sacrifices."

She had so much work to do at home she was always busy. And since Darren got mad when she went out or when someone came to visit, Jalene stopped seeing her friends.

She was sure they had long since given up on her. Then came the night when Jalene's oldest daughter was 11. She came to Jalene crying, saying Dad had hurt her "down there." Jalene was shocked. She had thought the children would not be affected by Darren's behavior. She knew it would do no good to confront him, but she would NOT let it happen again. When Jalene lost her last pregnancy, the health provider who examined her asked about her injuries. Jalene had made some excuse. The health provider nodded her head and gave Jalene a card with information on safe places to stay for women in her situation. She told her if Jalene ever needed to leave, she and her children could go there, but to make sure that she was ready to leave when she did. Jalene was ready now.

Why did Darren hit Jalene? These are some of the wrong ideas that people have:

A man can do whatever he wants to his wife.

The truth: No man has the right to beat his wife. Nothing a woman does gives a man the right to hurt her, even if he thinks she deserves it—even if she herself thinks she deserves it.

It's just because he drinks...

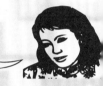

The truth: Alcohol does not cause violence, but it often makes it worse. Violence is also common in places where people do not drink alcohol.

It is best for the children if she stays with him. He can still be a good father to them.

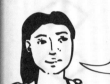

It's their business. It's not right to interfere with the private affairs of a couple.

The truth: It is not always better for the family when a woman stays with a violent man. He is teaching the children terrible, wrong ways to deal with their feelings, and about how women should be treated. He is not being good to his children if he is beating their mother—or them.

The truth: Violence is not just a family matter. Many women are hurt or killed. Violence is a social and community health problem.

Only poor, ignorant men beat their wives.

He wouldn't beat her if he didn't love her so much.

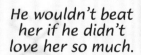

The truth: Beating is not a sign of love. Love means showing respect and kindness.

The truth: Violence is not just a problem of poverty or ignorance. Violence can happen in any home: rich or poor, educated or less educated, in the city or in rural areas.

Harmful Effects of Violence

Women

In women, men's violence can cause:

- lack of motivation or lack of a sense of self-worth.

- mental health problems, like anxiety and problems eating and sleeping. As a way to cope with the violence, women may begin harmful or reckless behavior—such as using drugs or alcohol, or having many sex partners.

- serious pain and injuries: broken bones, burns, black eyes, cuts, bruises, as well as headaches, belly pain, and muscle pains that may continue for many years after the abuse happens.

- sexual health problems. Many women suffer miscarriages from being beaten during pregnancy. They may also suffer from unwanted pregnancies, sexually transmitted infections (STIs) or HIV/AIDS as a result of sexual abuse. Sexual abuse often also leads to a fear of having sex, pain during sex, and lack of desire.

- death.

Children

In children, seeing their mothers abused can often cause:

- angry or aggressive behavior— copying the violence. Or they may become very quiet and withdraw to escape notice.

- nightmares and other fears. Children in abusive familes often do not eat well, grow and learn more slowly than other children, and have many illnesses, like stomach aches, headaches, and asthma.

- injury and worse if the violence is turned on them.

Community

In a community, violence can cause:

- the cycle of violence to continue into new generations.

- everyone's quality of life to suffers because women take part less in their communities when they are silenced or killed by the violence.

Violence not only hurts women. It also affects their children, and the whole community.

When a woman is abused at home, her children believe that this is how girls and women should be treated.

Warning Signs

One form of abuse often turns into another. In many cases, verbal abuse becomes physical abuse after a while. It may not seem like it at first, but the man may slowly begin to 'accidentally' push or bump the woman, or begin to sit down in the place the woman usually sits, so that she has to move. If this behavior works for him, it may get worse until he becomes violent.

When an abusive relationship becomes violent, it is much harder to leave. The longer a woman stays, the more control the man has over her, and the less faith she may have in herself.

Some men are more likely to become violent than others. There are certain signs that may mean a man will become violent. If you see these signs, and have a way to get out of the relationship, think carefully.

Ask yourself these questions:

• Does he act jealous when you see other people, or accuse you of lying to him? If you find you change your behavior to keep him from acting jealous, then he is controlling you.

• Does he try to keep you from seeing your friends and family, or from doing things on your own? It does not matter what reason he uses. He is trying to keep you from having their support. It will be easier for him to abuse you if you have nowhere else to go.

• Does he claim that alcohol, drugs, or stress are the reasons he acts the way he does? If he puts the blame on something else, he may say things will get better if he gets a new job, moves to a new town, or stops using drugs or alcohol.

• Does he blame you or someone else for the way he acts, or deny that he is doing anything wrong? He is less likely to want to change himself if he thinks that the way he acts is your fault.

It does not matter how much you love a person. Love cannot change someone. Only that person can choose to change himself.

Not all women who suffer other forms of abuse are beaten, but all women who have been beaten have suffered from other forms of abuse.

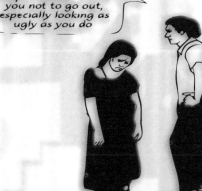

Stupid woman I told you not to go out, especially looking as ugly as you do

The first violent attack often seems like an isolated event. But in many cases, after the violence first happens the following pattern, or cycle, develops

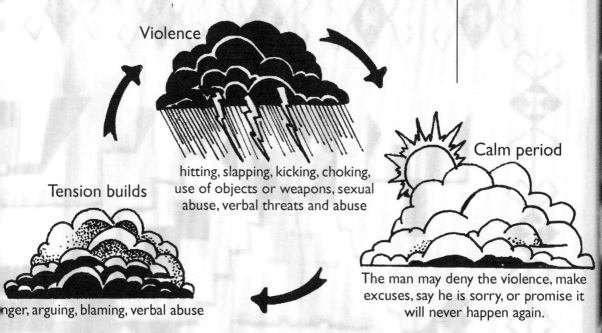

Violence

hitting, slapping, kicking, choking, use of objects or weapons, sexual abuse, verbal threats and abuse

Calm period

Tension builds

anger, arguing, blaming, verbal abuse

The man may deny the violence, make excuses, say he is sorry, or promise it will never happen again.

As the violence goes on, the calm period gets shorter and shorter for many couples. As the woman's will is broken, the man's control over her becomes so complete that it is no longer necessary for him to make promises that things will get better.

Some women try to make the violence happen so that it will be over with more quickly, and to get to the calm period sooner.

Some women are more likely to be abused

In many couples, the man becomes violent for the first time when the woman is pregnant. He may feel as though he is losing control because he cannot control the changes in her body. He may feel angry because she is paying more attention to the baby and less to him, or because she may not want to have sex with him. Also, many couples feel extra worried about money when they are expecting a new baby.

Women with disabilities are also more likely to be abused. Men may think a woman with a disability is easier to control because she may be less able to defend herself.

Why Women Stay with Men Who Hurt Them

"Why does she stay?" is the first question most people ask when they hear about a woman who is being abused. There are many reasons why a woman might choose to stay in an abusive relationship. They include:

• **fear and threats.** The man may have told her, "I will kill you, kill the children, kill your mother... if you try to leave." She may feel she is doing everything she can to protect herself and others by staying.

• **no money, and no place to go.** This is especially true if he has controlled all the money and not allowed her to see her family and friends.

• **no protection.** There may be nothing to stop him from coming after her and hurting or even killing her.

• **shame.** She may feel the violence is somehow her fault, or that she deserves it.

• **religious or cultural beliefs**. She may feel it is her duty to keep the marriage together, no matter what it costs her.

• **hope for change**. She may feel she loves the man and wants the relationship to continue. She may think there is some way to make the violence stop.

• **guilt about leaving the children with no father.** But perhaps a better question to ask is, "Why doesn't he go?" If we ask why she does not leave, it says that we think it is her personal problem to solve. It is wrong to think of the violence as only her problem.

The whole community needs to be responsible for the health and well-being of every person in that community.

It is the man who is committing a crime by violating the woman's right to live free from physical harm, or by killing her. His actions should be challenged and stopped.

If we ask why she does not leave, it says that we think the violence is her personal problem to solve. The whole community needs to be responsible for the health and well-being of every person in that community.

Find someone you trust who can help you sort out your feelings and think about your choices.

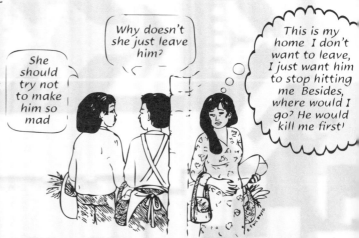

She should try not to make him so mad

Why doesn't she just leave him?

This is my home I don't want to leave, I just want him to stop hitting me Besides, where would I go? He would kill me first!

My Darling,

Your last words to me were, "I love you", and with that slight wave of your hand you bid me goodbye. I loved you so much that I would have done anything for you and I guess in many ways I did. Our goodbye in the ambulance never gave me the opportunity to tell you how much you meant to me as the love of my youth.

We were mean to each other in such exquisite ways. Do you remember, did we start out that way? It was so long ago I almost don't recall. Was it Indian love, you know the beating kind, or was it really spousal abuse that we both heaped upon one another and refused to accept as something other than the natural outpouring of our love? As I think of it now, so many years since your passing, I know that if it was love, it wasn't a good sort of love. Love doesn't have to hurt but ours did. I remember how we treasured those hurts as if they were jewels that we held in a velvet box as proof of our commitment to one another? It is still painful to remember those days even after all these years.

Frying pans and fists were our weapons of choice. Me, a raised voice and screams of frustration, hurt, and pain. You, silence always the silence and it was your very best weapon. In your last days you used it against me for the final time. The coma for six weeks as I sat at your bedside praying to hear your voice once again-even if it was to hear you telling me I had dandruff on my collar as we stood in the check out line at Fry's. I wanted you to tell me goodbye and that you really did love me. It never happened. I just prayed that it would.

I treasure every moment we had together. I treasure the things I learned from you both good and bad. But my darling as I have grown older, I have learned that pain and love are not synonymous. You were everything to me. But time has given me the wonderful gift of knowing who I can become. And the woman I have become no longer allows pain to be at the center of her love.

Backward glances hold mostly painful memories so I try to look forward most of the time. But when I do chance to look back for more than a second, I work so hard to remember the good parts of our life together- remember the three days in Bisbee camping by the stream. Just you and me. That is the time I choose to recall. But love of my youth, on days like today, I still weep for us.

One last thing I would like you to know, our life together gave me an eternal gift. Faith. I learned to have faith in God, because I so wanted us to work it all out; faith in prayer, because I wanted you to live and finally, faith in hope. Hope that I could carry on after you passed. I learned faith because of you and perhaps that is your greatest gift to me.

I can never forget you. You were everything to me then. Good bye and always remember that you were the love of my youth...

What to Do

Safety before the violence happens again

• Tell someone nearby about the violence. Ask that person to come or to get help if the person hears that you are in trouble. Perhaps a neighbor, male relative, or a group of women or men can come before you are seriously hurt .

• Think of a special word or signal that will tell your children or someone else in your family to get help.

• Teach your children how to get to a safe place. Safety during the violence

• If you can tell that he is going to become violent, try to have it happen where there are no weapons or objects that he can use to harm you, and where you can get away.

• Use your best judgement. Do whatever you need to do to calm him down so that you and your children are safe.

• If you need to get away from him, think about how you can escape. Where is the safest place to go? Safety when a woman gets ready to leave

• Save money any way that you can. Put money in a safe place (away from the house) or open a bank account in your own name so you can become more independent.

• If you can do so safely, think of other things you can do to become less dependent on him, such as making friends, joining a group, or spending more time with your family.

• See if there are 'safe houses' or other services for women who have been abused. These are special places in some towns and cities where abused women and their children can stay for a while. Try to find out before you leave if there is one that you can get to.

• Ask friends or relatives you trust if they would let you stay with them or lend you money. Be sure they will not tell your partner that you asked.

• Get copies of important documents, such as your identification or your children's vaccination records. Keep a copy at home and give a copy to someone you trust.

• Leave money, copies of your documents, and extra clothes with someone you trust so that you can leave quickly.

• If you can do it safely, practice your escape plan with your children to see if it would work. Make sure the children will not tell anyone.

If you decide to leave, you will need to be prepared for some of the new difficulties you will face:

If you leave

Safety. The most dangerous time for a woman is after she leaves. The man has lost control over her and will usually do anything to get it back. He may even try to follow through on his threat to kill her. She must make sure she is staying in a safe place that he does not know about or where she is protected. She should not tell anyone where she is staying. He may be able to force them to tell him where she is.

Surviving on your own. You need to find a way to support yourself and your children. If you can stay with friends or family, use that time to get more education or learn job skills. To save money, maybe you can share a place to live with another woman who also was abused.

Feelings. All the things you need to do to set up a new life may feel like too much to face. You may feel scared and lonely because you are not used to being alone in a strange place. You may miss your partner—no matter what he did to you. When things seem very difficult, you may not remember how bad it really was before you left. Give yourself time to feel sad about the loss of your partner and your former life. Try to stay strong. See if you can find other women in the same situation as you. Together you can support each other.

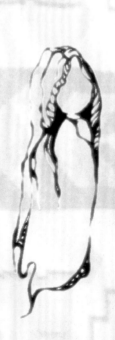
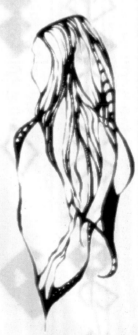

Standing Together Against Violence

Much of what has been gained in women's human rights so far has been thanks to the efforts of women themselves. They have organized themselves, broken taboos, spoken up - sometimes at great personal cost - and have led brave and inspiring campaigns against violence against women. They have achieved dramatic changes in laws, policies and practices.

Use social pressure

What are the pressures that prevent people where you live from doing things that most people believe are wrong?

In some places, it is the police. In others it may be the Tribal leaders, the family, or religion. In most places, it is a combination of these things.

For change to happen, people must stop thinking of violence against women as something that 'is just the way things are' or that is the woman's fault. Here are some ideas for helping stop violence in your community.

Raise your children to lead non-violent lives. You can work for change at home by helping your children find peaceful ways to solve problems.

Teach boys to respect themselves and to respect girls and women.

Encourage community leaders and other men to speak out against violence against women and to show their disapproval of men who beat women. Try and use all of the pressures that work where you live to keep men from abusing women.

Laws have been passed that punish men who abuse their wives. But laws do not always work well for abused women. In some places, the people who are supposed to enforce the laws—especially the police, the lawyers, and the judges—may be of limited support. But if the legal system and the police both work to protect women where you live, try to learn as much as you can about the laws and about women's rights.

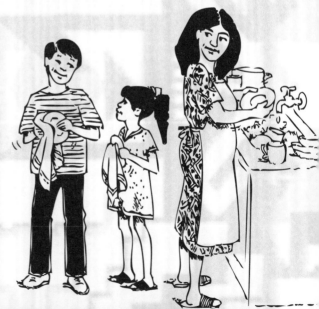

Resources:

The Department of Justice's Office on Violence Against Women (OVW)
www.usdoj.gov/ovw/

National Domestic Violence Hotline
1-800-799-SAFE (7233)
1-800-787-3224 (TTY)
Rape, Abuse, and Incest National Network (RAINN)
1-800-656-HOPE (4673)
National Sexual Violence Resource Center (NSVRC)
1-877-739-3895
National Center for Victims of Crime, Stalking Resource Center
1-800-394-2255
1-800-211-7996 (TTY)

www.now.org/issues/vio-lence/

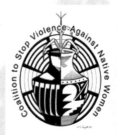

www.csvanw.org/
(505) 243-9199

http://toolkit.ncjrs.org/

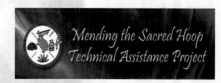

Mending the Sacred Hoop
STOP Violence Against Indian Women Techni-cal Assistance Project
Phone: 218-722-2781 or 1-888-305-1650
Fax: 218-722-5775
www.msh-ta.org

www.anjc.org/

www.4women.gov/violence/

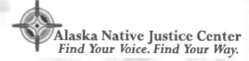

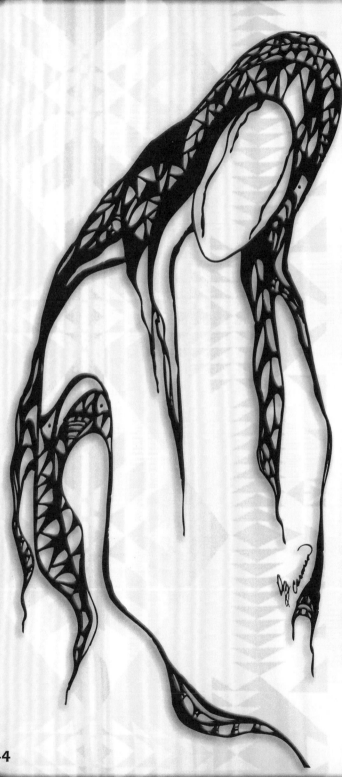

Sisters, in 2007 Amnesty International published a report on the conditions Native Women face called "Maze of Injustice; the failure to protect Indigenous women from sexual violence in the USA". In this report it is estimated that "one in three Native women will be raped during their lifetime....the comparable figure for the USA as a whole is less than one in five."

Sisters, we are at risk, as are our children. As you will learn in the Rape and Sexual Assault chapter, rape is a brutal form of violence and power. The rapist could be someone you love, a family member, a stranger, or a group. As written in **Maze of Injustice**, "sexual violence against women is not only a criminal or social issue, it is a human rights abuse. All women have the right to be safe and free from violence and the authorities have a responsibility to ensure that women can enjoy that right...the long history of abuse cannot be erased, but Indigenous women are working with determination and hope for a future where their rights to dignity and security is respected."

244

Rape and Sexual Assault

There are many different kinds of sexual assault. But only a few of them are seen by most people as rape. For example, sometimes life events can push a woman into having sex when she does not really want to. This can happen in a marriage. Some married women are made to feel that having sex is their duty, whether they want to or not. Although society does not punish this type of forced sex, it is still wrong.

For other women, having sex is a way to survive—to keep from being homeless, or to keep a job. No matter what the reason is, a woman should not be forced to have sex if she does not want to. In any relationship, a woman can choose to accept or refuse a sexual approach. If she refuses, the man then has a choice to either respect her and accept her decision, to try and change her mind, or to force her. Even if the woman knows the man and says "yes," if saying "no" was not really an option, then it is rape. Any time a woman is forced to have sex, whether or not there is other violence too, it can cause many problems with her health and emo-tions.

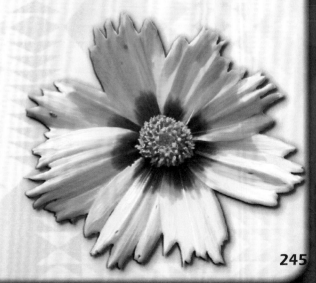

Using Sex as a Weapon

Rape and sexual assault both mean sexual contact that a woman does not want. Rape is any time a man puts his penis, finger, or any object into a woman's vagina, anus, or mouth without her consent. Rape is sometimes called sexual 'assault' because it is an act of violence, using sex as a weapon. Sexual assault can include rape as well as other kinds of unwanted sexual attention.

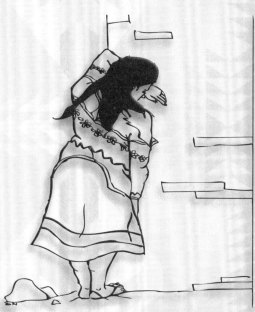

Some people think that forced sex is rape only if the man beats up a woman or leaves her unconscious. They think she must try hard to get away and risk being killed rather than be raped. But even if a woman does not fight back, it is still rape. No matter what she decides to do, if it was not her choice, it was rape, and it is never her fault.

> Rape is sexual violence. Women are not to blame for it.
>
> As with other kinds of violence, the goal of the rapist is to gain power over and control his victim.

Any woman can be raped, but there is an even greater risk if she:

- has a disability—if she is in a wheelchair, deaf, blind, or mentally slow.
- lives on the streets or is homeless.
- is a sex worker (prostitute).
- has been arrested or in prison.
- is being abused by her husband or boyfriend.

A rapist may see these women as easy victims—because of their disabilities, or because they have lost the protection of a community.

A woman often finds it harder to ask for help if the man is someone she knows.
It is also harder to feel safe if she must see him again.

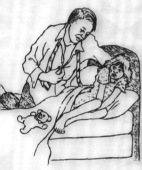

Touching a child sexually is rape.

Sometimes sexual abuse of children continues for many years. A girl may be told that she will be harmed or even killed if she tells anyone about it.

Rape by someone the woman knows:

Most women who are raped know the man who rapes them. If the woman must continue to have contact with him, it can make it very hard for her to recover from the rape and to tell others about it.

Rape by a husband or ex-husband:

If the law or traditional custom treats a woman as the property of her husband, he may think he has the right to have sex whenever he wants, even if the woman does not want it. A woman can be raped by her boyfriend. Her boyfriend may say he has the right to have sex because he has spent money on her, because they have had sex before, because she has teased him sexually, or because he has offered to marry her. But if he forces her, it is still rape. A woman may find it hard to talk about this kind of rape, because she fears others will blame her.

Sexual harassment:

A woman may be forced to have sex by a co-worker or by her supervisor or boss so that she can keep her job. She may be threatened with losing her job or other punishment if she tells anyone.

Rape by a stranger:

This is the kind of sexual assault that most people think of when they hear the word 'rape.' A woman may be grabbed on the street, or attacked in her home. This kind of rape is very frightening, but it is much less common than rape by someone the woman knows.

Sexual abuse of children

A girl or boy can be raped by a man in the family or any adult. If a father, stepfather, uncle, brother, cousin, or any other family member makes a child have sex, or touches her or him in a sexual way, this is rape. It is important to realize that children may be confused and may not understand what is happening to them, especially if they trust the person who is abusing them. Other members of the family may not know of the abuse, they may deny that it happens, or they may say it is the child's fault. It is never right to blame the person who has been raped, especially not a child.

I Only Wanted a Cup of Sugar

By Morning Star

This is a true story that happened a very long time ago, when I was 10 years old, but I still remember it like it happened yesterday. It is a story about what can happen to an innocent young Indian girl in a blink of an eye.

It happened to me.

When I was 10 years old, I lived with my family in an Indian community. Homes with families lived close to one another; it felt safe to live there.

One evening during supper time, we ran out of sugar at the dinner table. In those days, it was customary for families to borrow a cup of this and that from neighbors until we could get to the store. I was chosen to walk to my aunts to borrow a cup of sugar, which were several houses away.

I ran to my aunts and knocked on her door and was invited in, my aunt went to the store, I was told by her boyfriend. As he invited me to come in and asked me what I needed, I told him; "I need a cup of sugar" and handed him the cup. He went to the cupboard and filled my cup with sugar. He turned and gave me the filled cup. I thanked him as I started to walk out the back door with my cup.

Being innocent I didn't think anything as I started out the door, than all of a sudden I was grabbed from behind. I started scream-ing and he put his hand on my mouth to shut me up, but I started fighting and kicking, as he tried to drag me into the bedroom. All I can remember is if my grandfather was home, he could hear me. So I started screaming again, and I wiggled out from his grip, I started running out the back door. I heard him behind me, telling me that if I told anyone, he would hurt me.

I ran for my grandfather house (he lived away from the main house), but as I got close to it, I could see the padlock on his door, he was gone.

So I kept running until I ran into my parent's house and told them, I didn't get the cup of sugar, because the boyfriend tried to hurt me. I babbled out the story and they ran out of the house, telling me to lock the door.

They came home later and I was still scared, but they reassured me that everything is okay and that no one was going to hurt me again.

I never knew the whole story about what happened until much later. Later that evening my aunt had come home and her boyfriend was gone. You see, he was in the military on leave and came to see her and she assumed he went back early. She died soon after not knowing what happened. But, apparently not only did my folks go and teach him Indian justice; he was told to never come back to our community by the headman of our village. Older ladies told me when I grew up, what happened to him after he hurt me.

I suppressed my hurt for over 40 years, before I told anyone about it. It is a hard issue for Indian women to talk about what happened to them as children. My mother never mentioned it to me again, only to warn me to stay away from certain families, which I did. But, it was still there and I have learned to deal with it, so I could feel whole again. I could feel clean again. One needs to talk it out to a special friend, a person you can trust who can understand the pain that it has caused you, because I learned it wasn't something that I caused and I didn't need to feel bad about it anymore.

I still wake up at nights, thinking about that incident and what could have happened to me at the age of 10. You see, I felt that uneasiness, when he invited me in and told me that my aunt was gone, I should have left, but I needed that cup of sugar, so I stayed to get it.

I learned a big lesson from that incident; when your gut tells you that something is weird or strange, please get out and away. Listen to your gut feeling, it is trying to warn you. In a blink of an eye, your life can be changed forever. Today, I can't have anyone touch me around the neck it reminds me of that incident so many years ago.

In the end, the sugar was spilled and I never took the sugar home.

How to Avoid Rape

There is no one right or wrong way to behave to avoid rape. But there are some things a woman can do that may make her less likely to suffer some kinds of rape. What a woman does depends on how well she knows the man, how afraid she is, and how much danger she thinks she is in. Remember, if a woman is raped, it is not because she failed to avoid the rape, but because someone stronger forced himself on her.

These ideas may help any woman avoid rape

- Do not let anyone who makes you feel nervous into your home. Do not let him know if you are there alone.

- Try not to walk alone, especially at night. If you must go alone, hold your head up and act as though you feel confident. Most rapists will look for a woman who looks easy to attack.

- If you think you are being followed, try walking in another direction, or go up to another person, a house, or a store. Or, turn around and ask him very loudly what he wants.

Avoiding rape by someone you know

Learn to trust your feelings. Most women are taught from a very early age to always be polite and to try not to offend anyone. So when someone does something that makes a woman feel uncomfortable, she often has a hard time acting on her feelings. But be careful if you:

- Have a lasting feeling that something is not right.

- Feel afraid, or like you want to leave.

- Feel uncomfortable with comments or suggestions the person is making.

- Dislike the physical contact he makes.

- Carry something with you that will make a loud noise, like a whistle. Also, carry something that you can use to defend yourself. This could be a stick or something you can spray in his eyes.

- If you are attacked, scream as loudly as you can or use your whistle. If this does not work, hit back quickly to hurt him, so that you may be able to get away.

Trust your feelings. It is better to offend someone if you are wrong than to be raped.

It can be hard to act on these feelings because you may be afraid of what other people will think. In addition, if the person is someone you know or care about, you may not want to admit that he would do you harm. But it is always best to trust your feelings and get out of a situation that feels uncomfortable before anything bad happens.

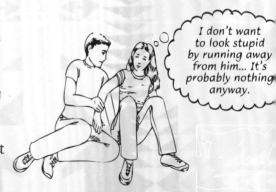

I don't want to look stupid by running away from him... It's probably nothing anyway.

Be prepared to get away:

- Avoid going somewhere alone with a person who makes you feel uncomfortable or who you do not know well.
- Always have a way to get home if you decide you need to leave. It is better not to go somewhere if you will not be able to get back without the person's help.
- Tell the person that his comments or touch make you uncomfortable. If he does not change the way he is acting you should get away from him as soon as possible.

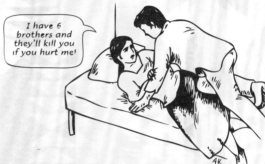

I have 6 brothers and they'll kill you if you hurt me!

If he has power over you

(for example if he is your boss, a teacher, or an official):

- The first time he does something that makes you feel uncomfortable, tell him to stop. If he is trying to take advantage of his power, he will look for someone who is easy to frighten. Let him know that you are not frightened. He is less likely to treat you badly (for example to fire you, or deny your request) if you can get him to stop bothering you before he has done anything that makes him look foolish.
- Talk to other women about him. You are probably not the only one he has bothered. If you must continue to deal with him, try to bring a friend with you so you are never alone with him. Warn other women to be careful.

Rape is about power, not sex. A rapist uses actual force or violence — or the threat of it — to take control over another human being.

Help children avoid sexual abuse

- Teach children about the possibility that they may be touched sexually, and how to tell the difference between touching that is affectionate and touching that is sexual.
- If possible, have girls and boys sleep separately, especially after age 10 or 11 years old.
- Make sure children know who they can talk to if something should happen to them.
- Believe a child who says he or she feels uncomfortable around an adult or older child—no matter who that person is.

Self Defense for Women

Practice these self defense movements with a friend, so that you will be prepared to fight off an attacker. Hit him as hard as you can. Do not be afraid to hurt him—he is not afraid to hurt you.

If you are attacked from behind

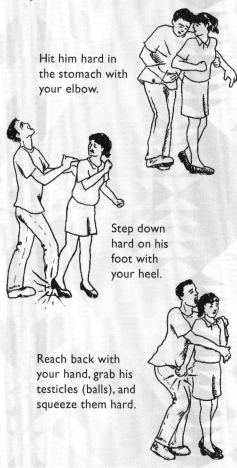

Hit him hard in the stomach with your elbow.

Step down hard on his foot with your heel.

Reach back with your hand, grab his testicles (balls), and squeeze them hard.

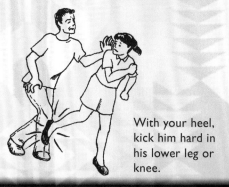

With your heel, kick him hard in his lower leg or knee.

If you are attacked from the front

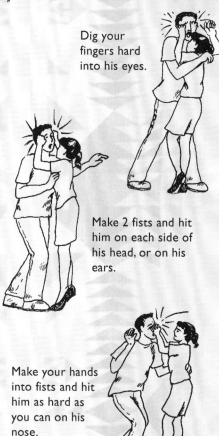

Dig your fingers hard into his eyes.

Make 2 fists and hit him on each side of his head, or on his ears.

Make your hands into fists and hit him as hard as you can on his nose.

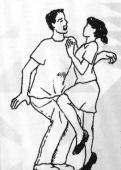

Lift your knee, and push it as hard and fast as you can into his testicles (balls).

If a woman is able to resist her attacker, she
will usually be able to avoid the rape, even
if the rapist has a weapon. The more different ways a woman tries to keep from being
raped, the more likely she is to be able to
avoid the rape, or to suffer fewer injuries and

If You Are Sexually Assaulted

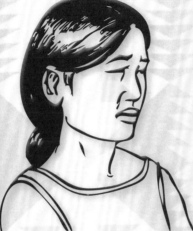

mental health challenges from the
rape afterward. It is impossible to
know ahead of time how a woman will react when someone is trying to rape her. Some women are
filled with rage and feel strength
they did not know they had. Others feel like they cannot move. If
this should ever happen to you,
know that you will do what you
can. Here are some ideas that may
help you during a sexual assault:

• Do not cry, plead, or give in. It
usually does not help. In fact, women who try this often suffer more injuries than women who fight back.

• Stay aware. Watch the rapist carefully. There may be times
when he is not watching you, or when he loses his control.

• Try different things. Kick, yell, bargain, trick him—do whatever you can think of to make him realize you are not an
easy victim. Try to make him realize that you are a person,
not an object.

• If you know the rapist, tell him how you feel. Do not let
him believe that women like to be raped. Make him be
aware of what he is doing to you.

• If the rapist is a stranger, try to memorize what he looks
like. How big is he? Does he have scars, marks, or tatoos?
What kind of clothes is he wearing? Try to remember them
so that you can tell the police and warn the other women in
your community.

What to Do if You Have Been Raped

Every woman's experience with rape is different. But there are a few things you need to do to help yourself recover.

First, ask yourself these questions:

- Who can you ask for help?
- Do you want to tell the police about the rape?
- Where can you go for medical care?
- Do you want to try to punish the rapist?

You need someone to talk to when you feel sad, hurt, scared, or angry, to go with you for medical care, and to help you figure out what to do. Choose someone who cares about you, who you trust will not tell others, and who is strong and dependable. Sometimes a woman's husband or parents are too upset themselves to be able to give much support.

If someone you know has been raped

- Reassure her that it is not her fault.

- Be supportive. Listen to her feelings, help her decide what she needs, and reassure her that she can go on with her life.

- Respect her wishes for privacy and safety. Do not tell anyone else unless she wants you to.

- Go with her to see a health care provider, to report the rape to the police, to talk with someone who is trained to listen and support her, to see a lawyer, and to go to court if she wants to do those things.

- Do not protect the rapist if you know him. He is a danger to every woman in the community.

> If you do not want to go to the police, or if you cannot go until later, you should see a health care provider anyway—even if you are not badly hurt.

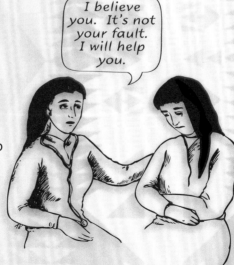

I believe you. It's not your fault. I will help you.

254

1. If you're injured, go straight to the emergency room - most medical centers and hospital emergency departments have doctors and counselors who have been trained to take care of someone who has been raped.

2. Call or find a friend, family member, or someone you feel safe with and tell them what happened. If you want to report the rape, call the police right away. Preserve all the physical evidence. Don't change clothes or wash.

3. If you aren't sure what to do, call a rape crisis center.

The decision to use the law must be made carefully.

- Can someone go with you to talk to the police?
- Has the law helped other women in your community who have been raped?
- Do you want the rape to remain private? Can the police keep others from learning about the rape?
- Did the rapist threaten to hurt you more if you reported the rape?
- If the rapist is caught and you can prove that he raped you, how will he be punished?

What Happens During the Medical Exam?

Tell the health care provider that you have been raped. She should then check you for cuts or tears, and give you some medicines to prevent pregnancy and sexually transmitted infections (STIs). Ask her to write down everything that she finds because it will help prove to the police or to others in the community that you were raped.

Go to do it as soon after the rape as possible. Do not wash before you go, and bring the clothes that you were wearing in a bag. These things can help you prove that you were raped. Take a friend with you, and ask to have a female health provider examine you, if possible.

If you go to the police

Rape is a crime. But it may take a long time and be very difficult to prove you were raped. The police will ask you what happened. If you know the rapist, tell them who it is. If you do not, you will need to describe what he looks like. This is not an exam to help you get well, but to help prove that you were raped. If the rapist is arrested, you will have to identify him, either in front of the police or in front of a judge in court. If there is a trial, try to find a lawyer who has worked with rape cases before. The lawyer will tell you what to expect and help you prepare for the trial. Always take someone with you. Going to court for a rape is never easy. Describing what happened may make you have the feelings of being raped all over again. Not everyone will be understanding. Some may try to blame you or say you are lying.

255

Pregnancy

Pregnancy can be prevented if you act quickly and use emergency family planning (see the "Family Planning" chapter). You must use it as soon as possible, but no later than 5 days after the rape.

Sexually transmitted infections (STIs)

STIs are passed more easily with violent sex because the skin in the vagina is often torn. If the man who raped you had an STI, he may have passed it to you. Since you cannot know if he was infected, you should be treated so you can avoid getting an infection and passing it on to others. Your health care provider may have you take medicines for gonorrhea, syphilis, and chlamydia, and watch for signs of other STIs. Take the medicines whether or not you think you were infected. You should also try to have an HIV test.

Tears and cuts

Sometimes rape damages the genitals by causing tears and cuts. These usually cause pain, but will go away in time. If there is a lot of bleeding, you may need to see a health care provider trained to stitch tears. For small cuts and tears:

> It may take a long time before you feel better, but talking with someone you trust, or who has also survived rape, can help you to heal.

- Soak your genitals 3 times each day in warm water that has been boiled and cooled. Putting chamomile leaves in the boiling water can help soothe the tears and help with healing. Or you can put gel from an aloe plant on the tears.

- Pour water over your genitals while passing urine so that it will not burn. Drinking a lot of liquid makes the urine weaker so it will burn less.

- Watch for signs of infection: heat, yellow liquid (pus) from the torn area, a bad smell, and pain that gets worse.
- After violent sex it is also common for women to have a bladder or kidney infection.

Sexual relations after rape

You can have normal sexual relations again after rape. You will need to wait until your genitals no longer hurt and any tears have healed. For many women, having sex makes them think about the rape. If this happens to you, talk with your partner about why you need to wait. Sometimes a woman's partner may reject her after she has been raped. He may feel ashamed or act as though he is angry with her. This can be very hard for a woman who is already dealing with many difficult feelings.

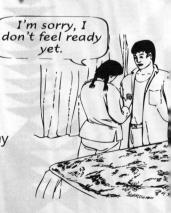

I'm sorry, I don't feel ready yet.

The rape may still bother you long after your body has healed. Here are some common reactions:

It is important for a woman who has been raped to talk to someone or to do something to help herself feel better after the rape—every woman needs to find her own way to heal. For some women, this can mean performing a ritual. For others it means trying to punish the rapist, or working to prevent other women from being raped. Whatever you do, be patient with yourself and ask others to be patient, too.

Dealing With Feelings

Rape isn't just physically damaging, it can be emotionally traumatic as well. The right emotional attention, care, and support can help a person begin the healing process.

Talking about rape in a safe environment is a good way to ensure long-term healing. Working through the pain sooner rather than later can help reduce symptoms like nightmares and flashbacks. It can also help people avoid potentially harmful behaviors and emotions, like major depression or self-injury.

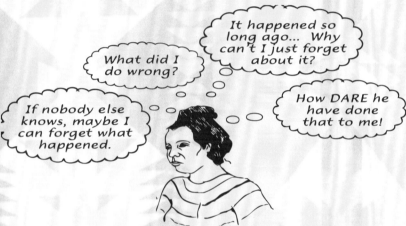

Resources

Rape, Abuse, and Incest National Network (RAINN)
1-800-656-HOPE (4673)

National Sexual Violence Resource Center (NSVRC)
1-877-739-3895

National Center for Victims of Crime, Stalking Resource Center
1-800-394-2255
1-800-211-7996 (TTY)

Sisters, we are blessed with the strength of the land below our feet, the great trees around us and the sky above. We hold in our hearts the wisdom of generations of Native Women. Together we are an example for all who walk this earth. We have the power to heal ourselves and others. We can dance, sing, and live in balance on our life journey.

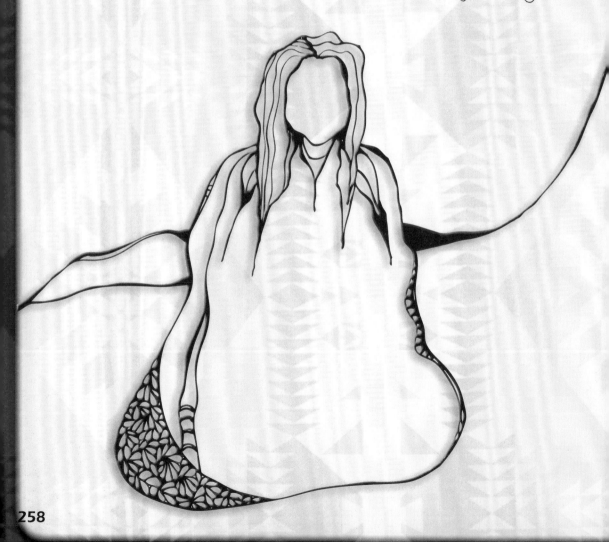

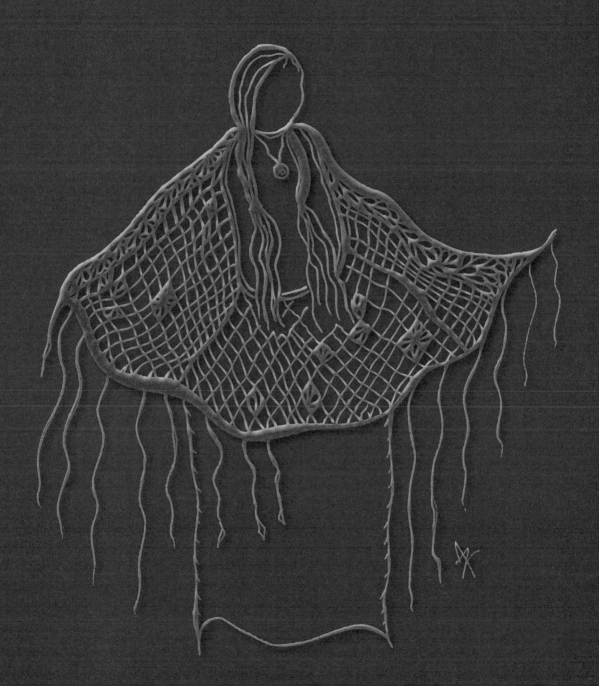

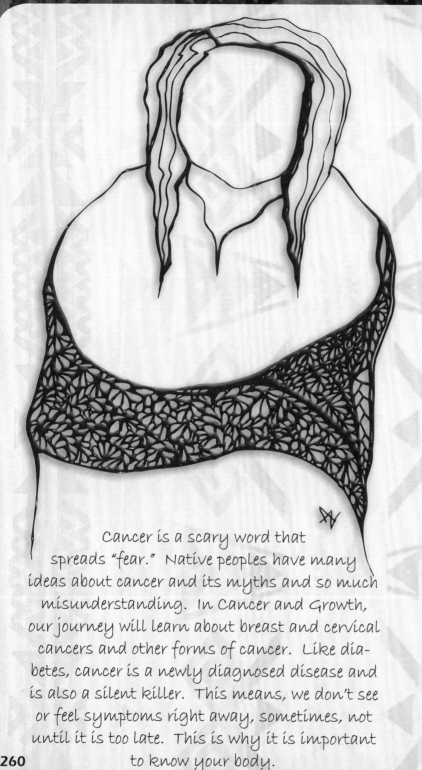

Cancer is a scary word that
spreads "fear." Native peoples have many
ideas about cancer and its myths and so much
misunderstanding. In Cancer and Growth,
our journey will learn about breast and cervical
cancers and other forms of cancer. Like diabetes, cancer is a newly diagnosed disease and
is also a silent killer. This means, we don't see
or feel symptoms right away, sometimes, not
until it is too late. This is why it is important
to know your body.

Cancer

Cancer cells were once healthy cells that have stopped listening to the body. They start to grow out of control and crowd out some of the healthy cells nearby. Cancers are named after the part of the body where the uncontrolled cell growth begins. When cancer cells grow so much that they get in the way of other cells, the healthy cells can't work like they should. When this happens, it is called cancer.

Cancer is continuing to increase in Indian Country. Eveyone's risk for cancer increases as they grow older. Most cancers happen in people over 40. Many types of cancers do not have symptoms. This is why it is important to get regular checkups, including cancer screening, even if you are feeling fine. People are at greatest risk for developing cancer if they use tobacco in a non-traditional way, are exposed to too much sunlight, are exposed to some viruses, drink 2 or more alcoholic drinks daily, do not get daily physical activity, have a family history of cancer or eat high fat foods.

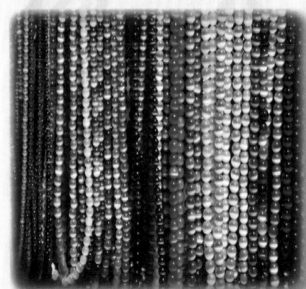

The "C" Word (Cancer)

Cancer is a serious sickness that can affect many different parts of the body. If it is treated early it is often curable, but if left too long it can cause death. Native Women often put other's needs before their own and may not see a health provider unless they are very sick. These women who get cancer are more likely to get very sick or die because the cancer is not found early enough.

In the past, women who got cancer were sometimes considered 'cursed' and sometimes shunned or feared by their families or communities. This isolation is not only bad for the women who are sick, but also for the whole community, since it keeps everyone from knowing about how cancer makes people sick.

What is cancer?

All living things, like the human body, are made up of tiny cells that are too small to see without a microscope. Life is a continuous cycle of cell growth and death as part of a balanced system. However, sometimes cells change and grow in an abnormal way, causing growths (tumors). Some growths go away without treatment. But some growths get larger or spread and may cause health problems. Most growths do not become cancer, but some do.

Cancer starts when some cells begin to grow out of control and take over parts of the body. They continue to grow and crowd out normal cells. Although there are many kinds of cancer, they all have in common this out-of-control growth of cells and ability to spread throughout the body if not stopped early.

When cancer is found early, it can often be removed by surgery, or treated with medicines or radiation, and the chance of it being cured may be good. Once cancer spreads, however, curing it is more difficult and eventually becomes impossible.

65% of adults diagnosed with cancer will be alive five years after diagnosis up from 50% in the 1970s.

Different kinds of cancer can behave very differently. For example, lung cancer and breast cancer are very different diseases. They grow at different rates and respond to different treatments. That's why people with cancer need treatment that is aimed at their kind of cancer.

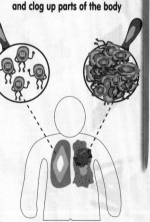

Cancer = cells that grow out of control and clog up parts of the body

Cancer cells are so small, you need a microscope to see them.

262

Tumors and cysts are growths that might interfere with normal function of the body.

A cyst is a sac that may contain air, fluid or semi-solid material. It can form in any part of the body, including in bones, organs and soft tissues. Most cysts are not cancer (benign).

Tumor refers to an abnormal mass of tissue that forms when cells divide more than they should or don't die when they should. Tumors can be cancerous (malignant) or noncancerous (benign).

The only way to be absolutely sure if a cyst or tumor is cancerous is to remove some of the affected tissue (biopsy) for examination under a microscope.

Metastasis

Sometimes cancer cells break away from a tumor and spread to other parts of the body through the blood or lymph system. They can settle in new places and form new tumors. When this happens, it is called metastasis (meh-tas-tuh-sis).

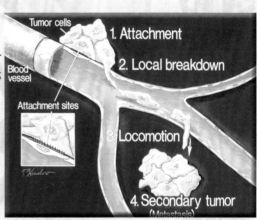

Cancer that has spread in this way is called metastatic cancer.

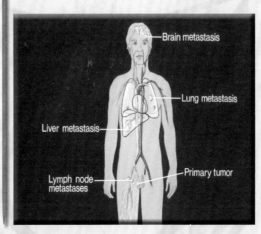

Even when cancer has spread to a new place in the body, it is still named after the part of the body where it started. For example, if prostate cancer spreads to the bones, it is still called prostate cancer. If breast cancer spreads to the lungs, it is still breast cancer.

Cancer cells from one part of the body can spread and take over other body parts like your lungs, liver, stomach, brain and bones. When the cancer spreads it is called metastasis.

Benign: does not grow in an unlimited, aggressive manner, does not invade surrounding tissues and does not metastasize (spread).

Malignant: malignancy is unlimited in its growth, is capable of invading neighboring tissues, and are capable of spreading to distant tissues

263

Finding and treating cancer early

Finding cancer early can often save a woman's life, because she can get early treatment, before the cancer spreads. Some cancers have warning signs that show something may be wrong. But usually, to find out if you have cancer, you must have a test that takes a few cells from the part of your body where the cancer may be. Then the cells must be examined with a microscope, by someone who is trained to recognize cancer. Cancers that do not have early signs can often be found with screening tests, routine tests given to people to see if everything is normal. A Pap test for cancer of the cervix is one kind of screening test. If you have warning signs, or a test shows something may be wrong, do not wait. Follow the advice in this chapter for finding and treating the problem as soon as possible.

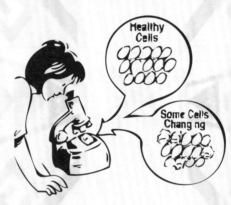

Healthy Cells

Some Cells Changing

Cancer is the second leading cause of death for American Indians.

Cancer is the leading cause of death for Alaska Natives.

All cancers are genetic, in that cancers are caused by genetic mutations (changes) in genes that lead to abnormal cell growth (malignancy).

Unhealthy cell changes, including genetic mutations that lead to cancer may be caused by things we are exposed to in our environment including pollution, chemicals, radiation, viruses, bacteria, tobacco smoke, and other harmful materials.

Early Detection - When Women Need to Be Screened For Cancer

Breast Cancer Screening:
- Clinical Breast Exam annually and Breast Self Exam each month starting at age 18
- Mammogram annually for women age 40 and older

Cervical Cancer Screening (women):
- Pap test each year starting at age 21 or within 3 years of your first sexual encounter

Colorectal Cancer Screening:
- Each Year starting at age 50 - Blood stool test
- Every 10 years starting at age 50 - colonoscopy

Cancer and American Indians and Alaska Natives

• Cancer rates which were previously reported to be lower in American Indian and Alaska Natives have been shown to be increasing in the past twenty years.

• Cancer is the second leading cause of death among American Indians and Alaska Natives over the age of 45.

• American Indians and Alaska Natives continue to have the poorest survival from "all cancers combined" than any other racial group.   from ICCnetwork.org/cancerfacts

Cancer of the breast, ovaries, cervix and womb (uterus) are the most common 'women's' cancers. Other common cancers that both men and women get are cancer of the lung, colon, liver, stomach, mouth, and skin.

Cancer Risk Factors

The direct causes of most cancers are not known. But these things may make you more likely to get cancer :

• smoking tobacco, which is known to cause lung cancer, and also increases the risk of getting many other cancers
• certain viral infections, like HIV, Hepatitis B & C or HPV
• eating foods with too much fat or with harmful chemicals
• using some medicines, like hormones, incorrectly
• working with or living around certain chemicals (like pesticides, dyes, paints, and solvents)
• living or working near nuclear power plants or nuclear waste facilities.

Also, if others in a woman's family (blood relatives) have had a certain kind of cancer, this may mean she is more likely to get that same kind of cancer (this is called a hereditary risk).

Healthy living can prevent many cancers. This means eating nutritious food and avoiding things that may cause cancer.
For example:

• Do not smoke or chew tobacco.
• Try to avoid harmful chemicals in your home or workplace, including foods grown or preserved with them.
• Protect yourself from sexually transmitted infections (STIs).
• Avoid alchohol
• Be active and maintain a healthy weight

Causes of Cancer

The leading cause of changes to the cells that lead to cancer include tobacco use, exposure to radiation, diet. However, much of what causes cancer cannot be determined. A leading scientist once responded that the main cause of cancer is "bad luck".

Those diagnosed with cancer may have feelings that they have "brought on" the cancer in some way. No one is to blame for most cancers, especially the person diagnosed with the cancer. A positive mental and spiritual attitude by those diagnosed with cancer and their loved ones is a critical part of successful healing. Feelings of guilt or blame won't help the healing process.

How Cancer may be Diagnosed

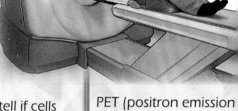

Diagnosis is not the same as detection. Cancer may be detected when symptoms or abnormalities, such as a lump or growth, are recognized by a patient or doctor. After a cancer is detected, it still must be carefully diagnosed.

PET (positron emission tomography) scan

Diagnosing cancer can include a variety of tests that tell if cells found in a lump or growth are normal or not. The doctor must run tests to find out if these cells are malignant (cancerous) or non-malignant (non-cancerous). If they are malignant, your doctor will need to determine how serious (aggressive) the particular cancer cells are. Aggressive cancers grow and spread more quickly than less-aggressive or "indolent" (slow growing) cancers which tend to grow more slowly and not cause symptoms. There are many types of tests specifically designed to evaluate cancer. Here are examples of possible tests:

- Cells examined under a microscope
- X-rays, computed tomography (CT), positron emission test (PET), magnetic resonance imaging (MRI), and combined PET/CT .
- Blood tests to measure substances in the blood that may indicate how advanced the cancer is or other problems related to the cancer.
- Tumor marker tests detect substances in blood, urine, or other tissues that occur in higher than normal levels with certain cancers.
- Special laboratory evaluation of DNA of the abnormal cells.

Cancer Staging

Following a diagnosis of cancer, the most important step is to accurately determine the stage of cancer.

Stage describes the extent of the original tumor and how far the cancer has spread. (Some cancers, such as leukemia, may not be staged.) Each stage of cancer may be treated differently. In order for you to begin evaluating and discussing treatment options with your doctors, you need to know the correct stage of your cancer.

There are many staging systems, but TNM is the most common. "T" refers to the size of the tumor, "N" to the number of lymph nodes involved, and "M" to metastasis. TNM staging measures range from 0 to 4. Generally, the lower the stage, the better the treatment prognosis (outcome).

Stage 0 – precancer

Stage 1 – small cancer found only in the organ where it started

Stage 2 – larger cancer that may or may not have spread to the lymph nodes

Stage 3 – larger cancer that is also in the lymph nodes

Stage 4 – cancer in a different organ from where it started

The stage of a cancer describes how much the cancer has spread. The stage may takes into account:
• the size of a tumor,
• how deep it has gone into an organ
• whether it has invaded neighboring organs,
• how many lymph nodes it has metastasized to (if any), and
• whether it has spread to distant organs.

Staging of cancer is important because treatments are often based on the stage.

Cancer Staging (TNM Model)	
Stage	**Definition**
Stage 0	**Carcinoma in situ** (early cancer that is present only in the layer of cells in which it began).
Stage I, Stage II, and Stage III	Higher numbers indicate more extensive disease: greater tumor size, and/or spread of the cancer to nearby lymph nodes and/or organs next to the primary tumor.
Stage IV	Cancers have often **metastasized**, (spread to other organs or throughout the body).

Types of Cancer (most common)

Lung cancer is a growing problem that is most often caused by smoking tobacco. It is more common in men because they usually smoke more than women. But because many women now smoke as much as men, they are starting to get more lung cancer. In some parts of Indian Country, more women now die from lung cancer caused by smoking than from any other kind of cancer. And in many places, girls are starting to smoke as early and as much as boys. As more girls and women smoke, even more women will end up getting lung cancer.

Lung cancer does not usually affect people until they are over 65 years old. If a woman stops smoking, her risk of getting lung cancer becomes much less. The signs (coughing up blood, losing weight, difficulty breathing) appear when the cancer is advanced and difficult to cure.

Lung cancer that forms in tissues of the lung, usually in the cells lining air passages. The two main types are small cell lung cancer and non-small cell lung cancer. These types are diagnosed based on how the cells look under a microscope.

Lung cancer causes the most common cancer death in Indian County.

87% of all lung cancer deaths can be linked to tobacco smoking.

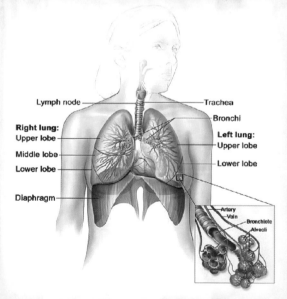

Lymph node
Trachea
Bronchi
Right lung:
Upper lobe
Left lung:
Upper lobe
Middle lobe
Lower lobe
Lower lobe
Diaphragm

Artery
Vein
Bronchiole
Alveoli

Surgery to remove part of the lung, medicines, and radiation therapy are all used to treat lung cancer.

www.cancer.go
cancertopics

Some people who become infected with hepatitis B or C develop cancer of the liver years later. Signs of liver cancer are a swollen abdomen and general weakness. See a health provider if you think you may have liver cancer. Hepatitis

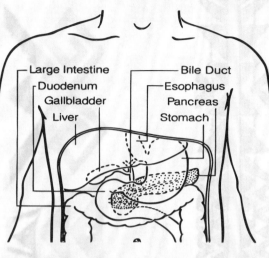

Large Intestine
Duodenum
Gallbladder
Liver
Bile Duct
Esophagus
Pancreas
Stomach

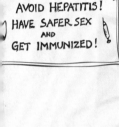

Cancer of the liver can be caused by hepatitis B and C

AVOID HEPATITIS!
HAVE SAFER SEX AND
GET IMMUNIZED!

B and C can be prevented by having safer sex & by not sharing needles. There is a vaccine for hepatitis B. Adults can be vaccinated at any time. There currently is no vaccine for hepatitis C.

Stomach cancer

This type of cancer forms in tissues lining the stomach. It is also called gastric cancer. Cancer of the stomach can occur in women and men over age 40, but typically in those over 65. Risk factors include smoking, H. Pylori bacteria, and smoke, salted or pickled foods. Usually there are no signs until it is advanced. Surgery is the only treatment and may not be successful.

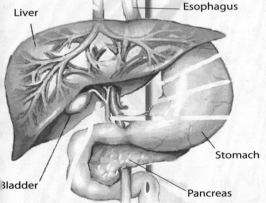

Liver
Esophagus
Stomach
Bladder
Pancreas

Pancreatic cancer

Studies have found that age, smoking, diabetes, and being male may increase the risk for pancreatic cancer. Pancreatic cancer is one of the most serious of cancers. It develops when cancerous cells form in the tissues of your pancreas. Pancreatic cancer spreads rapidly and is seldom detected in its early stages. But, as the cancer grows, symptoms may include pain in the upper abdomen, yellow skin and eyes, weakness and weight loss. At this time, pancreatic cancer can only be cured when caught at an early stage. Those diagnosed late may want to consider enrolling in clinical trials.

Colon and Rectal Cancer

Not counting skin cancers, colorectal cancer is the third most common cancer found in men and women in this country and the second leading cause of cancer death.

If caught early, it can be treated and even cured! Screenings can detect not only when it's small, but even before its cancer. Current Rates of Screening within Indian Health Service show low rates of colorectal cancer screening. Screening rates are consistently less than 10 % for most areas of Indian Health Service. Screening methods that rely on sigmoidoscopy and/or colonoscopy are consistently less than 5%.

Colorectal cancer is common, lethal, an preventable disease 90% of cases occu after age 50.

Colorectal Cancer Screening
Starting at Age 50 for most

Indian Health Service is recommending the following:
1. Renewed emphasis on colorectal cancer screening
2. Improved patient education about colorectal cancer screening
3. Fecal occult blood testing (FOBT) every year if possible; every 2 years at a minimum
4. Appropriate follow-up for positive FOBT results
5. Additional screening options if available
    a. Flexible sigmoidoscopy within the last 5 years
    b. Annual FOBT plus flexible sigmoidoscopy every 5 years
    c. Double contrast enema every 5 years
    d. Colonoscopy within the last 10 years

Medicare and many private insurance companies will cover colonoscopies or sigmoidoscopies - but yo may have to ask to be refered for this testing from your health care provider.

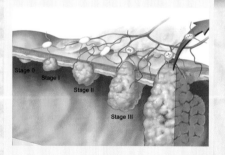

Colorectal cancer screening looks for signs of blood in the stool and ultimately for "polyps" in the colon (see picture on left). If the polyps are found early and removed, colon cancer will not develop. Treatment for advanced colon cancer may include surgery to remove of a section of the colon, chemotherapy and/or radiation therapy. Success of treatment depends, in part, on 1)the stage of the cancer 2)whether the cancer has blocked or created a hole in the colon and whether the cancer has recurred.

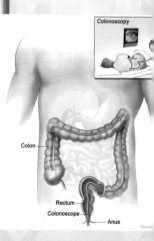

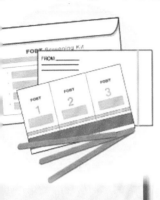

"My Doctor Wants Me to do WHAT!?!"

This may be your first response when you hear how you can be screened for colon and rectal cancer. If you're over FIFTY years old, your doctor may ask you to take an envelope home with you. This envelope contains three popsicle sticks, a sheet of directions, and three stool cards. "Stool Cards!" That's right... little cards about the size of credit card on which we want you to stool. Then we want you to put the three cards back in the envelope and mail them back to us.

The Blood Stool Test

"Why am I sending stool to my doctor?"
These cards are the way doctors perform what is called the Fecal Occult Blood Test (FOBT, for short). This can detect blood in your stool.

"I can tell the difference between blood and stool, so can't I just look at my stool to see if there's any blood in it?"
Actually these cards can detect amounts of blood much smaller than you would be able to see. It is important because blood in the stool may be an early sign that something's not right.

"Like what?"
Well, hemorrhoids can bleed and so can an ulcer, which is a sore in the lining of your gut. Blood in your stool can also be an early sign of colon cancer. In fact, this is one of the easiest, most inexpensive, and most effective ways to detect colon cancer.

"You mean my stool can predict the future?"
Well, not exactly, but it can detect some polyps (little growths in your colon that may turn into cancer). So we may be able to remove these polyps and prevent cancer from ever even starting!

"OK, it sounds like a good thing to do, but I'm worried about those popsicle sticks. What are they for again?"
Nothing uncomfortable, trust us... We just need you to place a little bit of stool from three bowel movements in a row on the three separate stool cards. We include three popsicle sticks to help you take some stool from the toilet paper and place it on the cards. Your doctor or nurse will show you how. It takes just a minute.

"Three bowel movements! But I only have one at a time."
You don't have to stay in the bathroom or even a home, in between these three bowel movements. These don't have to be on the same day. In fact some people may take three or four days to move their bowels three times. That's fine, as long we get a sample from three bowel movements in a row.

"So if you find blood in my stool, what do I have to do next?"
If your stool cards have blood on them, your doctor will most likely have you make an appointment to see specialist. This doctor will want to take a closer look at your colon to determine where the blood is coming from.

Apapted from a publication by the IHS Colorectal Cancer Screening Initiative

Cancer of the Kidney

Cancer that forms in tissues of the kidneys. Kidney cancer includes renal cell carcinoma (cancer that forms in the lining of very small tubes in the kidney that filter the blood and remove waste products) and renal pelvis carcinoma (cancer that forms in the center of the kidney where urine collects). Kidney cancer develops most often in people over 40, but no one knows the exact causes of this disease. Risk factors include obesity, smoking, high blood pressure and long-term dialysis. Males also have a higher risk of cancer of the kidney. Common symptoms include blood in the urine (making the urine slightly rusty to deep red), pain in the side that does not go away, a lump or mass in the side or the abdomen, weight loss and fever. Most often, these symptoms do not mean cancer, see health care provider for more information. People with kidney cancer may have surgery, arterial embolization, radiation, biological, or chemotherapy. Some may have a combination of treatments.

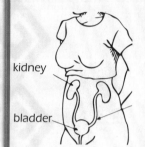

kidney

bladder

Lymphoma

Cancer that begins in cells of the immune system. There are two basic categories of lymphomas 1)Hodgkin lymphoma, 2)non-Hodgkin lymphomas, which includes a large, diverse group of cancers of immune system cells. Non-Hodgkin lymphomas can be further divided into cancers that are slow-growing & fast-growing. These subtypes behave and respond to treatment differently. Both Hodgkin and non-Hodgkin lymphomas can occur in children and adults, and prognosis and treatment depend on the stage and the type of cancer. Lymphomas may spread from one site to other parts of the body.

The Immune System

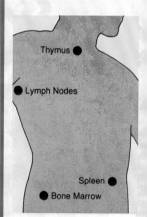

Thymus

Lymph Nodes

Spleen

Bone Marrow

Leukemia (loo-KEE-mee-uh)

Cancer that starts in blood-forming tissue such as the bone marrow and causes large numbers of blood cells to be produced and enter the bloodstream. In people with leukemia, the bone marrow produces abnormal white blood cells. The abnormal cells are leukemia cells. At first, leukemia cells function almost normally. In time, they may crowd out normal white blood cells, red blood cells, and platelets. This makes it hard for blood to do its work.

The terms lymphocytic or lymphoblastic indicate that the cancerous change takes place in a type of marrow cell that forms lymphocytes.

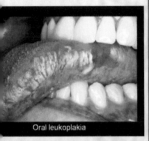

Oral leukoplakia

Mouth and throat cancer

Mouth and throat cancer may appear as white or red spots inside the mouth, loose teeth, bleeding in the mouth, a lump in the neck or difficulty swallowing. Smoking and chewing tobacco as well as alcohol use can increase your risk for mouth and throat cancer. If you smoke or chew tobacco, and have sores in your mouth that do not heal, get medical advice.

Skin Cancer

When cancer forms in the cells of the skin that make pigment, it is called melanoma. Melanoma often begins in a mole and is the most serious type of skin cancer. When cancer forms in cells that do not make pigment it may begin in basal cells (small, round cells in the base of the outer layer of skin) or squamous cells (flat cells that form the surface of the skin). Both types of skin cancer usually occur in skin that has been exposed to sunlight, such as the skin on the face, neck, hands, and arms. Treatment for skin cancer depends on the type and stage of the disease, the size and place of the growth, and your general health and medical history. Some-times all of the cancer is re-moved during the biopsy. In such cases, no more treatment is needed. If you do need more treatment, your doctor will describe your options.

symmetry   Border irregularity   Color   Diameter: ¼ inch or 6mm

The ABCDs of Skin Cancer

Ovarian Cancer

Risk factors include being over the age of 55, a family history of ovarian cancer, a personal history of cancer, and never being pregant. Early ovarian cancer may not cause obvious symptoms. But, as the cancer grows, symptoms may include pressure or pain in the abdomen, pelvis, back, or legs, a swollen or bloated abdomen, nausea, indigestion, gas, constipation, or diarrhea or feeling very tired all the time. Treatment choices for most women consist of surgery and chemotherapy. Rarely, radiation thera-py is used.

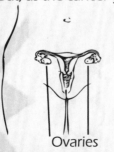

Ovaries

Questions you can ask the doctor before you or a loved one is treated for cancer:

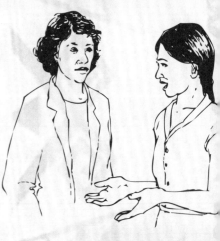

- What is my diagnosis?

- Has the cancer spread? If so, where? What is the stage of the disease?

- What is the goal of treatment? What are my treatment choices? Which do you recommend for me? Why?

- What are the expected benefits of each kind of treatment?

- What are the risks and possible side effects of each treatment? How can side effects be managed?

- Will infertility be a side effect of my treatment? Can anything be done about that? Should I consider storing sperm or eggs?

- What can I do to prepare for treatment?

- How often will I have treatments? How long will my treatment last?

- Will I have to change my normal activities? If so, for how long?

- What is the treatment likely to cost? Will my insurance cover the costs?

- What new treatments are under study? Would a clinical trial be appropriate for me?

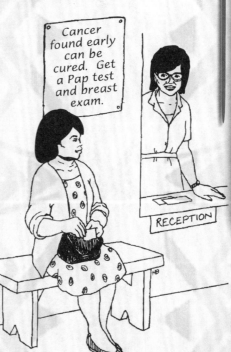

Cancer found early can be cured. Get a Pap test and breast exam.

RECEPTION

Cancers you can screen for

Women only:
- Breast Cancer
- Cervical Cancer

Men only:
- Prostate Cancer

Everyone:
- Colon/rectal Cancer

Unfortunately, screening tests are not available to detect other cancers.

Many unnecessary deaths from cancer could be prevented if more cancers were found and treated earlier.

Cancer Treatment

Radiation therapy is the use of high energy x-rays and other sources to kill cancer cells and shrink tumors. Radiation may come from a machine outside the body or it may come from a radioactive material placed in the body near the cancer cells

Chemotherapy is treatment with drugs that kill cancer cells.

Surgery is a procedure (operation) to remove or repair a part of the body or to find out whether disease is present.

Alternative Treatment Methods are used in place of standard treatment.

Complimentary Care is used along with standard medical treatment.

Traditonal Healing the values, belief and practices that may include the use of traditional plants and herbs, medicine from a traditional healer, or other traditions in healing passed down through generations.

Clinical Trials are a type of research study that tests how well new medical approaches work in people. Clinic trials test new methods of screening, prevention, diagnosis, or treatment of disease.

Palliative Care
In some cases, palliative treatments may be used to alleviate the side effects of curative treatments, such as relieving the nausea associated with chemotherapy. Palliative care also refers to the use of medical treatment to relieve pain symptoms rather than to cure. See "End of Life" chapter for more information on palliative care.

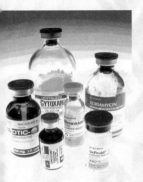

Chemotherapy

Cancer is more than 100 diseases characterized by uncontrolled abnormal growth of cells.

Different cancers are treated differently.

Complimentary and Alternative Medicine (CAM)

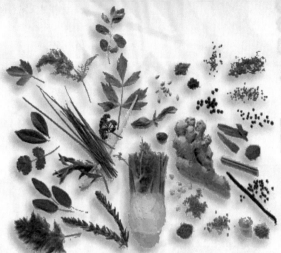

Complimentary medicine and Alternative medicine are choices for maintaining healing and treatment.

- Complementary medicine is used together with conventional medicine.
- Alternative medicine is used in place of conventional medicine.

Talk with Your Doctor Before You Use CAM

Some people with cancer are afraid that their doctor won't understand or approve of the use of CAM. But doctors know that people with cancer want to take an active part in their care. They want the best for their patients and often are willing to work with them. Your doctor will make sure that all aspects of your cancer care work together. This is important because things that seem safe, such as certain foods or pills, may interfere with your cancer treatment. If you decide to try a CAM therapy, ask your doctor if it will interfere with your treatment or medicines .

Complimentary or Alternative Medicine may include:

- **Whole Medical Systems**, such as Chinese medicine, Homeopathy or Naturopathic medicine.

- **Mind-Body Medicines** include practices that focus on the minds ability to influence the body including meditation, biofeedback, hypnosis, yoga, imagery and creative outlets such as music or dance.

- **Biologically Based Practices** uses things found in nature, examples include vitamins, herbs, foods and special diets.

- **Manipulative and Body-Based Practices** might include massage, Chiropractic care or Reflexology.

- **Energy Medicine** examples include Tia Chi, Reiki and Therapeutic touch.

A note about nutrition:

It's common for people with cancer to have questions about different foods to eat during treatment. Yet it's important to know that there is no one food or special diet that has been proven to control cancer. Too much of any one food is not helpful, and may even be harmful. Because of nutrition needs you may have, it's best to talk with the doctor in charge of your treatment about the foods you should be eating.

Living Long as a Cancer Survivor

The National Coalition for Cancer Survivorship (NCCS) defines a cancer survivor as from the time of diagnosis and for the balance of life, a person diagnosed with cancer is a survivor. The definition also includes family, friends and caregivers who are affected by the diagnosis in any way.

The **Native People's Circle of Hope** is a coalition of Native American cancer support groups. We have chapters in Alaska, Idaho, Oklahoma, Oregon, Arizona, Montana and nationwide affiliates. NPCOH's mission is to provide hope, an improvement of communication, support, education and advocacy for the cancer survivor.

www.nativepeoplescoh.org/

From: Native People's Circle of Hope (NPCOH)

Cancer is the second leading cause of death for American Indians over the age of 45 and the leading cause of death for Alaska Natives. Although the incidence (the number of people who actually get cancer) is relatively low, death from cancer is high because Natives are generally diagnosed in the later stages of their disease.

So, for many Natives cancer is seen as a death sentence. This does not have to be so. Cancer treatment is better than it once was. People are starting to hear the message that "early detection" is the key to surviving a cancer diagnosis. But for the survivor, their family members or caretakers the fight to defeat the disease can be a lonely, scary, traumatic experience. NPCOH's mission is to provide hope, an improvement of communication, support, education and advocacy for the cancer survivor.

Cancer found late

Many cancers can be cured, but others cannot, especially if the cancer has spread to several parts of the body.

Sometimes, when cancer is found late, the treatment may not work. Then it may be best to stay at home in the care of your family. This time can be very difficult. Eat as well as you can and get enough rest. Medicines for pain, anxiety, and sleeping problems can make you more comfortable. Talking with someone close to you can help you prepare for death, and help plan for your family's future after you are gone. See "End of Life" chapter on resources for pain relief and end of life.

Working Together to Control Cancer

Many unnecessary deaths from cancer could be prevented if more cancers were found and treated earlier. Making sure treatment is followed, whether it is modern medicine treatment and traditional healing or both, is also extremely important. The body is under attack and needs all the help it can get.

To help control cancer we can work together to:
- ask for cancer screening in Urban Indian Clinic, Tribal Clinic, Indian Health Service, or other health agency. Many states require private health insurance to cover breast, cervical and colorectal cancer screening. If we keep asking, IHS or the federal government may ensure that all Native peoples receive cancer screening services.

- You may be eligible for free breast and cervical cancer screening. Contact you local clinic or your state health department to find out more.

- better education and more community awareness about how cancer can be prevented, who is at risk, what the warning signs are, and the benefits of cancer screening.

It is also important for women to:
- learn to do breast self-examinations.

- know the signs of cancer, especially cancer of the womb, breast, and cervix.

When people in the community know more about the things that are likely to cause cancer, they may be better able to avoid them. This could prevent many cancers from starting. Help people in your community learn that they can prevent many unnecessary deaths from cancer if they avoid smoking or chewing tobacco, and if women are able to protect themselves from STIs.

Awareness is Key

Together we can work to control cancer through better education and more community awareness about how cancer can be prevented, who is at risk, what the warning signs are, and the benefits of cancer screening.

STRONG PARTNERSHIPS

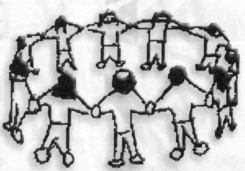

Unified + Mobilized Community

Resources

The National Cancer Institute's (NCI's) Cancer Information Service (CIS) is a national information and education network.

cis.nci.nih.gov/
1-800-4-cancer
www.cancer.gov/

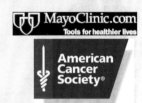

www.mayoclinic.com/health/cancer/CA99999

American Cancer Society
www.cancer.org
1-800-ACS-2345

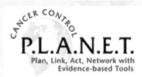

Lance Armstrong Foundation
www.livestrong.org
(512) 236-8820

cancercontrolplanet.cancer.gov/

www.cdc.gov/cancer/
1 (800) CDC-INFO

www.gildasclub.org/
888-GILDA-4-U

cancer support
for the whole family,
the whole time

Native American Cancer Research
www.natamcancer.org/

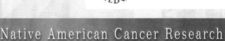

Native People's Circle of Hope
www.nativepeoplecoh.org

National Center for Complementary and Alternative Medicine (NCCAM)
nccam.nih.gov/health/camcancer/
1-888-644-6226

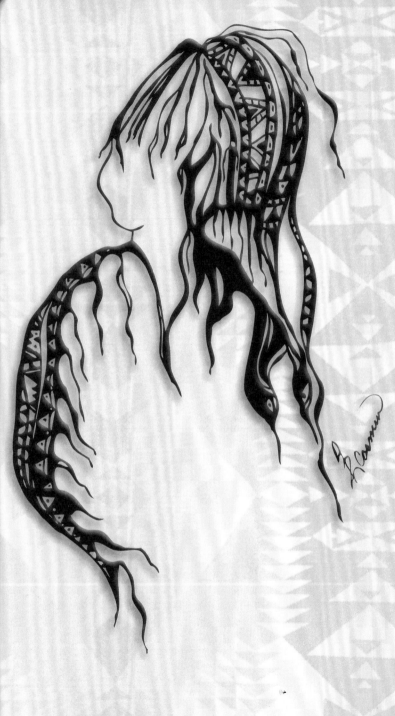

Sisters, our cervix serves as our passageway for delivering children. It is a miracle that this tiny circle can expand for life to pass through, but like our breast, the cervix can also harm us. The cervix cells sometimes change and become abnormal or precancerous due to infections, inflammations, cysts, and other causes. These cells if left untreated can become precancerous and over time, develop into cancer of the cervix. Cervical cancer is one of the cancers that can be prevented through annual PAP testing. We can achieve a day when changes in the cervix are caught early and no more women die from cervical cancer.

This "Cervical Cancer" chapter will journey into early detection and prevention, HIV, HPV, and other risk factors for developing cervical cancer. Sisters, please advocate for your family and friends; once a year over the age of 18 or first sexual activity.

Cervical Cancer

Cancer of the cervix (also known as cervical cancer) begins in the lining of the cervix. The cervix is another name for the neck of the womb. Cervical cancers do not form suddenly. Normal cervical cells gradually develop pre-cancerous changes that turn into cancer.

Only some women with pre-cancerous changes of the cervix will develop cancer. This process usually takes several years but sometimes can happen in less than a year. For most women, pre-cancerous cells will remain unchanged and go away without any treatment. But if these precancers are treated, almost all true cancers can be prevented.

Cervical screening is very important because we can stop cervical cancer from developing in the first place. This is one of the few cancers that is preventable because pre-cancerous cell changes can be picked up before they have a chance to grow into a full blown cancer.

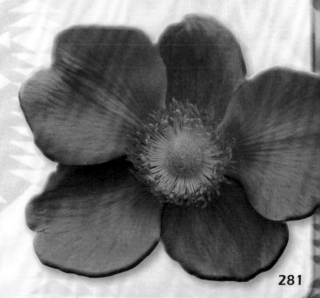

Problems of the Cervix
(the Opening of the Womb)

Cancer of the cervix is the most common cause of death from cancer in many parts of the world where women have no cervical cancer screening resources. Fortunately, cervical cancer screening has been available in the United States since the 1960s, preventing many cervical cancers from developing. The main cause of cervical cancer is a different strain of the same virus—Human Papilloma Virus (HPV)—that causes genital warts. This cancer grows slowly for about 10 years, and if it is treated early it can be completely cured. But many women die every year from cancer of the cervix because they never knew they had HPV, cell changes on their cervix or possibly cervical cancer.

A woman is at greater risk of getting cancer of the cervix if she:
- is positive for HPV
- has not had "regular" Pap tests
- is older than 40
- began to have sex at a young age (within only a few years of starting her monthly bleeding)
- has had many sex partners, or has a partner who has had many sex partners
- has had frequent STIs
- has HIV/AIDS
- smokes tobacco
- has had many children
- has used birth control for many years
- though rare, exposure to DES*

Warning signs:
There are usually no outward signs of cancer of the cervix until it has spread and is more difficult to treat. (There are often early signs on the cervix, which can be seen during a pelvic exam. This is why regular exams are so important.) Abnormal bleeding from the vagina, including bleeding after sex, or an abnormal discharge or bad smell from the vagina can all be signs of a serious problem, including advanced cancer of the cervix. If you have any of those signs, try to get a pelvic exam and a Pap test.

282

Nicotine from cigarette smoking concentrates in the cells of your cervix, increasing your risk for cervical cancer. Think of it this way - for every one cigarette a woman smokes, her cervix is smoking four!

Important: If you are treated with medicines for a vaginal discharge and do not get better, you should try to have your cervix examined and get a Pap test to look for cancer.

*In the early 1970's, it was discovered that women whose mothers took an estrogen drug during pregnancy called DES (diethylstilbestrol) are at risk of a rare form of cervical and vaginal cancer. This drug was used from 1938 until 1971, and was sometimes combined with prenatal vitamins in the mistaken belief that it prevented miscarriages.

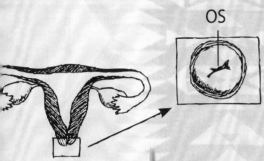

OS

The cervix is the lower third portion of the uterus which forms the neck of the uterus that opens into the vagina. The narrow opening of the cervix is called the os. The os allows menstrual blood to flow out, and widens during labor to allow the passage of the baby through the vagina during childbirth.

The Cells of the Cervix

Cervical cancer develops in the lining of the cervix. This condition usually develops over time. Normal cervical cells may gradually undergo changes to become precancerous and then cancerous.

The vagina is the tube from the outside of the body to the entrance to the womb. The skin-like cells that cover the cervix join with the skin covering the inside of the vagina. So even if you have had your womb and cervix removed, you can still have smear tests taken from the top of the vagina.

The area where cervical cells are most likely to become cancerous is called the transformation zone. It is the area just around the opening of the cervix that leads on to the birth canal. The endocervical canal is the narrow passageway that runs up from the cervix into the womb. The transformation zone is the area that your doctor or nurse will concentrate on when taking a cervical smear.

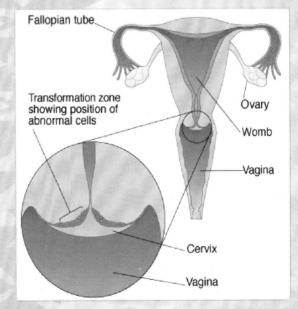

Fallopian tube

Transformation zone showing position of abnormal cells

Ovary

Womb

Vagina

Cervix

Vagina

283

Cervical Cancer Can Be Prevented!!

You can prevent most precancers of the cervix by avoiding exposure to the Human Papilloma Virus (HPV).   Risk factors for HPV can be avoided by the following:

- Delaying having sexual intercourse if you are young can help you avoid HPV.

- Limiting your number of sexual partners can help you avoid HPV.

- Avoiding sex with people who have had many other sexual partners lowers your risk of exposure to HPV.

- Remember that HPV does not always cause warts or other symptoms, so a person may have the virus and pass it on without knowing it. HPV can be present for years with no symptoms.

- Condoms (rubbers) provide some protection. Although the protection is not complete, condoms reduce the infection rate by about 70% when used regularly and correctly. Condoms do not protect completely because HPV can be passed from person to person through skin-to-skin contact with any HPV-infected area of the body, such as skin of the genital or anal area not covered by the condom.

- Not smoking is another important way to reduce the risk of cervical precancer and cancer.

Most invasive cervical cancers are found in women who have not had regular Pap tests.

Cancer found early can be cured. Get a Pap test and breast exam.

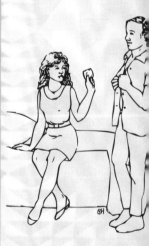

The Pap test

A way to look at cells collected from the cervix. This test can find cancer or abnormal cells that lead to cancer. For this test, a health provider scrapes some cells from the cervix (this is not painful) during a pelvic exam and sends them to a laboratory to be examined with a microscope. Low cost and free Pap tests are available at clinics that offer maternal and child health services, family planning, or treatment for STIs.

The second way to prevent cervical cancer is to have regular testing (including a Pap test) to detect abnormal cell changes. Treatment of precancers can stop cervical cancer before it is fully developed.

All women should begin getting an annual women's exam, which includes a Pap test, about 3 years after they begin having vaginal intercourse, but no later than when they are 21 years old. Testing should be done every year with the regular Pap test or every 2 years using the newer liquid-based Pap test.

Women 70 years of age or older who have had 3 or more normal Pap tests in a row and no abnormal Pap test results in the last 10 years may choose to stop having cervical cancer testing. Women with a history of cervical cancer, DES exposure before birth, HIV infection, or a weakened immune system should continue to have testing as long as they are in good health.

Women who have had a total hysterectomy (removal of the uterus and cervix) may also choose to stop having cervical cancer testing, unless the surgery was done as a treatment for cervical cancer or precancer. Women who have had a hysterectomy without removal of the cervix (simple hysterectomy) should continue to follow the guidelines above.

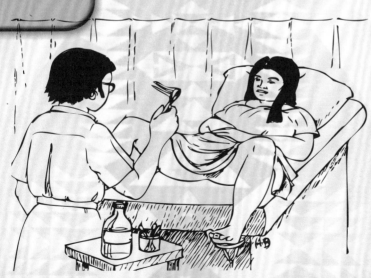

Some women believe that they do not need exams by a health care professional once they have stopped having children. This is not correct. They should continue to have an annual women's exam, including a Pap test.

What Every Woman Should Know About Cervical Cancer and the HPV (Human Papilloma Virus)

Changes in the cervix are often caused by a virus called HPV, which is short for human papilloma virus. HPV infections can lead to cervix cancer.

What is cervical cancer?
Cancer of the cervix is cancer that begins in the cervix, the part of the womb (or uterus) that opens to the vagina.

How common is it?
Cervical cancer is rare in this country today because most women get Pap tests that find it early or before it starts.

What is a Pap test?
The Pap test helps doctors find early changes in the cervix that might lead to cancer. It is done during a pelvic exam. Abnormal results on a Pap test are common.

What causes cervical cancer?
Cervix cancer is caused by a virus called HPV.

What is HPV?
HPV is short for human papilloma (pap-ah-LO-mah) virus. This virus can cause changes in the cervix. HPV is NOT the same as HIV. HPV is not a new virus, but we are learning more about this virus. Almost everyone who has ever had sex has had HPV at some time in his or her life.

How does HPV cause cervical cancer?
HPV is spread through sex and it can cause an infection in the cervix. The infection usually doesn't last very long because your body is able to fight the infection. If the HPV doesn't go away, the virus may cause cervix cells to change and become precancer cells. Precancer cells are not cancer. Most cells with early precancer changes return to normal on their own. Sometimes, the precancer cells may turn into cancer if they are not found and treated. Very few HPV infections lead to cervix cancer.

Are there any symptoms of HPV?
No. Most people will never know they have HPV. But if the HPV does not go away on its own, it can cause changes in the cervix cells. These changes usually show up on your Pap test.

How is HPV treated?
There is no treatment for the type of HPV that causes cervix cell changes, but most HPV infections go away without treatment. Antibiotics or other medicines do not treat HPV. There are treatments for the cell changes in the cervix that HPV can cause. If your Pap test shows cervix changes, your doctor or nurse will discuss these treatments with you, if you need them.

Will a Pap test tell me if I have HPV?
A Pap test will usually tell you if you have any cervix cell changes that could be caused by HPV. If a Pap test does not find cell changes that are in the cervix, then usually those changes will be found during the next Pap test. So it is important to get regular Pap tests.

HPV Vaccine

Approximately 20 million people are currently infected with HPV in the United States. At least 50 percent of sexually active men and women acquire genital HPV infection at some point in their lives. By age 50, at least 80 percent of women will have acquired genital HPV infection. About 6.2 million Americans get a new genital HPV infection each year.

Vaccines have been developed that can protect women from HPV infections. This vaccine can only be used to prevent HPV infection – before an abnormal Pap test develops. It cannot be used to treat an existing infection.

The vaccine has been approved by the FDA and should be covered by most medical insurance plans. It should also be covered by government programs that pay for vaccinations in children under 18.

To be most effective, the HPV vaccine should be given before a person becomes sexually active. The American Cancer Society recommends that the vaccine be routinely given to females aged 11 to 12 and as early as age 9 years at the discretion of doctors. The Federal Drug Administration (FDA) has approved the vaccine for use in females 9 to 26 years of age.

The vaccine requires 3 injections over a 6 month period. The injections are given every two months until all 3 are completed.

The vaccine doesn't protect against all cancer-causing types of HPV, so it is important that you still have routine Pap tests.

When to get vaccine: age 11 to 12 - or ask your doctor

How many shots: 3 shots, two months apart

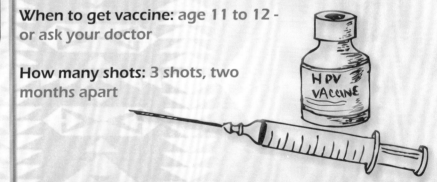

• Almost all women who have had sex will have HPV at some time, but very few women will get cervical cancer.
• Most HPV infections go away without causing cervix changes. HPV does not have any symptoms and cannot be treated. But the cell changes that HPV can cause in the cervix can be treated.
• HPV that does not go away over many years can lead to cervix cancer.

The Annual Women's Exam

Along with routine monitoring of your height, weight and blood pressure, an annual women's exam may include:

- talking about your personal, family, sexual, and medical history; laboratory tests and screening for sexually transmitted infections and other conditions (at your own or your doctor's request)
- counseling and education, such as how to perform a breast self exam
- a clinical breast exam
- a pelvic exam
- a Pap test

Nearly half of the women in the Uni[...] States who develo[...] cervical cancer ha[...] never had a Pap te[...]

Regular Pap tests decrease a woma[...] risk for developing cervical cancer be-cause they can de[...] precancerous cerv[...] lesions at early, tre[...] able stages.

Pap Test Versus Pelvic Exam

The Pap test is usually done just before the pelvic exam, when the doctor removes cells from the cervix by gently scraping or brushing with a special instrument.

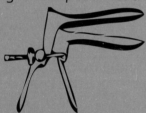

It is a simple and quick test. While you lie on an exam table, the doctor puts an instrument called a speculum into your vagina, opening it to see the cervix. She will then use a special stick or brush to take a few cells from inside and around the cervix. The cells are placed on a glass slide or in a tube and sent to a lab for examination. While usually painless, a Pap test is uncomfortable for some women.

The pelvic exam is part of a woman's routine health care. During a pelvic exam, the doctor looks at and feels the reproductive organs, including the uterus and the ovaries and may screen for sexually transmitted illnesses. But the pelvic exam will not find cervical cancer at an early stage and cannot find abnormal cells of the cervix.

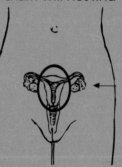

Pelvic exams may help find other types of cancers and reproductive problems, but only Pap tests give information on early cervical cancer or precancers.

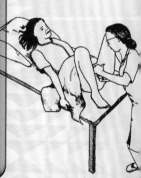

Pelvic Exam

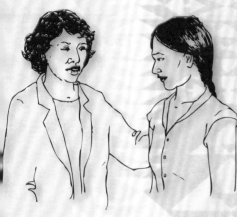

1. Schedule your annual women's visit and exam for a time when you will not have your period — unless you have bleeding problems that your health provider wants to check. Menstrual fluid can affect the results of some lab tests. Let your health provider know if it turns out that you will be having your period during the exam. You may want to reschedule.

2. Make a list of all the questions and problems you want to talk about. It's easy to forget these things during your appointment.

3. Women shouldn't douche. If you do, however, don't douche for at least 24 hours before the appointment.

4. Do not use tampons, birth control foams, jellies, or other vaginal creams or vaginal medications for 48 hours before the Pap test.

5. Don't have vaginal intercourse or insert anything into your vagina for between 24–48 hours before your visit.

Other tests used to diagnose cervical cancer

These tests many be used to diagnose abnormal cell changes of the cervix. They are explained later in this chapter.

- Biopsy
- Colposcopy
- LEEP
- Conization or Cone Biopsy

Checklist for things I want to talk to the doctor about during my annual exam:

___ bleeding after sex

___ heavier than usual flow

___ abdominal or pelvic pain

___ spotting between periods

___ vaginal discharge

___ unpleasant vaginal odors

___ family planning

___ STD protection and testing

___ breast lump or breast pain

___ nipple discharge

___ Other:_____

Pap Test Results

Doctors use several terms to describe abnormal and precancerous changes of the cervical cells, including cervical intraepithelial neoplasia (CIN), squamous intraepithelial lesion (SIL), and dysplasia. If abnormal cells are present, the Pap test will detect it most of the time. Pap testing is effective if it is done routinely; cell changes can take up to 10 years to turn into a cancer, so a yearly test will probably find it in time.

Pap testing has cut cervical cancer rates by 75 percent or more in nations with thorough screening. In the United States, there are now about 10,000 cases of cervical cancer each year and 4,000 deaths. More than half the cases are in women who do not undergo screening.

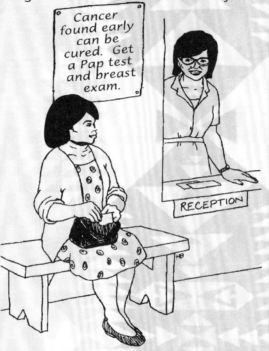

Cancer found early can be cured. Get a Pap test and breast exam.

RECEPTION

The most important thing to understand is that dysplasia is limited to the "skin" of the cervix, and has not invaded into other tissues. Even "carcinoma-in-situ" (meaning is "in place" and has not spread) is not invasive cancer.

Atypical squamous cells (ASCs); these a further divided into ASC-US and ASC-H Low-grade squamo intraepithelial lesion (SILs)
High-grade SILs
Squamous cell carci noma

What is cervical dysplasia?

The term "plasia" means growth. Cervical dysplasia means disordered growth. When we look at the lining of the normal cervix under a microscope we see layers of cells. The normal distribution is that the bottom layer is made of round young cells. As the cells mature they rise to the surface and flatten out, so that on the surface the cells are flat.

Surface

Flat Squamous C

Normal Cells

Normal Cervix

Cervical dysplasia is considered to be pre-cancerous, but not cancer.

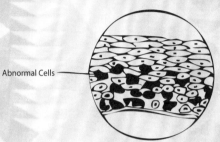

In cervical dysplasia there is a lack of this organized growth process. In **mild dysplasia** (CIN I) only a few cells are abnormal, while in **moderate dysplasia** (CIN II) the abnormal cells involve about one-half of the thickness of the surface lining of the cervix.

Abnormal Cells

Moderate Dysplasia is also called CIN II

Moderate Dysplasia

In **severe dysplasia** or **carcinoma-in-situ** (CIN III) the entire thickness of cells is disordered, but the abnormal cells have not yet spread below the surface. Carcinoma-in-situ means "cancer in place". If this condition is not treated, it often will grow into an invasive cervical cancer.

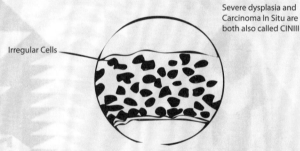

Irregular Cells

Severe dysplasia and Carcinoma In Situ are both also called CINIII

Severe Dysplasia, or Carcinoma-In-Situ

In dysplasia and carcinoma-in-situ all of the abnormalities are confined to the surface lining (or "skin") of the cervix. In **invasive cancer** the cells are not only disordered throughout the entire thickness of the lining, but they invade the tissue underlying the surface. Invasive cancer is treated entirely differently than dysplasia.

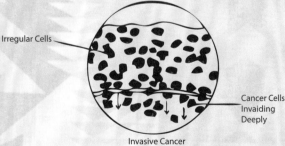

Irregular Cells

Cancer Cells Invaiding Deeply

Invasive Cancer

© 2003 Emily Shaw

291

How Pap Test Results Are Reported

The most widely used system for describing Pap test results is The Bethesda System (TBS, 2001). The general categories are:

Negative for intraepithelial lesion or malignancy (Normal): This means that no signs of cancer or pre-cancerous changes or other significant abnormalities were found.

ASC—atypical squamous cells. Squamous cells are the thin flat cells that form the surface of the cervix. This term is used when it is not possible to tell (from how the cells look under a microscope) whether the abnormal cells are caused by an infection, another cause of irritation, or by a precancer. The Pap test is usually repeated after several months, or other tests, such as colposcopy (explained below) and biopsy may be recommended, depending on the patient's history. Most doctors recommend having an HPV test in this situation. If this shows no HPV, then only usual follow-up is needed. If it does show HPV, colposcopy is recommended. This category has two groups:

- **ASC–US—atypical squamous cells of undetermined significance.** The squamous cells do not appear completely normal, but doctors are uncertain about what the cell changes mean. Sometimes the changes are related to human papillomavirus (HPV) infection. ACS–US are considered mild abnormalities.
- **ASC–H—atypical squamous cells cannot exclude a high-grade squamous intraepithelial lesion.** The cells do not appear normal, but doctors are uncertain about what the cell changes mean. ASC–H may be at higher risk of being precancerous.

AGC—atypical glandular cells. Glandular cells are mucus-producing cells found in the endocervical canal (opening in the center of the cervix) or in the lining of the uterus. The glandular cells do not appear normal, but doctors are uncertain about what the cell changes mean.

AIS—endocervical adenocarcinoma in situ. Precancerous cells are found in the glandular tissue.

Have you ever felt like the doctor was talking in a different language than you?

Sometimes we get results back from our Pap test that we don't understand - and sometimes we hear that the test was "abnormal" without hearing more.

The information on these pages may be technical, but some women may want to have a better understanding of our bodies and what the doctor finds - knowledge is power.

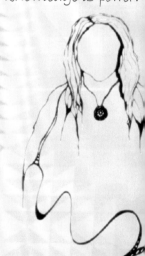

SIL–squamous intraepithelial lesions: Changes are seen in the cells that may show signs of precancer. All patients with SIL should have a colposcopy.

• **LSIL—low-grade squamous intraepithelial lesion.** Low-grade means there are early changes in the size and shape of cells. The word lesion refers to an area of abnormal tissue. Intraepithelial refers to the layer of cells that forms the surface of the cervix. LSILs are considered mild abnormalities caused by HPV infection.

• **HSIL—high-grade squamous intraepithelial lesion.** High-grade means that there are more marked changes in the size and shape of the abnormal (precancerous) cells, meaning that the cells look very different from normal cells. HSILs are more severe abnormalities and have a higher likelihood of progressing to invasive cancer.

Cancer or Squamous cell carcinoma: Diagnostic testing results show that the woman is likely to have an invasive squamous cell cancer. More testing will be done to be sure of the diagnosis before doctors recommend treatments such as radiation therapy, chemotherapy, or radical surgery.

Pap Test Terms		
Cervical changes may be called CIN or SIL. Both of these terms also are referred to as dysplasia.		
Term	CIN	SIL
Human papillomavirus	1	Low-grade
Mild dysplasia	1	Low-grade
Moderate dysplasia	2	High-grade
Severe dysplasia	3	High-grade
Carcinoma in situ	3	High-grade

Diagnostic tests for Cervical Cancer

Because the Pap test is a screening test rather than a diagnostic test, if you have an abnormal result, you will need to have other tests (colposcopy and biopsy, and sometimes an endocervical scraping) to find out whether a precancerous change or cancer is present.

Colposcopy: In this procedure you will lie on the exam table as you do with a pelvic exam. A speculum is placed in the vagina to expose the cervix. The doctor will use the colposcope to examine the cervix. The colposcope is an instrument with magnifying lenses very much like binoculars. With the colposcope, doctors can see the surface of the cervix closely and clearly. The doctor will usually "treat" your cervix with a weak solution of acetic acid (similar to vinegar).This will highlight any abnormal areas.

Colposcopic biopsy: For this type of biopsy, a doctor or other health care professional first examines the cervix with a colposcope to find the abnormal areas. Using a biopsy forceps, he or she will remove a small (about 1/8-inch) section of the abnormal area on the surface of the cervix. The biopsy procedure may cause mild cramping or brief pain, and you may have light bleeding afterward. A local anesthetic may be used to numb the cervix.

LEEP: The tissue is removed with a thin wire loop that is heated by electrical current and acts as a scalpel. For this procedure, a local anesthetic is used, and it can be done in your doctor's office. It takes only about 10 minutes. You may have mild cramping during and after the procedure, and mild to moderate bleeding may persist for several weeks. See the following pages for more information.

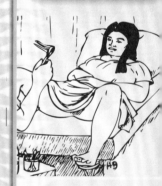

Common tests used to find cervical cancer
• **Biopsy.** A piece of tissue is taken from the cervix and sent to a laboratory to be examined for cancer cells.
• **Colposcopy.** This tool magnifies the cervix (makes it look bigger) so it is easier to see signs of cancer.

Endocervical curettage (endocervical scraping): This procedure is usually done at the same time as the colposcopic biopsy. A narrow instrument (the curette) is inserted into the endocervical canal (the passage between the outer part of the cervix and the inner part of the uterus). Some of the tissue lining the endocervical canal is removed by scraping with the curette. This tissue sample is sent to the laboratory for examination.

Cone biopsy: In this procedure, also known as conization, the doctor removes a cone-shaped piece of tissue from the cervix. The base of the cone is formed by the ectocervix (outer part of the cervix), and the point or apex of the cone is from the endocervical canal. This procedure is usually done in a hospital. Your health care provider will give you anesthesia.

Cold knife cone biopsy: A surgical scalpel or a laser as a scalpel is used rather than a heated wire to remove tissue. It requires general anesthesia (you are asleep during the operation) and is done in a hospital, but no overnight stay is needed. After the procedure, cramping and some bleeding may persist for a few weeks.

Finding and treating cancer of the cervix

Because cancer of the cervix does not have early warning signs, but can be cured if it is found early, it is good to be tested for it regularly. The tests are designed to look for abnormal tissue on the cervix which may be slightly abnormal (mild dysplasia), more abnormal (severe dysplasia), or early cancer (before it has spread).

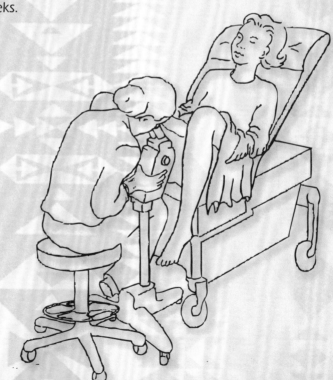

The LEEP

LEEP stands for Loop Electrosurgical Excision Procedure. This is a procedure designed to treat and/or diagnose the cervix with abnormal Pap Smear tests. This may also be called a Loop Cone Biopsy of the cervix. A fine wire loop which is attached to a high-frequency electrical generator allows very precise removal of abnormal tissue from your cervix. Because the procedure is so exact, and the loop very thin, there is very little damage to the tissue surrounding the area that needs to be removed, and the procedure allows for the blood vessels surrounding the area to be sealed.

You will be placed in the room, with your legs in stirrups or supports. The speculum will be inserted as for a pap smear. A local anesthetic will be injected (similar to the anesthetic you would get at a dental office). At the time of the injection, you may experience a cramp, like a mild menstrual cramping until the anesthesia has been injected. You may also experience some increase in your heart rate with some of the local anesthesia, and possibly some shakiness of your legs. These symptoms are normal and related to the medication. A solution is applied to the cervix to show the abnormal area that needs to be removed. You will hear a sound like a vacuum cleaner from what is known as the smoke evacuator and a humming sound when the electrosurgical generator is being used. It is VERY important that you do not move when the electrosurgical generator is making a sound. You may feel a dull cramp, however if you feel anything sharp, you should let the person performing the procedure know immediately. The removal of the tissue is over within a few seconds. The cautery portion of the procedure (burning of vessels after the procedure to prevent bleeding) takes a few minutes. Monsel's Solution (a green paste to assist in prevention of bleeding) is often applied, and the speculum is removed. The paste will cause a dark brown-black vaginal discharge for several days after the procedure.

The major benefit to LEEP is that the procedure allows safe removal of abnormal tissue, which can be thoroughly evaluated by the pathologist. Since cells are removed, the LEEP can diagnose and treat abnormal cervical tissue with this one procedure.

What should be expected afte a LEEP (cone biopsy)?

After the procedure, there may be some cramping or discomfort for a week or so. Activities including heavy lifting (over 15 lbs.) should be limited up to 10-14 days to avoid post operative bleeding. Avoid sexual intercourse, douching and use of tampons, for about 4 to 6 weeks. Take Motrin as needed for mild cramping. You may have heavy, bloody or a yellow-colored discharge for 2 to 3 weeks after the procedure. If you experience heavy bleeding (soaking a pad in 1 to hours), fever or worsening pain, you should contact your health care provider.

Treatment

If a test shows that you have severe dysplasia or advanced cancer, you need treatment. Together, you and your doctor can decide what treatment is best. Treatment in the early stages can be simple, using methods that remove or destroy the cancer tissue.

If an area of abnormal cells is seen during the colposcopy and usually confirmed by biopsy, your doctor will be able to remove the abnormal area by using such techniques as listed here:

- The **LEEP** (LLETZ procedure) *see previous page*

- A **cone biopsy** is a procedure that removes a small part of the cervix. During a cone biopsy, tissue is removed from the cervix while you are anaesthetized and sent to the laboratory to be studied. Cutting away the tissue also removes the abnormal cells. The tissue that grows back is likely to be normal, in which case no more treatment is needed.

- During **cryosurgery**, the doctor uses a metal probe cooled with liquid nitrogen to kill the abnormal cells by freezing them.

- In **laser surgery**, the doctor uses a focused beam of high-energy light to vaporize (burn off) the abnormal tissue. This is done through the vagina, with local anesthesia.

These outpatient treatments can be done in a doctor's office or clinic. After treatment, you may have a watery brown discharge for a few weeks. If it is available, these treatments may be best if you still want to have children and the cancer has not spread, because you can keep your womb. These treatments are almost always effective in destroying precancers and preventing them from developing into true cancers. You will need follow-up exams to make sure that the abnormality does not come back. If it does, treatments can be repeated.

When cancer is found and treated before it spreads, it can be cured. If the cancer is found after it has grown for a long time, it may have spread beyond the cervix to other parts of the body. In this case you will usually need surgery to remove both the cervix and womb (hysterectomy). Sometimes radiation therapy can help.

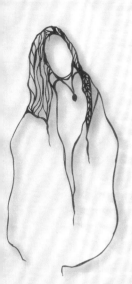

When I had cervical cancer in my late twenties (1978) doctors were fairly new at using colbalt radiation and radiation implants. I was given way too much of both. The test they performed were very invasive and painful. I felt like I was a guinnea pig. But I also have the satisfaction that they found new methods for doing these tests, and have realized they can use less radiation. I am still cancer free after 30+ years.

Wendy Kinswa
Cowlitz Tribe

Cervical Cancer Can be Prevented

To reduce the risks for cancer of the cervix by finding and treating more cancers early, we can:

• learn what increases a woman's risk, and work together on finding ways to reduce these risks. It is especially important for girls to be able to wait until they are grown women before having sex. All women also need to be able to protect themselves from STIs, including HIV/AIDS.

• avoid or quit non-traditional tobacco use (smoking).

• learn about cancer screening and tell your sisters, mothers, daughters, aunties and girlfriends of the importance of regular screening.

• work with your clinic to help reduce barriers to screening such as asking that a female health provider be available. Ask for childcare and transportation assistance if needed.

How can you take care of everyone else if you don't take care of yourself first!

Resources:

National Cervical Cancer Coalition

www.nccc-online.org/
(800) 685-5531
(818) 909-3849

www.cancer.gov/cancertopics/types/cervical

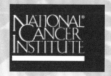

www.4women.gov/FAQ/ccervix.htm

www.cdc.gov/cancer/cervical/

womens*health.gov*
The Federal Government Source for Women's Health Information

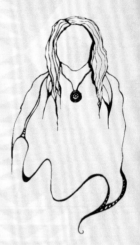

Native Women in and near Portland!

NARA's Women's Wellness Program provides breast and cervical cancer screening services to American Indian and Alaska Native women served at the NARA Indian Health clinic.

Contact the Women's Wellness Program at:
NARA INDIAN HEALTH CLINIC
15 N. Morris
Portland, Oregon
97227
503.230.9875

How to get free or low cost Pap tests:

Many Indian Health Service, Tribal and Urban Indian Health Clinics provide no or low cost annual women's exams including a Pap test. See the "Health System" chapter for contact information for American Indian and Alaska Native clinics.

Programs funded by the National Breast and Cervical Cancer Early Detection Program (NBCCEDP) offer free or low-cost Pap tests to women in need. These and other programs are available throughout the United States. To find contact information for a program near you, visit the NBCCEDP website at http://www.cdc.gov/cancer/nbccedp/ or call **1-888-842-6355** (select option 7). Also, your state or local health department can direct you to places that offer free or low-cost Pap tests.

Planned Parenthood offers low-cost Pap tests as well. To find the Planned Parenthood office in your area, call 1-800-230-7526 or visit their website at: http://www.ppfa.org

National Women's Health Information Center (NWHIC)
Phone Number: (800)-994-9662

Cancer Information Service, NCI, NIH, HHS
Phone Number: (800) 422-6237
Internet Address: http://cis.nci.nih.gov/

American College of Obstetricians and Gynecologists (ACOG) Resource Center
Phone Number: (800) 762-2264 x 192 (for publications requests only)
Internet Address: http://www.acog.org/

American Cancer Society
Phone Number: 1-800-227-2345
Internet Address: http://www.cancer.org

National Cervical Cancer Coalition (NCCC)
Phone Number: (800) 685-5531
Internet Address: http://www.nccc-online.org/

Centers for Disease Control
National Breast and Cervical Cancer Early Detection Program
Phone Number: (888) 842-6355
Internet Address: http://www.cdc.gov/cancer/nbccedp/

More information on American Indian and Alaska Native Breast and Cervical Cancer Early Detection Programs can be found at the front of this manual.

National Breast and Cervical
Cancer Early Detection Program

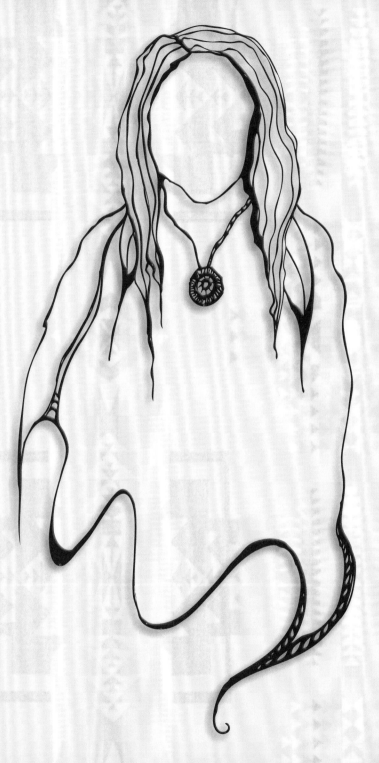

Mothers and Grand
mothers, our breasts
give life and there
is nothing better
in this world than
to hold your child
in your arms and
watch them drink
of your body. But
our breasts also can
harm us. Breast
cancer is a type of
cancer that occurs
when cells in breast
tissue divide and
grow out of control.
Breast cancer can
also travel to other
parts of your body,
such as the liver, an
strangely, is still
called breast can-
cer. Native women,
once diagnosed with
breast cancer have t
lowest survival rate
of any ethnic group
race. Breast Can-
cer will look at how
you can help care fo
yourself and look
into the breast itself

Breast Wellness

Small, large, young, old - we are women and we are gifted with breasts. Breast tissue to produce milk as well as to celebrate our feminity, this tissue supports life. At the same time, we women need to keep track of changes in our breasts.

Sometimes breast cells grow out of control. The extra cells form a mass called a tumor. Some tumors are "benign" or not cancer. These tumors usually stay in one spot in the breast and do not cause big health problems. Other tumors are "malignant" and are cancer. Breast cancer often starts out too small to be felt. As it grows, it can spread throughout the breast or to other parts of the body.

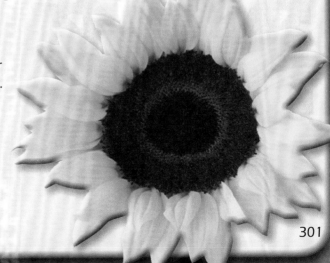

What Are My Breasts Made Of?

A breast is made up of glands, ducts, and connective tissue. The glands include the lobules and ducts that help women make milk when they are breast feeding. The lobules produce milk. The ducts are passages that carry milk to the nipple. The connective tissue (which consists of fibrous and fatty tissue) connects and holds everything together.

Every woman's breast are different. What is normal for you may not be normal for another woman. Most women say their breasts feel lumpy or uneven. The way your breasts look and feel can be affected by getting your period, having children, losing or gaining weight, and taking certain medications. Breasts also tend to change as you age.

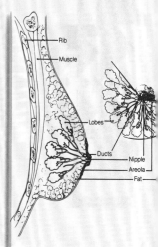

Breast Changes

Breast changes occur in almost all women. You might notice different kinds of breast changes at different times in your life. Many of these are caused by changes in your hormone levels and are a normal part of getting older. Most of these changes are not cancer. However, some breast changes may be signs of cancer. Breast changes that are not cancer are called benign.

Younger women may have more glandular (more dense, less fatty) breast tissue than older women who have stopped having their period (menopause). This kind of tissue is where breast changes usually occur.

Breast Changes Due to Your Period: Many women have swelling, tenderness, and pain in their breasts before and sometimes during their periods. You may also feel one or more lumps during this time because of extra fluid in your breasts. The lumpiness and pain usually go away by the end of your period. Because some lumps are caused by normal hormone changes, you may want to watch the lump for a month or two to see if it goes away. Before or during your period, you might have lumpiness, tenderness, and pain in your breasts.

During pregnancy, your breasts may feel lumpy, as the glands that produce milk increase in number and get larger. Still, breast cancer has been found in pregnant women, so talk with your doctor if you have questions about any breast lumps.

Fibroadenomas

Fibroadenomas are movable, solid, rounded lumps made up of normal breast cells. While not cancerous, these lumps may grow. And any solid lump that's getting bigger is usually removed to make sure that it's not a cancer. Fibroadenomas are the most common kind of breast mass, especially in young women.

Cysts

Unlike cancerous tumors which are solid, cysts are fluid-filled masses in the breast. Cysts are very common, and are rarely associated with cancer. Ultrasound is the best way to tell a cyst from a cancer, because sound waves pass right through a liquid-filled cyst. Solid lumps, on the other hand, bounce the waves right back to the film

Lumpiness:

Most women have some type of lumpiness in their breasts. Some areas may be more dense than others and can feel lumpy in an exam. Breast lumps are very common in most women, especially soft, fluid-filled ones (called cysts). These usually change during a woman's monthly cycle, and sometimes feel sore or painful when pressed. Single lumps can appear at any time and come in many types and sizes. Most lumps are not cancer, but your health care provider should always check the lump carefully. He or she may do more tests to make sure the lump is not cancer.

What causes breast lumps?

Many different conditions can cause lumps in the breast, including cancer. But most breast lumps are caused by other medical conditions. The two most common causes of breast lumps are fibrocystic breast condition and cysts. Fibrocystic condition causes noncancerous changes in the breast that can make them lumpy, tender, and sore. Cysts are small fluid-filled sacs that can develop in the breast.

Breast infection

If a woman is breastfeeding a baby and gets a hot, red sore area on the breast, she probably has mastitis, or an abscess. This is not cancer and is easily cured. If the woman is not breastfeeding, it may be a sign of cancer.

Discharge from the nipple

Nipple discharge is common for some women. It is fluid that comes from the nipple in different colors or textures. Usually, it is not a sign of cancer. For example, birth control pills can cause a little discharge. Milky or clear discharge from one or both nipples is usually normal if a woman has breastfed a baby within the last year. Certain infections also cause nipple discharge. However, for women who are going through or have passed menopause, nipple discharge can be a sign of cancer. See your doctor if you have nipple discharge for the first time, or a change in your discharge's color or texture. He or she may send a sample of the discharge to be checked at a lab. Brown, green, or bloody discharge—especially from only one nipple—could be a sign of cancer. Get it checked out.

Cancer of the Breast

Risk increases with age because the wear and tear of living increases the risk that a genetic abnormality, or "mistake," will develop that your body doesn't find and fix.

The risk of getting breast cancer over the course of an entire lifetime, assuming you live to age 90, is **one in 7**, with an overall lifetime risk of 14.3%.

Growing older is the biggest risk for breast cancer. The longer you live, the higher your risk:

- From birth to age 39, 1 woman in 231 will get breast cancer (<0.5% risk).
- From ages 40–59, the chance is 1 in 25 (4% risk).
- From ages 60–79, the chance is 1 in 15 (nearly 7%).

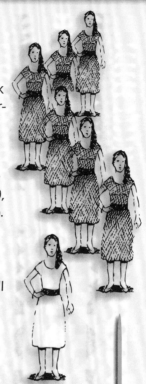

Breast cancer usually grows slowly. If it is found early, it can sometimes be cured. It is hard to tell who will get breast cancer. The risk might be greater for a woman whose mother or sisters have had breast cancer. Breast cancer is more common in women over age 50.

Facts on Breast Cancer

- Not counting some kinds of skin cancer, breast cancer in the United States is the most common cancer in women, no matter your race or ethnicity.

- Each year, approximately 200,000 women will be diagnosed with breast cancer and more than 40,000 women will die from it.

- The second most common cause of death from cancer among white, black, Asian/Pacific Islander, and American Indian/Alaska Native women (2003)

- Men can also get breast cancer. In men, breast cancer can happen at any age, but is most common in men who are between 60 and 70 years old. Male breast cancer is not very common. For every 100 cases of breast cancer, less than 1 are in men.

- As a woman gets older, her chance of getting or dying from breast cancer increases.

Different people have different warning signs for breast cancer. Some people do not have any signs or symptoms at all. A person may find out they have breast cancer after a routine mammogram.

Risk Factors

What causes breast cancer?

As with many types of cancer, medical experts do not know exactly what causes breast cancer. Almost all breast cancer, however, occurs in women. Breast cancer can develop in men, but it is very rare and accounts for less than half of 1 percent of all breast cancers. Researchers do know that bumping, bruising, pinching, or touching the breast does not cause breast cancer. They also know that you cannot "catch" breast cancer from another person.

As scientists continue to research possible causes of breast cancer, they have identified certain factors that increase a woman's risk for breast cancer.

No one knows the exact causes of breast cancer. Doctors often cannot explain why one woman develops breast cancer and another does not. They do know that bumping, bruising, or touching the breast does not cause cancer. And breast cancer is not contagious. You cannot "catch" it from another person.

Research has shown that women with certain risk factors are more likely than others to develop breast cancer. A risk factor is something that may increase the chance of developing a disease.

- Age: The chance of getting breast cancer goes up as a woman gets older. Most cases of breast cancer occur in women over 60. This disease is not common before menopause.
- The older a woman is when she has her first child, the greater her chance of breast cancer.
- Women who had their first menstrual period before age 12 are at an increased risk of breast cancer.
- Women who went through menopause after age 55 are at an increased risk of breast cancer.
- Women who never had children are at an increased risk.
- Women who have never breastfed are at an increased risk.
- Personal history of breast cancer or some non-cancerous breast diseases. A woman who had breast cancer in one breast has an increased risk of getting cancer in her other breast.
- Treatment with radiation therapy to the breast/chest.
- Being overweight after menopause.
- Drinking alcohol (more than one drink a day).
- Not getting regular exercise.
- Family history: A woman's risk of breast cancer is higher if her mother, sister, or daughter had breast cancer. The risk is higher if her family member got breast cancer before 40.
- Gene changes: Changes in certain genes increase the risk of breast cancer. These genes include BRCA1, BRCA2, and others.
- Women who take hormone therapy with estrogen & progestin after menopause appear to have an increased risk.

305

Staying Healthy and Lowering your Risk for Breast Cancer

Scientists are studying how best to prevent breast cancer. Staying healthy may help. To protect your overall health and to prevent many kinds of cancer:

- Aim for a healthy weight. Make healthy choices in the foods you eat and the kinds of drinks you have each day.

  - Eat five or more servings of fruits and vegetables every day.

  - Stay Active. Get regular physical activity. 30 minutes 5 days a week is a great start.

  - Do not smoke; if you do smoke, quit. Talk to your doctor about help in quitting smoking.

- Know your family history of breast cancer. If you have a mother, sister, or daughter with breast cancer, ask your doctor what is your risk of getting breast cancer and how you can lower your risk.

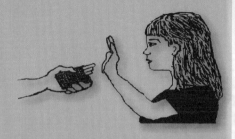

- Talk to your health provider about the risks and benefits of hormone replacement therapy. Some women use hormone replacement therapy (HRT) to treat the symptoms of menopause.

- Limit the amount of alcohol you drink.

- Get screened for breast cancer regularly. By getting the necessary exams, you can increase your chances of finding out early on, if you have breast cancer.

Having a risk factor does not mean you will get the disease. Most women have some risk factors and most women do not get breast cancer. If you have breast cancer risk factors, talk with your doctor about ways you can lower your risk and about screening for breast cancer.

Warning Signs

Most of the time, early breast cancer does not have any symptoms. As it grows, however, breast cancer can cause changes in how the breast looks or feels. Symptoms include:

- a hard painless lump with a jagged shape, that is in only one breast and does not move under the skin
- a new lump in the breast or thickening in the under-arm area
- a lump that has changed
- redness, or a sore on the breast that does not heal
- skin on the breast that is pulled in, or looks rough and pitted, like orange or lemon peel
- sometimes, a painful swelling under the arm
- A change in the size or shape of the breast
- pain in the breast or nipple that does not go away
- A nipple that is very tender or that suddenly turns inward
- fluid coming from the nipple when not nursing a baby

See your health provider if you notice any of these symptoms. If you have a question about any breast lump, if you notice a new lump, or if a lump has changed, talk with your health provider.

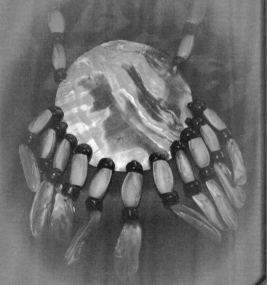

You can't be sure that a new lump is also benign.

Check with your doctor if you notice any kind of lump. Even if you had a lump in the past that turned out to be benign, you can't be sure that a new lump is also benign

Myths about Breast Cancer

Rumors and myths can do harm if they keep you from getting the very best possible care. Arm yourself with the facts (information from www.breastcancer.org). Here are common myths about breast cancer:

Breast cancer only affects older women.   No.
While it's true that the risk of breast cancer increases as we grow older, breast cancer can occur at any age. From birth to age 39, one woman in 231 will get breast cancer (<0.5% risk); from age 40–59, the chance is one in 25 (4% risk); from age 60–79, the chance is one in 15 (nearly 7%). Assuming you live to age 90, the chance of getting breast cancer over the course of an entire lifetime is one in 7.

If you have a risk factor for breast cancer, you're likely to get the disease.   No.
Getting breast cancer is not a certainty, even if you have one of the stronger risk factors, like a breast cancer gene abnormality. Of women with a BRCA1 or BRCA2 inherited genetic abnormality, 40–80% will develop breast cancer over their lifetime; 20–60% won't. All other risk factors are associated with a much lower probability of being diagnosed with breast cancer.

If breast cancer doesn't run in your family, you won't get it.   No.
Every woman has some risk of breast cancer. About 80% of women who get breast cancer have no known family history of the disease. Increasing age – just the wear and tear of living – is the biggest single risk factor for breast cancer. For those women who do have a family history of breast cancer, your risk may be elevated a little, a lot, or not at all. If you are concerned, discuss your family history with your physician or a genetic counselor. You may be worrying needlessly.

Only your mother's family history of breast cancer can affect your risk.   No.
A history of breast cancer in your mother's OR your father's family will influence your risk equally. That's because half of your genes come from your mother, half from your father. But a man with a breast cancer gene abnormality is less likely to develop breast cancer than a woman with a similar gene. So, if you want to learn more about your father's family history, you have to look mainly at the women on your father's side, not just the men.

Using antiperspirants causes breast cancer.   No.
There is no evidence that the active ingredient in antiperspirants, or reducing perspiration from the underarm area, influences breast cancer risk. The supposed link between breast cancer and antiperspirants is based on misinformation about anatomy and a misunderstanding of breast cancer.

Myths about Breast Cancer

Birth control pills cause breast cancer.   **No.**
Modern day birth control pills contain a low dose of the hormones estrogen and progesterone. Many research studies show no association between birth control pills and an
increased risk of breast cancer. However, one study that combined the results of many
different studies did show an association between birth control pills and a very small increase in risk. The study also showed that this slight increase in risk decreased over time.
So after 10 years, birth control pills were not associated with an increase in risk. Birth
control pills also have benefits including decreasing the risk of ovarian and endometrial
cancer, relieving menstrual disorders, pelvic inflammatory disease, and improving bone
mineral density.

Eating high-fat foods causes breast cancer.   **No.**
Medical research has not been able to show a clear connection between eating high-fat
foods and a higher risk of breast cancer. We can say that avoidance of high-fat foods is
a healthy choice for other reasons: to lower the "bad" cholesterol (low-density lipoproteins), increase the "good" cholesterol (high-density lipoproteins); to make more room in
your diet for healthier foods, and to help you control your weight. Excess body weight,
IS a risk factor for breast cancer, because the extra fat increases the production of estrogen outside the ovaries and adds to the overall level of estrogen in the body. If you are
already overweight, or have a tendency to gain weight easily, avoiding high-fat foods is
a good idea.

A monthly breast self-exam is the best way to diagnose breast cancer.   **No.**
High quality screening mammography is the most reliable way to find breast cancer as
early as possible, when it is most curable. By the time a breast cancer can be felt, it is
usually bigger than the average size of a cancer first found on mammography. Breast
examination by you or your healthcare provider is still very important. About 25% of
breast cancers are found only on a clinical breast examination (not on the mammogram), about 35% are found on mammography alone, and 40% are found by both
physical exam and mammography. Keep both bases covered.

A breast cancer diagnosis is an automatic death sentence.   **No.**
Fully 80% of women diagnosed with breast cancer have no signs of metastases (no cancer has spread beyond the breast and nearby lymph nodes). Furthermore, 80% of these
women live at least five years, most longer, and many live much longer. Even women
with signs of cancer metastases can live a long time. Plus promising treatment break-
throughs are becoming available each day.

Screening Tests for Breast Cancer

Breast cancer screening means checking a woman's breasts for cancer before there are signs or symptoms of the disease. Three main tests are used to screen the breasts for cancer.

Mammogram (each year after age 40). A mammogram is an X-ray of the breast. Mammograms are the best method to detect breast cancer early when it is easier to treat and before it is big enough to feel or cause symptoms. Having regular mammograms can lower the risk of dying from breast cancer.

Clinical breast exam (each year). A clinical breast exam is an examination by a doctor or nurse, who uses his or her hands to feel for lumps or other changes. The exams involve checking the look and feel of the breasts and underarm for any changes. The breasts are checked while a woman is sitting up and lying down.

Breast self-exam (each month). A breast self-exam is when you check your own breasts for lumps, changes in size or shape of the breast, or any other changes in the breasts or underarm (armpit).

Tips for getting a mammogram

Try not to have your mammogram the week before you get your period or during your period. Your breasts may be tender or swollen then.

On the day of your mammogram, don't wear deodorant, perfume, or powder. These products can show up as white spots on the x-ray.

Some women prefer to wear a top with a skirt or pants, instead of a dress. You will need to take your clothes off from your waist up for the mammogram.

Before you get a mammogram, you may want to ask the following questions:

What will happen? How long will I be there? Do you have my previous mammograms? When will my doctor get the results? When and how will I learn about the results? When will I need to have my next mammogram?

Breast Self-Exam
A woman should examine her breasts every month, even after her monthly bleeding has stopped forever.

Breast Self Exam (BSE)

How to examine your breasts

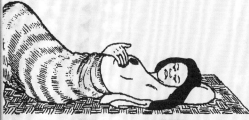

· Look at your breasts in a mirror. Raise your arms over your head. Look for any change in the shape of your breasts, or any swelling or changes in the skin or nipple. Then put your arms at your sides and check your breasts again.

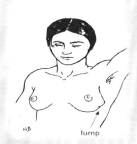

HB   lump

Early breast cancer usually does not cause pain. Still, a woman should see her health care provider about breast pain or any other symptom that does not go away. Most often, these symptoms are not due to cancer. Other health problems may also cause them. Any woman with these symptoms should tell her doctor so that problems can be diagnosed and treated as early as possible.

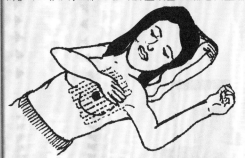

Lie down. Keeping your fingers flat, press your breast and feel for any lumps.

Be sure to touch every part of your breast. It helps to use the same pattern every month.

What to do if you find a lump

If the lump is smooth or rubbery, and moves under the skin when you push it with your fingers, do not worry about it. But if it is hard, has an uneven shape, and is painless, keep watching it—especially if the lump is in only one breast and does not move even when you push it. See a health care provider if the lump is still there after your next monthly bleeding. This may be a sign of cancer. You should also get medical help if there is a discharge that looks like blood or pus.

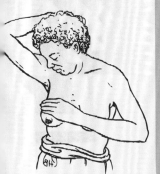

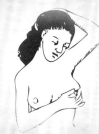

311

Screening mammograms

Screening mammograms are used to check women who have no signs or symptoms of breast cancer. It usually involves two x-rays of each breast. The goal of a screening mammogram is to find cancer early, when it is too small to be felt by a woman or her doctor. Finding breast cancer early greatly increases a woman's chance for successful treatment.

What happens if my mammogram is normal?

Continue to get regular mammograms. Mammograms work best when they can be compared with previous ones. This allows your doctor to compare them to look for changes in your breasts.

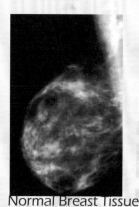

Normal Breast Tissue

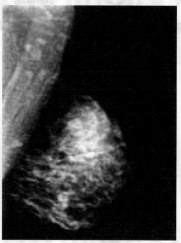

Normal left mammogram of heterogeneously dense breast. Cancer can be difficult to detect in a woman with this type of breast tissue because the fibroglandular tissue (whiter areas) may hide the tumor.

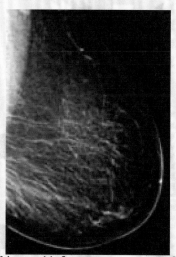

http://www.radiologyinfo.org/en/photocat/photos_more_pc.cfm?pg=mammo

Normal left mammogram of fatty breast. Breast cancer is relatively easy to detect in a woman with this type of breast tissue.

Understanding Mammograms

What is a mammogram?
A mammogram is an x-ray picture of the breast. Doctors use a mammogram to look for early signs of breast cancer.

Why should I get a mammogram?
Regular mammograms are the best tests doctors have to find breast cancer early, sometimes up to three years before it can be felt. When their breast cancer is found early, many women go on to live long and healthy lives.

When should I get a mammogram?
Most women should have their first mammogram at age 40 and then have another mammogram every one or two years. Talk to your health professional if you have any symptoms or changes in your breast, or if breast cancer runs in your family. He or she may recommend that you have mammograms before age 40 or more often than usual.

How is a mammogram done?
You will stand in front of a special x-ray machine. A technologist will place your breast on a clear plastic plate. Another plate will firmly press your breast from above. The plates will flatten the breast, holding it still while the x-ray is being taken. You will feel some pressure. The other breast will be x-rayed in the same way. The steps are then repeated to make a side view of each breast. You will then wait while the technologist checks the four x-rays to make sure the pictures do not need to be re-done.

What does having a mammogram feel like?
Having a mammogram is uncomfortable for most women. Some women find it painful. A mammogram takes only a few moments and the discomfort is over soon. What you feel depends on the skill of the technologist, the size of your breasts, and how much they need to be pressed. Your breasts may be more sensitive if you are about to get or have your period.

What does a mammogram look like?
An example of a normal mammogram is shown here. Each woman's mammogram may look a little different because all breasts are a little different. A doctor with special training, called a radiologist, will read the mammogram. He or she will look at the x-ray for early signs of breast cancer or other problems.

When will I get the results of my mammogram?
You will usually get the results within a few weeks, although it depends on the facility. A radiologist reads your mammogram and then reports the results to you or your doctor. If there is a concern, you will hear from the mammography facility earlier. Contact your doctor or the mammography facility if you do not receive a report of your results within 30 days.

What if my mammogram is abnormal?

Do not panic. Mammograms find many conditions that are not cancer. Most women who need more exams or testing do not have cancer. Some of the usual follow-up exams and tests are described below. The tests your doctor recommends will depend on what showed up on your mammogram.

Additional Diagnostic Mammograms

A doctor may ask for additional diagnostic mammograms to get different or bigger views of a particular area of a breast. In most cases, special images magnify a small area of the breast, making it easier to read. These views give a better look at what a doctor sees on a regular mammogram. Sometimes a woman will receive a diagnostic mammogram shortly after her screening mammogram. It is used to look more closely at abnormalities found on the first mammogram.

Ultrasound

An ultrasound is a test that can be used in addition to a mammogram. It uses sound waves to make pictures of the breast. This test is more commonly used in younger women or women with dense breast tissue. It also helps distinguish between cysts and solid masses and between benign and cancerous tumors. The doctor or technician views the picture on a monitor.

Exams by Specialists (Consultation)

Your doctor may send you to a specialist, such as a breast specialist or surgeon, for a physical exam or other tests. It does not necessarily mean you have cancer or need surgery. Breast specialists are experienced in conducting physical exams of the breasts, diagnosing breast problems, and performing biopsies (described on the next page).

Breast Cancer screening with an MRI ?

For women at high risk – those with a strong family history of the disease or with a genetic mutation associated with breast cancer the American Cancer Society guidelines advise discussing with their doctor other screening methods – like MRI or ultrasound. These procedures might be used instead of regular mammography or in addition to mammography. Screening at a younger age and screening more frequently are also options. Also make sure to ask if your insurance or other health care payer will cover each procedure.

You may want to ask your doctor the following questions before having a biopsy:

What kind of biopsy will I have? Why? How long will it take? Will I be awake? Will it hurt? Will I have anesthesia? What kind? Are there any risks? What are the chances of infection or bleeding after the biopsy? How soon will I know the results? If I do have cancer, who will talk with me about the next steps? When?

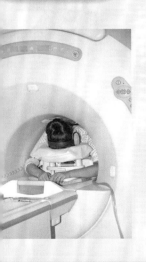

Biopsy

A biopsy is removal of small samples of breast tissue, which can be done with a needle or through surgery. A needle biopsy is usually performed in the doctor'soffice. A woman receives a shot in the breast to numb the area, and the doctor inserts a needle to withdraw some tissue. A surgical biopsy is usually performed at a surgical center, the doctor's office, or a hospital. Typically, a woman will receive medication to help her feel relaxed and drowsy before the surgeon makes a smallcut in the skin of the breast. He or she removes a small piece of breast tissue in the suspicious area and sends it to a laboratory. A doctor who specializes in diagnosing diseases (pathologist) examines the sample under a microscope to see if there are any cancer cells.

Steriotactic Core Breast Biopsy

A stereotactic core needle biopsy uses x-ray equipment and a computer to analyze the pictures (x-ray views). The computer then pinpoints exactly where in the abnormal area to place the needle tip. This procedure is often used to biopsy microcalcifications (calcium deposits).

Fine Needle Aspiration (FNA)

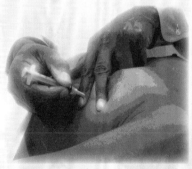

A procedure in which your doctor inserts a very thin needle into your breast and the suspected cyst and withdraws (aspirates) any fluid and/or tissue with a syringe. This is often done when the doctor finda a lump that appears to be a cyst.

Magnetic Resonance Imaging(MRI)

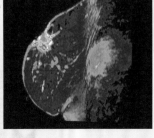

MR imaging uses a powerful magnetic field, radio waves and a computer to produce detailed pictures of organs, soft tissues, bone and other internal body structures. The images can then be examined on a computer monitor or printed. MRI does not use ionizing radiation (x-rays).

Breast Cysts

Cysts are fluid filled sacs within the breast. These sacs form when normal milk producing glands enlarge. Cysts are oval or round, smooth and firm, and they move slightly when you press them. Breast cysts may be solitary but are most commonly multiple and can vary in size from microscopic to larger than a ping pong ball.

Breast cysts are common, particularly in women age 40-60. Your doctor can't determine from a clinical breast exam alone whether you have a cyst, so you'll need further evaluation. Most likely, your doctor will perform fine-needle aspiration to drain the cyst and check for the presence of cancer.

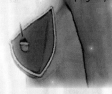

Fluid filled sac (Cyst)

Solid Lump (Fibroademoma)

Fibroadenomas

Fibroadenomas are round, firm, rubbery masses that arise from excess growth of glandular and connective tissue. These masses can grow to the size of a small plum, but they're benign and usually painless. Fibroadenomas respond to hormonal changes and tend to enlarge during pregnancy and shrink after menopause. Women of any age may have them, but they're usually detected in women in their 20s or 30s. Your doctor can't tell from a clinical breast exam alone whether a breast lump is a fibroadenoma. Mammography and ultrasound may help with the diagnosis, but the only way to be certain of a fibroadenoma is to take a sample of tissue for lab analysis (biopsy). Your doctor may also recommend surgery to remove the lump completely.

Breast calcification can be caused by:

- Calcium in a cyst o fiboradenoma (no cancer)
- Calcifications from milk duct
- An injury to the breast happened while ago
- Inflammation due infection
- Skin calcifications from metallic parti in powders, ointments and deodo ants
- Radiation therapy breast cancer
- Calcification of the arteries

Breast Calcifications

Breast calcifications are tiny white spots - like grains of salt - that might show up on a mammogram. These spots are made up of calcium that is in the breast tissue. Breast calcifications are common. Many women have at least one calcification that can be seen on a mammogram. Calcifications can't be felt. Although breast calcifications are usually not cancer (benign), some patterns of calcifications — such as tight groups of white spots with irregular shapes — may indicate breast cancer.

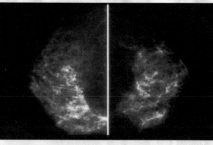

X-ray with microcalcifications

Calcium in your diet d NOT cause calcificatio

Possible Mammogram Results and Follow-Up Care

Conditions	Features	What Your Doctor May Recommend
Cysts	Fluid-filled lumps Usually not cancer Occur most often in women ages 35-50 Often in both breasts Some too small to be felt	Doctors often watch cysts over time or use fine-needle aspiration to remove the fluid from the cyst. Ultrasound may be used to see whether a lump is solid or filled with fluid.
Fibroadenoma	Hard, round, benign growth Feels like rubber; moves around easily Usually painless Often found by the woman herself Appears on mammogram as smooth, round lumps with clearly defined edges Can get bigger when the woman is pregnant or nursing	Sometimes diagnosed with fine-needle aspiration If the fibroadenoma does not appear normal, the doctor may suggest taking it out to make sure it is benign.
Macro-calcifications	Appear on a mammogram as large calcium deposits Often caused by aging Usually not cancer	Have another mammogram to have a closer look at the area A biopsy may be used for diagnosis
Mass	May be round and smooth or have irregular borders May be caused by normal hormone changes	A mammogram and/or ultrasound may be used to see whether a lump is solid or filled with fluid A biopsy may be used for diagnosis
Micro-calcifications	Appear on a mammogram as tiny specks of calcium that might be found in an area of rapidly dividing cells If they are found grouped together in a certain way, they may be a sign of cancer.	Have another mammogram to have a closer look at the area A biopsy may be used for diagnosis

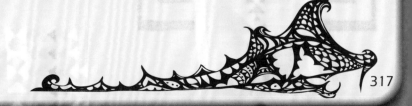

What happens if they find breast cancer?

For many women, treatment for breast cancer begins within a few weeks after the diagnosis. Usually, a woman has time to learn about her options and doesn't have to make an immediate decision. She can discuss her treatment choices with her doctor, get a second opinion, talk to friends, or learn from other women with cancer. Not all breast cancers are treated the same way, and different treatments have different advantages and disadvantages. It is normal to feel some shock and stress, making it hard to process information at first or even to ask questions. Some women find it helps to make a list of questions, take notes, or have a family member or friend with them when they talk to the doctor. The most important thing is that a woman feels informed of her options and comfortable with her decision.

How is breast cancer treated?

There are many different types of treatments available for breast cancer. A woman will most likely be sent to a doctor who is an expert in a particular type of treatment. This may be an oncologist (doctor specializing in cancer treatment), surgeon, or other kind of specialist. Each of these doctors has extra training and experience in the type of treatment they offer. Understanding all the options and talking to her primary doctor may help a woman choose the treatment that is best for her. Common treatments for breast cancer include one or more of the following:

• Surgery involves an operation in which some of or the entire breast is removed. Several types of surgeries are used in breast cancer, so ask your doctor to explain your options, the pros and cons of each, and how they will affect how your breast looks. Surgery is the most common treatment for breast cancer.

• Radiation therapy uses special high-energy x-rays and other types of radiation to kill cancer cells.

• Chemotherapy uses drugs to kill or stop the growth of cancer cells.

• Hormone therapy removes hormones or blocks their action to stop cancer cells from growing.

Staging

If breast cancer is diagnosed, tests are done to find out if cancer cells have spread within the breast or to other parts of the body. This process is called staging. Whether the cancer is only in the breast, is found in lymph nodes under your arm, or has spread outside the breast determines your stage of breast cancer. The type and stage of breast cancer tells doctors what kind of treatment will be needed. See page 267 for more information on staging.

Options for Breast Cancer Treatment

from www.breastcancer.org

For every stage of breast cancer, you and your treatment team can consider three broad types of treatment:

1. **Local/regional treatment** is directed to the breast and to lymph nodes around the breast. ("Regional" here refers to the lymph nodes in the region of the body surrounding the breast—these are also called "adjacent" lymph nodes.) In the case of metastatic disease, local treatment may be given to specific areas of metastasis (places where cancer may have spread, such as bones or lungs). The whole breast can be treated by mastectomy or breast preservation therapy:

> Mastectomy involves removal of the entire breast. Mastectomy may be followed by radiation to the area where the breast used to be.
>
> Breast preservation therapy removes the breast cancer by lumpectomy (also called "wide resection," "partial mastectomy," or "quadrantectomy") and is also followed by radiation to the remainder of the breast tissue.

2. **Systemic treatments** are directed to the whole body or "system." They include hormonal therapies, chemotherapy and possibly immune therapies.

> The goal of systemic therapy is to get rid of any cancer cells that may have spread to another part of the body. It's an "insurance policy" that may be used even if there is no direct proof that cancer has spread. If the cancer HAS spread and formed tumors elsewhere, systemic treatment can help shrink the cancer and, it is hoped, lead to remission.

> Systemic treatment decisions are made based on "personality features" of the cancer. The "meaner" the cancer's personality, the higher the risk of cancer spread, and the greater the need for systemic treatment. The milder the personality, the lower the risk of spread, and the smaller the need for systemic management.

3. **Complimentary, Alternative and Holistic Therapies** are directed to the whole person, including mind and spirit as well as body.

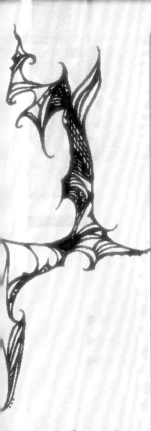

The goal of complementary medicine is to balance the whole person — physically, mentally, and emotionally — while conventional medicine does its work. For many people diagnosed with breast cancer, complementary medicine has helped to:

• relieve symptoms

• ease treatment side effects

• improve quality of life

319

At the end of January this year, I discovered a lump in my breast. After moving quickly to Doctor, then mammogram, then biopsy, it was confirmed that I had invasive ductile carcinoma. After one more procedure to determine if the lymph nodes were involved, surgery was scheduled.

Several years ago, I woke with pain in my left breast that felt like I had been run over by a truck. I went to the doctor, but nothing was discovered. It was at that time that I knew that I might lose that breast. I thought about it, and knew that, at that point, I could willingly give it up. I had nursed my babies; comforted my men and I could go forward with that knowledge.

While I knew I must have the surgery, and the loss of the breast would be the sacrifice for new life, I didn't want my breast tissue to be thrown away or discarded without thought or dignity. That was my greatest worry. I guess it came from reading about being whole when one dies. So, I asked if I could freeze the tissue and have it buried with me when it was indeed time to go. But I was told that because of the disease, it was State law that the breast be incinerated. That avenue being closed, I knew that I had to find a fitting ceremonial for my breast, so that I would not live with remorse over the loss. I needed to be proactive so my being would be honored in spite of State laws and sterile operating procedures.

After much thought, I had two of the strongest, most intelligent women that I know write me a prayer of thanks for my left breast. When I received the prayers, I was in awe of the intellect and intention that went with them.

I asked the Surgeon for two favors. The one that related to the prayers was to have these prayers accompany the breast tissue and be incinerated with it. He took this request seriously, assuring me that he knew the pathologist and would convey how important it was that this happen. Immediately, I felt better. I knew that I have found the right ceremonial and my grief over the loss would be short. My tissue would be put to rest honorably.

The days before my surgery, I printed the prayers out on beautiful, hand-made paper. I included the Sioux-English version of the Four Directions prayer and a really touching version of the Lord's Prayer. Then I made small packets of sage, cedar, sweet grass and tobacco (covering all my native spiritual bases), wrapped them in ribbons the colors of the Four Directions (black, red, white, yellow), and folding everything together in a packet, tied it with a red ribbon. I put this packet in a plastic storage bag with the instructions on both sides: "These are to go with and be burned with the breast tissue."

When I had made the decision that I would have a mastectomy instead of other options, I needed to push for a second request. But that request was dependent upon the doctor's knowledge and sensitivity to my need to honor my heritage. So, I asked him if he knew what a Sun Dance was. He said yes, he did know. So my second request was that he put two ceremonial piercing scars over the long scar that would go across my chest. The purpose to be my own legend that I had defied tradition and done the Sun Dance, whirling and dancing so hard that not only did I pull out the skewers and thongs, but that I pulled my breast off in the process.

My surgeon said he would be willing to do the ceremonial scarification. We talked about how that would have been done in the past. My assumption was an obsidian knife. He said he has a friend who is a flint knapper, and he would have him make him some knives for the surgery. I smiled. How nice to have such a caring medical professional who could sense the importance of those two little scars. Before surgery, when I finally saw my doctor, I asked him if he had the knives, expecting to be disappointed. He said that they were sterilized and ready to go. As I went to surgery, I took two packages with me. One was the packet to go with the tissue; the other was for the doctor and held sweet grass, the Lakota Christian Prayer to the Four Directions and the Four Directions prayer in Sioux and English. The smudging did not happened, but the sweet grass was hung over the surgical table in a gesture that affirmed my spirit.

At eight o'clock the next morning, the doctor appeared in my room for a post-surgical observation. He brought me the obsidian knives he had used and gave them to me. He said that, after he figured out how to hold them, it was easy, and he had done the whole surgery with the obsidian knives. That was a complete surprise and one that did indeed honor my spirit. Bless this man and his sensitivity!

The surgeon talked about how amazed he was at how easily and sharply the obsidian knives cut.

I was pleased that the surgeon could be mindful of my requests. Somehow, the need for some tradition familiar to my soul seemed to bubble up and asked to be heard; and it was. I was not raised on a reservation; my parents were neither Traditional nor Christian. Where this need came from, I didn't know. But I knew it was there and that it was from deep within my soul and I knew it had to be honored.

Two weeks after the surgery, I can say that it was fairly easy with minimal pain and little fatigue. As I looked upon my scar for the first time, I had no regrets, no sorrow. Each time, I look at my piercing scars, I smile. I give myself credit that I had made a good decision and had honored my breast and my needs in an intentional, thoughtful, spiritual way.

My teaching to others is this: Know what is good for your soul. Have faith that there is a God, Holy Spirit or Creator that is with us and embraces us in our humanness. Have faith that all things happen for a reason, and we are to learn and teach lessons from them. Honor your traditions, know yourself, be your best advocate. Take care of yourself. If you can't take care of yourself, you can't take care of others who are counting on you. Like the airlines say: "Put your own oxygen mask on first, next help those in need." First and last, pray for those you love and those who love you, the earth and its bounty. And give thanks for all the goodness in life. It is there waiting to be discovered.

Aho,
Rev. Anne Scissions, Rosebud Sioux

Types of breast cancer

Determining what type of breast cancer you have is an important step in treating the disease. Get the facts on types of breast cancer and how they differ.

If your doctor suspects that you have breast cancer, as part of the diagnosis process, your doctor will send a tissue sample (biopsy) to the lab for analysis. After the test results come in, you'll learn whether or not you have breast cancer and, if so, what type of breast cancer you have. Knowing what type of breast cancer plays a big role in selecting the type of treatment. Understand the differences among types of breast cancer, including common and less common types.

Common types of breast cancer

The most common types of breast cancer originate in either your breast's milk ducts (ductal carcinoma) or lobes (lobular carcinoma).

In situ breast cancer

In situ breast cancer is a type of cancer where the cells have not spread beyond the tissue where they began — they haven't invaded breast tissue around the duct or lobule.

Ductal carcinoma in situ (DCIS)

DCIS is abnormal cells in the lining of a milk duct that haven't spread. This is early-stage breast cancer. Some experts call DCIS a "precancerous" condition. Almost all women with DCIS can be successfully treated. However, if left untreated, DCIS could develop into invasive breast cancer.

Lobular carcinoma in situ (LCIS)

LCIS is abnormal cells in the lobule of your breast, but they haven't spread. According to the National Cancer Institute LCIS is NOT breast cancer, or a marker for the future development of cancer. If you have LCIS, you're at an increased risk of developing breast cancer in either breast in the future. In the breast that had the LCIS, you're more likely to develop invasive lobular breast cancer. If cancer develops in the other breast, it's equally likely that it could be invasive lobular or invasive ductal carcinoma.

Is breast cancer the most common cause of death for women?

No. Although many women get breast cancer, it is not a common cause of death. Heart disease is the number one cause of death among women age 40 and above, followed by stroke, lung cancer, and lung diseases. Breast cancer is the fifth leading cause of death. Each year, about 200,000 women are diagnosed with breast cancer. Many fewer women, around 40,000 each year, die from breast cancer.

Invasive breast cancer

Invasive (infiltrating) breast cancers are those that break free of where they originate and have spread beyond the layer, invading the surrounding tissues that support the ducts and lobules of your breast. The cancer cells can travel to other parts of your body, such as the lymph nodes.

Invasive ductal carcinoma (IDC).

IDC accounts for the majority of invasive breast cancers. If you have IDC, cancer cells form in the lining of your milk duct, break free of the ductal wall and invade surrounding breast tissue. The cancer cells may remain localized — staying near the site of origin — or they can spread (metastasize) even farther throughout your body, carried by your bloodstream or lymphatic system.

Invasive lobular carcinoma (ILC).

Although less common than IDC, this type of breast cancer acts in a similar manner. ILC starts in the milk-producing lobule and invades the surrounding breast tissue. It can also spread to more distant parts of your body. With ILC, you might not be able to detect a breast lump. You may perceive only a general thickening — or a sensation that your breast tissue feels different. ILC can be harder to detect by touch, and it's also less likely to appear on a mammogram.

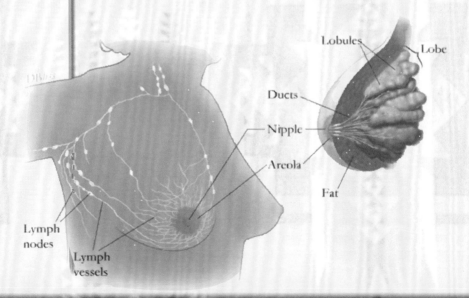

Lobules

Lobe

Ducts

Nipple

Areola

Fat

Lymph nodes

Lymph vessels

Less common types of breast cancer

Not all types of breast cancer originate in a duct or lobule. Less common types of breast cancer include:

Inflammatory breast cancer

This is a rare but aggressive type of breast cancer. The skin on your breast becomes red and swollen and may take on a thickened, pitted appearance — similar to an orange peel. This results from cancer cells blocking lymph vessels located near the surface of your breast.

Medullary carcinoma

This is a specific type of invasive breast cancer where the tumor's borders are clearly defined, the cancer cells are large, and immune system cells are present around the tumor.

Mucinous (colloid) carcinoma

With this type of invasive breast cancer, the cancer cells produce mucus and grow into a jelly-like tumor. The prognosis for mucinous carcinoma is better than for other, more common types of invasive breast cancer.

Paget's disease of the breast

This rare type of breast cancer affects your nipple and the dark area of skin surrounding your nipple (areola). It starts in a milk duct, as either an in situ or invasive cancer. If associated with carcinoma in situ, the prognosis is very good.

Tubular carcinoma

This rare type of breast cancer gets its name from the appearance of the cancer cells under a microscope. Though it's an invasive breast cancer, the outlook is more favorable than it is for invasive ductal carcinoma or invasive lobular carcinoma.

Cystosarcoma Phyllodes

A large, bulky tumor may be an indication of a phyllodes tumor. Phyllodes tumors develop in the connective tissue of the breast, rather than in a duct or lobule. The outlook for a phyllodes tumor is uncertain. If the tumor can't be removed, it's difficult to treat. This is a rare sarcoma of the breast.

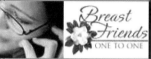

Metaplastic carcinoma

Metaplastic carcinoma represents less than 1 percent of all newly diagnosed breast cancers. This lesion tends to remain localized and contains several different types of cells that are not typically seen in other forms of breast cancer. Prognosis and treatment is the same as for invasive ductal carcinoma.

Sarcoma

A sarcoma is a tumor that develops in the connective tissue of the breast. This type of tumor is usually cancerous (malignant).

Micropapillary carcinoma

This invasive type of breast cancer tends to be relatively aggressive, often spreading to the lymph nodes even when very small.

Adenoid cystic carcinoma

This type of breast cancer is characterized by a large, local tumor. It's an invasive but slow-growing type of breast cancer that's unlikely to spread.

 National Breast and Cervical Cancer Early Detection Program

The Centers for Disease Control and Prevention (CDC) provides low-income, uninsured, and underserved women access to timely, high-quality screening and diagnostic services, to detect breast and cervical cancer at the earliest stages, through the National Breast and Cervical Cancer Early Detection Program (NBCCEDP).

The CDC contracts with states and tribal organizations to provide these services. For breast and cervical cancer screening services in your area call: 1 (800) CDC-INFO or go to:

http://apps.nccd.cdc.gov/cancercontacts/nbccedp/contacts.asp

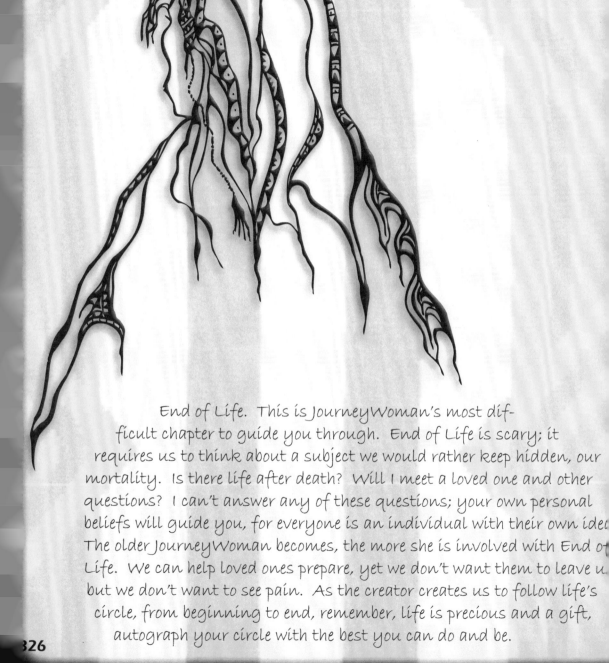

End of Life. This is JourneyWoman's most difficult chapter to guide you through. End of Life is scary; it
requires us to think about a subject we would rather keep hidden, our
mortality. Is there life after death? Will I meet a loved one and other
questions? I can't answer any of these questions; your own personal
beliefs will guide you, for everyone is an individual with their own idea.
The older JourneyWoman becomes, the more she is involved with End of
Life. We can help loved ones prepare, yet we don't want them to leave u.
but we don't want to see pain. As the creator creates us to follow life's
circle, from beginning to end, remember, life is precious and a gift,
autograph your circle with the best you can do and be.

End of Life

Every culture has a system of beliefs about death and ideas about life after death. These ideas, beliefs, and traditions may comfort a person facing death. But she also needs support, kindness, and honesty from her loved ones. You can help a dying person most by listening to her feelings and needs. If she wants to die at home—surrounded by the people she loves—rather than in a hospital, try to respect her wishes. If she wants to talk about death, try to be honest. Anyone who is dying usually knows it, partly by what her body tells her, and partly by the reactions she sees in those she loves. Let her talk openly about her fears, and about the joys and sorrows in her life. This way, when death comes, she may more easily accept it as the natural end of life.

Helping a loved one prepare for end of life may be the last great gift you can give to someone you care for. Making sure that they are not in pain and are comfortable, and helping make sure they have quality health care, including palliative care, are steps that help all involved face end of life.

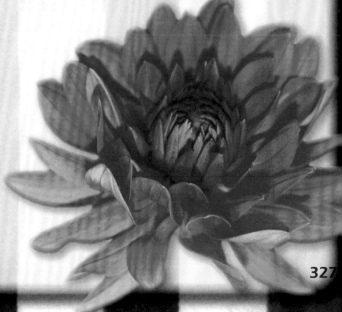

Caring for Someone Who Is Near Death

At some point there is nothing more that can be done for a person with a disease such as cancer. You may know this time has come when:

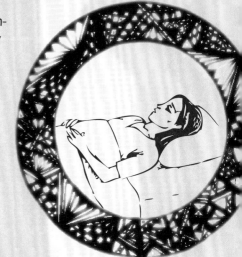

- the body starts to fail.
- medical treatment is no longer effective or is not available.
- the person says she is ready to die.

If the sick person wants to remain at home, you can help her die with dignity by:

- giving comfort.
- having family and friends stay with her.
- allowing her to make decisions.
- helping her prepare for death. It may help her to talk about death, about fears of dying, and about worries for the family's future. It does not help to act as if she is not dying. Assure her that you will do what you can to prevent pain and discomfort. Talk about funeral arrangements if she wishes.

End of Life Care Questions & Answers
(from www.cancer.gov)

At the end of life, care continues. The care focuses on making the your loved one comfortable. Medications and treatments to control pain and other symptoms , such as constipation, nausea, and shortness of breath continue to be needed for many. Some people remain at home during this time, while others enter a hospital or other facility. Either way, services are available to help your loved one and their families with the medical, psychological, and spiritual issues surrounding dying. A hospice often provides such services.

The time at the end of life is different for each person. Each individual has unique needs for information and support. The patient's and family's questions and concerns about the end of life should be discussed with the health care team as they arise.

The following information can help answer some of the questions that many patients, their family members, and caregivers have about the end of life.

How long is your loved one expected to live?

Patients and their family members often want to know how long a person is expected to live. This is a hard question to answer. Factors such as whether your loved one has other illnesses can affect what will happen. Although doctors may be able to make an estimate based on what they know about the patient, they might be hesitant to do so. Doctors may be concerned about over- or under-estimating one's life span. They also might be fearful of instilling false hope or destroying a person's hope.

What are some ways that caregivers can provide emotional comfort to the patient?

Everyone has different needs, but some emotions are common to most dying patients. These include fear of abandonment and fear of being a burden. They also have concerns about loss of dignity and loss of control. Some ways caregivers can provide comfort are as follows:

- Keep the person company—talk, watch movies, read, or just be with your loved one.
- Allow your loved one to express fears and concerns about dying, such as leaving family and friends behind. Be prepared to listen.
- Be willing to reminisce about your loved one's life.
- Avoid withholding difficult information. Most people prefer to be included in discussions about issues that concern them.
- Reassure your loved one that you will honor advance directives, such as living wills.
- Ask if there is anything you can do.
- Respect the person's need for privacy.

When caring for a loved one at home, when should the caregiver call for professional help?

When caring for a loved one at home, there may be times when the caregiver needs assistance from the health care team. A caregiver can contact your loved-one's doctor or nurse for help in any of the following situations:

- The patient is in pain that is not relieved by the prescribed dose of pain medication,
- The patient shows discomfort, such as grimacing or moaning,
- The patient is having trouble breathing and seems upset,
- The patient is unable to urinate or empty the bowels,
- The patient has fallen,
- The patient is very depressed or talking about committing suicide,
- The caregiver has difficulty giving medication to the patient,
- The caregiver is overwhelmed by caring for the patient, or is too grieved or afraid to be with the patient, or
- At any time the caregiver does not know how to handle a situation.

Palliative Care

Palliative care is an approach that improves the quality of life of people and their families facing the problem associated with life-threatening illness, through the prevention and relief of suffering by means of early identification and assessment and treatment of pain and other problems, physical, psychosocial and spiritual. Palliative care:

- provides relief from pain and other distressing symptoms;

- affirms life and regards dying as a normal process;

- intends neither to hasten or postpone death;

- integrates the psychological and spiritual aspects of patient care;

- offers a support system to help loved ones live as actively as possible until death;

- offers a support system to help the family cope during the patients illness and in their own bereavement;

- uses a team approach to address the needs of patients and their families, including bereavement counselling, if indicated;

- will enhance quality of life, and may also positively influence the course of illness;

- can be used early in an illness along with other therapies that are meant to prolong life, such as chemotherapy or radiation therapy.

Hospice care is a type of palliative care for those facing the end of life.

The goal of palliative care i to prevent and relieve sufferin and to improve quality of life fo people facing serious, comple illness.

330

How to get Palliative Care

The first step is to talk to your own doctor. Most of the time, you have to ask your health care provider for a palliative care referral to get palliative care services. Whether you are in the hospital or at home, a palliative care team can help you. Following are some tips to help you talk to your doctor:

- Tell your health care provider you are considering palliative care and ask what palliative services are available in your area.

- Ask your health care provider to explain your illness as well as past, current, and future treatments and procedures.

- Explain to your health care provider what quality of life means to you. This list may include being able to spend time with loved ones, having pain and other distressing symptoms aggressively treated, the ability to make your own decisions for care and your preferred location of treatments (home vs. in the hospital).

- Be sure your health care provider is aware of any personal, religious, or cultural beliefs, values, or practices that are important to consider in your care and treatment decisions.

- Tell your health care provider what curative treatments you may or may not want, such as resuscitation if your heart were to stop, being placed on a mechanical ventilator if your lungs were to fail, undergoing dialysis if your kidneys were to fail, and artificial nutrition by a feeding tube if you were unable to eat.

- If you have completed a living will or health care proxy, be sure to inform your health care team and provide him or her with a copy.

- If you are suffering with pain and other symptoms due to a serious illness, ask your health care provider for a palliative care referral.

Pain

In the later stages of life (and other serious illnesses like cancer), pain may become a part of daily life. Pain can be caused by many things, such as:

- not being able to move
- pressure sores
- infections
- headache
- nerve pains
- swelling of the legs and feet

Many health care providers are trained in taking care of the pain when it is most important to make someone comfortable (less pain), especially if they are nearing the end of life. This is called "Palliative Care". If you or a loved one in need of palliative care, talk to your doctor.

The following medicines may be used to control pain that comes day after day (chronic pain). Take the medicines regularly, according to instructions. If you wait until the pain has become very bad, the medicines will not work as well.

- mild pain medicine
- ibuprofen or codeine—if you need something stronger
- oral morphine—if the pain is very bad

Treatment for pain, without medicines:

- Try relaxation exercises, meditation, or prayer.
- Try to think about other things.
- Play music, or have someone read aloud or tell stories.
- For pain from swelling in the hands and feet, try raising the swollen part. For headache, keep the room dark and quiet.
- Acupressure may help some kinds of pain.
- For a burning feeling in the hands and feet caused by nerve pain, put the body part in water.
- For skin that hurts to touch, line the bed with soft covers and pillows. Be gentle when touching the person.

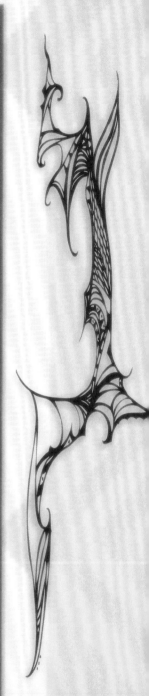

Accepting Death

Elders are often more ready to accept their own approaching death than are those who love them. Persons who have lived fully are not usually afraid to die. Death is, after all, the natural end of life. We often make the mistake of trying to keep a dying person alive as long as possible, no matter what the cost. Sometimes this adds to the suffering and strain for both the person and their family. There are many occasions when the kindest thing to do is not to hunt for 'better medicine' or a 'better doctor' but to be close to and supporting of the person who is dying. Let them know that you are glad for all the time, the joy and the sorrow you have shared, and that you, too, are able to accept her death. In the last hours, love and acceptance will do far more good than medicines.

Old or chronically ill persons would often prefer to be at home, in familiar surroundings with those they love, than to be in a hospital. At times this may mean that the person will die earlier. But this is not necessarily bad. We must be sensitive to the person's feelings and needs, and to our own. Sometimes a person who is dying suffers more knowing that the cost of keeping her barely alive causes their family to go into debt or children to hunger. She may ask simply to be allowed to die —and there are times when this may be the wise decision. Yet some people fear death. Even if they are suffering, the known world may be hard to leave behind. Every culture has a system of beliefs about death and ideas about life after death. These ideas, beliefs, and traditions may offer some comfort in facing death. Death may come upon a person suddenly and unexpectedly or may be long-awaited. How to help someone we love accept and prepare for his approaching death is not an easy matter. Often the most we can do is offer support, kindness, and understanding.

The death of a younger person or child is never easy. Both kindness and honesty are important. A child—or anyone—who is dying often knows it, partly by what her own body tells her and partly by the fear or despair she sees in those who love her. Whether young or old, if a person who is dying asks for the truth, tell her, but tell her gently, and leave some room for hope. Weep if you must, but let her know that even as you love her, and because you love her, you have the strength to let her leave you. This will give her the strength and courage to accept leaving you. To let her know these things you need not say them. You need to feel and show them.

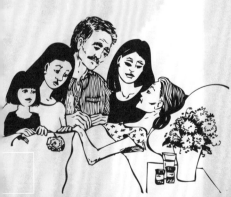

We must all die. Perhaps the most important job of the healer is to help people accept death when it can or should no longer be avoided, and to help ease the suffering of those who still live.

What are the signs that death is approaching?
What can the caregiver do to make your loved-one comfortable?

Families and friends often find themselves as the main caregiver for someone who is facing death. Certain signs and symptoms can help a caregiver anticipate when death is near. They are described below, along with suggestions for managing them. Not every person experiences each of the signs and symptoms and having one or more of these symptoms does not necessarily indicate that the patient is close to death.   If possible, contact a local hospice service or your doctor or clinic if you have questions.

Drowsiness, increased sleep, and/or unresponsiveness (caused by changes in metabolism). The caregiver and family members can plan visits and activities for times when the loved one is alert. It is important to speak directly to your loved one and talk as if the person can hear, even if there is no response. Most people are still able to hear after they are no longer able to speak. They should not be shaken if they do not respond.

Confusion about time, place, and/or identity of loved ones; restlessness; visions of people and places that are not present; pulling at bed linens or clothing (caused in part by changes in metabolism). Gently remind your loved one of the time, date, and people who are with them. If the patient is agitated, do not attempt to restrain the patient. Be calm and reassuring. Speaking calmly may help.

Decreased socialization and withdrawal (caused by decreased oxygen to the brain, decreased blood flow, and mental preparation for dying). Speak to your loved one directly. Let the him or her know you are there for them. She may be aware and able to hear, but unable to respond. Professionals advise that giving the patient permission to "let go" can be helpful.

Decreased need for food and fluids, and loss of appetite . Allow your loved one to choose if and when to eat or drink. Ice chips, water, or juice may be refreshing if the patient can swallow. Keep the patient's mouth and lips moist with swabs and lip balm.

Loss of bladder or bowel control (caused by the relaxing of muscles). Keep your loved one as clean, dry, and comfortable as possible. Place disposable pads on the bed beneath their body and remove them when they become soiled.

Turning the head toward a light source (caused by decreasing vision). Leave soft, indirect lights on in the room.

Darkened urine or decreased amount of urine (caused by slowing of kidney function and/or decreased fluid intake). Caregivers can consult a member of the patient's doctor or health care team about the need to insert a catheter to avoid blockage. A member of the health care team can teach the caregiver how to take care of the catheter if one is needed.

Skin becomes cool to the touch, particularly the hands and feet; skin may become bluish in color, especially on the underside of the body (caused by decreased circulation). Blankets can be used to warm the your loved one. Although the skin may be cool, he or she are usually not aware of feeling cold. Caregivers should avoid warming your loved one with electric blankets or heating pads, which can cause burns.

Rattling or gurgling sounds while breathing, which may be loud; breathing that is irregular and shallow; decreased number of breaths per minute; breathing that alternates between rapid and slow (caused by congestion from decreased fluid intake, a buildup of waste products in the body, and/or a decrease in circulation to the organs). Breathing may be easier if the patient's body is turned to the side and pillows are placed beneath the head and behind the back. Although labored breathing can sound very distressing to the caregiver, gurgling and rattling sounds do not cause discomfort to the patient. An external source of oxygen may benefit some people. If your loved one is able to swallow, ice chips also may help. In addition, a cool mist humidifier may help make the patient's breathing more comfortable.

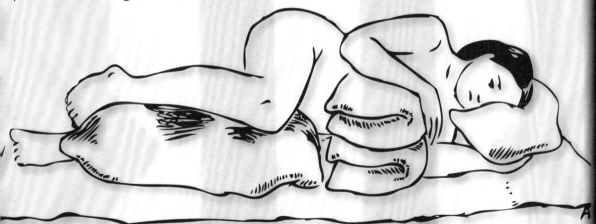

Increased difficulty controlling pain (caused by progression of the disease). It is important to provide pain medications as the patient's doctor has prescribed. The caregiver should contact the doctor if the prescribed dose does not seem to relieve the pain. With the help of the doctor and health care team, caregivers can also try alternative pain relief such as massage and relaxation techniques to help with pain.

What needs to be done after someone has died?

After the someone has passed away, there is no need to hurry with arrangements. Family members and caregivers may wish to sit with their loved one, talk, or pray. When the family is ready, the following steps can be taken.

- Place the body on its back with one pillow under the head. If necessary, caregivers or family members may wish to put the love one's dentures or other artificial parts in place.

- If the loved one is in a hospice program, follow the guidelines provided by the program. A caregiver or family member can request a hospice nurse to verify the patient's death.

- Contact the appropriate authorities in accordance with local regulations. If the loved one has requested not to be resuscitated through a Do-Not-Resuscitate (DNR) order or other mechanism, do not call 911.

- Contact the loved one's doctor and funeral home.

- When the family is ready, call other family members, friends, and clergy.

- Provide or ask for emotional support for family members and friends to cope with their loss.

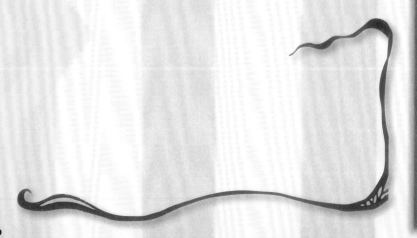

Resources:

The National Cancer Institute (NCI)'s Cancer Information Service (CIS) at 1–800–4–CANCER (1–800–422–6237).

www.cancer.gov

Aging With Dignity, Five Wishes Project
http://www.agingwithdignity.org/5wishes.html

http://www.getpalliativecare.org/

http://www.nlm.nih.gov/medlineplus/endof-lifeissues.html

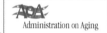

http://www.aarp.org/families/end_life/

http://www.agingwithdignity.org/

http://www.aoa.gov/eldfam/How_To_Find/Agencies/Agencies.asp

www.scu.edu/fow
Finding Our Way: Living with Dying in America - The Online Course.

www.painfoundation.org
Online resourse for people with pain, their families, friends, care-givers.

www.aarp.org/confacts/cargive
- Help for Caregivers
.

www.lastacts.org
resource for families/consumers.

List of Words

Here is a list of words that may be difficult to understand. Knowing what these words mean can help you use the book better. Some of the words included here are explained in the chapters, but many are not.

A

Abdomen =The part of the body that contains the stomach, liver, guts and reproductive organs. The belly.

Abdominal (ab-dom-in-uhl) = The area right below your stomach.

Abnormal bleeding = Bleeding that is different from what is usual, natural, or average. Not normal.

Abortion = When a woman does something to end a pregnancy.

Abscess = A raised, red, painful lump on the skin that is filled with pus (for example, a boil).

Abstinence (ab-stu-nuns) = Not having sex of any kind.

Abuse = When someone hurts another person's body (physical abuse), humiliates or insults a person (emotional abuse) or makes a person do sexual things against her will (sexual abuse).

Access (to health services) = When health services are available, and a woman has the freedom, the money, and the time to use them.

Access = The ability of people to reach or use health services. Barriers to access may be influenced by: (1) a person's locality, income or knowledge of services available; (2) the availability or acceptability of existing services.

Acne (ak-nee) = Bumps on the skin caused by hormone changes during puberty.

Acute = When something happens suddenly, lasts for a short time, and is usually serious or strong—for example, acute pain or acute infection. Compare with chronic.

Addiction = This is a condition where you become dependent on, or can't do without, physical substances or an activity to the point that stopping it is very hard and causes severe physical and mental reactions. Substances you can become addicted to include tobacco, alcohol, and drugs (both illegal and prescription drugs). Activities that can be addicting include lying, stealing, and gambling. Addiction can be treated with counseling and, in some cases, medication.

Addiction = When the body feels a strong need for alcohol or a drug.

Adenocarcinoma (AD-in-o-kar-sin-O-ma) = Cancer that begins in cells that line the inside of organs. These organs make substances like hormones or milk. Most breast cancers are of this type. They begin in cells that make milk or in the cells that drain the breast milk.

Adolescence (add-ul-ess-ence) = The period of life from puberty to adulthood when a young person "grows up."

Adrenal glands (a-dree-nal) = A pair of small glands, each of which sits on top of the kidneys. These glands produce hormones that help to control the body's heart rate, blood pressure, the way food gets used, and other functions. They make the hormone adrenaline, which the body releases in response to stress.

Adrenal glands = The adrenal glands are two small glands that sit on top of the kidneys. They make hormones that help control heart rate, blood pressure and the way the body uses food.

Advanced Care Directives = These are written documents meant to communicate the conditions under which individuals wish to receive or refuse certain treatment or stop life-support treatment, in the event that they are no longer legally competent to make their own decisions.

Aerobic exercise (uh-roh-bick ex-er-syze) = Aerobic exercise burns fat, gets your heart rate going (you will be able to feel it beating faster) and makes your heart muscle stronger. It also increases the number of blood cells you have, which helps your blood carry more needed oxygen to blood vessels throughout your body.

Age of consent = The minimum age for marrying and sexual contact (varies from state-to-state).

AIDS = This disease hurts the immune system, (the body's way of protecting itself), so that it becomes easy to get dangerous infections and cancers. It is caused by the HIV infection. Learn more about HIV and AIDS.

AIDS (acquired immune deficiency syndrome) = A disease caused by the HIV virus usually passed through sex. A person has AIDS (rather than just being infected with HIV) when the immune system gets so weak it can no longer fight off common infections and illnesses.

Alkylating chemotherapy drugs = Alkylating chemotherapy drugs kill cancer cells by stopping them from dividing. Commonly used alkylating chemotherapy drugs include cyclophosphamide, busulphan, melphalan, mytomycin-C, and the platinum-based (cis-platinum, carboplatin) drugs. These drugs are used to treat slow-growing cancers.

Allergies (al-ur-jee) = When someone has an allergic reaction to something, the body's immune system (which protects the body from outside substances), gives off a much bigger response than it normally would. The result is to have a reaction, such as sneezing or trouble breathing, to things that are usually not harmful, such as certain foods or animals.

Allergy, allergic reaction, allergic shock = A problem—such as itching, sneezing, hives or rash, and sometimes difficult breathing or shock—that affects certain people when specific things are breathed in, eaten, injected, or touched.

Amenorrhea (uh-men-or-ee-uh) = When a woman does not have periods, either ever (after age 16) or they stop as a result of: pregnancy, too much exercise, extreme obesity or not enough body fat, or emotional distress.

Americans with Disabilities Act (ADA) = The ADA is a federal law that prohibits employers from discriminating against qualified individuals with disabilities in the job application process, hiring, firing, advancement, compensation, job training, and other privileges provided in the workplace.

Anaerobic exercise = Anaerobic exercise involves building muscle strength in different parts of your body. This type of exercise goes along well with aerobic exercise because having stronger muscles helps you to burn more calories. This will also help you look toned and feel strong.

Analgesics (ah-nuhl-jee-zicks) = Analgesics are meant to relieve pain. These pain relievers don't get rid of what causes your pain, rather they block the nerve pathways that send pain signals from the body part to the brain so that you don't hurt as much.

Anatomic pathology -The study and diagnosis of disease based on structural changes in cells, tissues and organs.

Anemia = A disease in which the blood gets weak and thin because it lacks red blood cells. This happens when blood is lost or destroyed faster than the body can replace it.

Anemia (uh-nee-mee-uh) = When there are fewer red blood cells in the blood, it can cause health problems. This is measured by a decrease in what is called hemoglobin, which both provides the red color and moves oxygen through

339

List of Words

the body. There are many different types of anemia.

Anesthesia = General anesthesia is when you are given medicine to make you sleep during an operation so you will not feel pain. Local anesthesia is when you are given an injection in one place so that you will not feel pain in that area.

Anorexia nervosa (an-or-eck-see-uh nur-vo-suh) = An eating disorder causes people to refuse to stay at a healthy body weight by not eating. People with anorexia have a fear of gaining weight and a picture of what their body looks like in their mind that is not what it really is.

Antacid = Medicine used to control too much stomach acid and to calm stomach upset. See heartburn.

Antibiotic (an-ty-by-ah-tiks) = Antibiotics fight bacterial infections by killing bacteria or stopping it from growing. Antibiotics can help your body's immune system fight off infections. If you have ever had strep throat, your doctor probably gave you an antibiotic to take.

Antibiotic = Medicine used to fight infection caused by bacteria.

Antibodies (an-ty-bod-eez) = Proteins produced by white blood cells to fight bacteria, viruses, and other foreign substances.

Antibodies = Substances the body makes to fight infection.

Antiretrovirals = Medicines used to help people with AIDS stay healthier and live longer. They do not cure AIDS.

Anus = The opening of the intestine where waste (stool) leaves the body.

Anxiety = Feeling nervous or worried.

Appendicitis = An infection of the appendix.

Appendix = A finger-like sac attached to the large intestine.

Areola = The dark, bumpy area around the nipple.

Aromatase inhibitors = These medicines stop the body from producing the hormone estrogen. Aromatase inhibitors are used to treat most women with breast cancer, because estrogen makes the tumor grow. Aromatase inhibitors can also be used to treat infertility.

ART = AntiRetroviral Therapy ART is a combination of 3 or more antiretroviral medicines taken every day by people with AIDS. (It is also called HAART or Triple Therapy.)

Arteries (ar-tuh-reez) = Thick-walled blood vessels that carry blood away from the heart to other parts of the body.

Artery = A thin, tube-like vessel that carries blood from the heart through the body. Arteries have a pulse. Veins, which return blood to the heart, have no pulse.

Arthritis = Pain and swelling in the joints.

Asphyxiation (as-fix-eeh-ay-shun) = Suffocation or smothering.

Aspiration -(ass-per-AY-shun) = Taking out fluid or cells from a lump with a hollow needle and a syringe. This may be done to see if the lump is just a fluid-filled cyst. It can also remove cells to see if they are normal cells or cancer cells.

Asthma (az-muh) = When your airways are inflamed, causing you to wheeze, feel shortness of breath, cough and feel a tightness in your chest.

Asthma = A disease of the lungs, which causes attacks of difficult breathing. There is often a hissing or wheezing sound when a person breathes out.

Asymptomatic (AY-simp-tuh-MAT-ik) = Having no signs or symptoms of disease. For example, an asymptomatic lump has no associated pain, swelling, or bleeding.

Atrophy = A decrease in size or wasting away of cells, tissue, organs or muscle.

List of Words

Attention Deficit Disorder (say: A-D-D) = A behavioral condition that makes it hard for people to pay attention and concentrate.

Autism (ah-tiz-em) = Disorder in the brain that affects both verbal and nonverbal communication (speaking and non-speaking) skills.

Autonomic nervous system = The autonomic nervous system is a branch of the peripheral nervous system that controls most body functions that happen automatically. Examples include: blood pressure, heart rate, sweating, bowel and bladder function.

Axilla = The axilla is commonly known as the armpit. The lymph nodes that filter lymph fluid for the upper part of your body are located in the axilla. For the lower limbs, the filtering lymph nodes are located in the groin.

Axillary (AK-sil-air-ee) = This refers to the underarm area, including the lymph nodes in that area.

Axillary lymph nodes (AK-sil-air-ee LIMF nodes) = Lymph nodes found in the armpit area. They filter the lymph fluid that drains from the breast through the lymph vessels and goes back to the heart.

Axon = The long, hairlike extension of a nerve cell that carries impulses from the cell body to another nerve cell.

B

Bacteria = Germs that cause many different infectious diseases. Bacteria are too small to see without a microscope.

Bacterial vaginosis = An infection of the vagina caused by bacteria.

Bag of waters = The sac (or amniotic sac) inside the womb that holds the baby. When the sac breaks and releases fluid, this usually means that labor has begun.

Barrier methods = Family planning methods that prevent pregnancy by keeping the sperm from reaching the egg.

Bartholin's glands = Small glands on either side of the vaginal opening that make a liquid to keep the vagina wet.

Behavioral Therapy = A psychological technique used to help individuals change negative behavior.

Benign (beh-NINE) = Has no signs of cancer. The growth of the cells in the tumor, cyst, lump, tissue, or cells is under control. There is no spread to nearby tissue or to other parts of the body.

Benign = Generally applied to a tumor or neoplasm that is not malignant. Benign tumors don't spread to other organs, which is their main distinction from malignant tumors (cancer).

Bilateral (by-LAT-uh-rul) = Affecting both the right and left sides of body.

Bilateral mastectomy (by-LA-ter-ul mass-TECK-tum-ee) = Surgery that removes all of both breasts.

Bile = A liquid found in the gallbladder that helps digest fatty foods.

Biopsy = A biopsy is a procedure where cells or tissues are removed from the body so they can be examined under a microscope to look for unhealthy cells. During a biopsy, a doctor can remove an entire lump or remove a sample of tissue. A doctor can also use a needle to remove fluid or a small tissue sample. This procedure is called a needle biopsy.

Biopsy = When a piece of tissue or fluid is taken from somewhere on or in the body and examined to see if it is healthy or diseased.

Birth canal See vagina.

Birth control pills = A hormonal family planning method.

Birth control See family planning.

List of Words

Birth defects = Physical or mental problems a child is born with, like a cleft lip or cleft palate, or an extra finger or toe.

Birth spacing = Using family planning methods to space your children.

Bisphosphonates = Bisphosphonates are medicines that can be used to treat osteoporosis. These drugs prevent cells that cause bone decay from being absorbed into the bones.

Blackouts = When you are using too much alcohol or other drugs and wake up not knowing what happened.

Bladder = The bag inside the abdomen that stores urine. As the bladder fills, it stretches and gets bigger. It is the organ that stores urine produced by the kidneys.

Blood clots = Soft, dark red, shiny lumps in the blood that look like liver.

Blood pressure = As blood is pumped from your heart through your body, the blood exerts force or pressure against the blood vessel walls. Your blood pressure reading is a measure of this pressure. When that reading goes above a certain point, it is called high blood pressure or hypertension, which can be lowered and controlled with medication and changes in lifestyle and diet.

Blood pressure = The force or pressure of the blood upon the walls of the blood vessels (arteries and veins). Blood pressure varies with the age and health of the person.

Blood test = This is either done by using a finger prick to get a few drops or by using a needle to get a larger amount of blood. Blood tests are used to check for many different diseases and viruses.

Blood transfusion = When someone's blood is given to another person, in a vein and using a special needle, to replace blood the person may have lost.

Bone marrow = Soft tissue found inside bones from which blood cells are produced and released into the bloodstream.

Bowel = The bowel is part of the digestive system and includes the small and large intestine. The small intestine is where most food is digested and absorbed into the body. The large intestine absorbs water into the body and prepares feces to leave the body.

BRCA1 = A gene that maintains normal cell growth. If the gene becomes abnormal, then cell growth can become abnormal. The cells can grow out of control, forming a cancer. A woman who inherits an abnormal version of BRCA1 has a higher risk of getting breast and ovarian cancer.

BRCA2 = A gene that normally helps to prevent cell growth, especially the growth of abnormal or defective cells. A person who inherits an abnormal version of BRCA2 has a higher risk of getting breast, ovarian, or prostate cancer.

Breakthrough pain = Pain that shows up in between doses of regular pain control medicine. It can happen for no reason that we know of. It can come from activity. Or it can happen because the dose of regular medicine is not strong enough.

Breast exam = Checking the breasts for lumps that might be a sign of cancer.

Breast infection (mastitis) = An infection inside the breast that can be very painful for the mother, and make it difficult for the baby to suck the nipple.

Breast reconstruction = Surgery to rebuild the breast's shape after a mastectomy.

Breast-conserving surgery = An operation that completely removes the breast cancer along with a rim of normal breast tissue around it. Most of the normal breast is saved. There are 3 main ways this surgery is done: lumpectomy, quadrantectomy, and segmental mastectomy.

Breech = When a baby is born feet or buttocks first, instead of head first. This can be dangerous for the baby.

Bronchitis = An infection of the large tubes in the lungs.

Bulimia nervosa (buh-lee-mee-uh nur-vo-suh) = An illness defined by uncontrollable overeating, usually followed by making oneself throw up or purge (get rid of food) in other ways.

C

CA-125 = A protein that can be made by abnormal ovary cells. It can be a tumor marker. If it is present in high levels in the blood or in other body fluids or tissues, it may be a sign of ovarian cancer.

Caffeine = A drug found in coffee, tea, and cola drinks that causes the heart to beat faster and makes a person feel more awake.

Calcification = Calcium that builds up in the tissues of the breast. It looks like grains of salt and can be seen on a mammogram. It cannot be found by touch. Calcifications are tiny flecks of calcium—like grains of salt—in the soft tissue of the breast that can sometimes indicate the presence of an early breast cancer. Calcifications usually can't be felt, but they appear on a mammogram. Depending on how they're clustered and their shape, size, and number, your doctor may want to do further tests. Big calcifications— "macrocalcifications"—are usually not associated with cancer. Groups of small calcifications huddled together, called "clusters of microcalcifications," are associated with extra breast cell activity. Most of the time this is non-cancerous extra cell growth, but sometimes clusters of microcalcifications can occur in areas of early cancer.

Calcium = A mineral found in some foods that helps make bones and teeth strong.

Cancer = Cancer is a group of diseases in which cells divide without control. Cancer cells can spread through the bloodstream and lymphatic system to other parts of the body. There are at least 200 different kinds of cancers, which can grow in almost any organ of the body. Cancers are usually defined by the name of the organ from which they arise, e.g., breast cancer, but sometimes by the type of cells comprising the cancer (e.g. leukemia, arising from primitive blood cells).

Cancer continuum = The spectrum of cancer-related experience, including prevention, early detection, diagnosis, treatment, living with cancer, and end of life.

Cancer control = The totality of measures taken to reduce the impact of cancer, including prevention, early detection and screening, treatment, rehabilitation, and palliative care.

Cancer treatment = Specific treatment measures taken to cure cancer, or ameliorate its major effects. Cancer treatment includes surgery, radiation therapy, chemotherapy, hormone therapy, and pain relief measures.

Capillaries (kap-il-air-eez) = Tiny blood vessels that branch through body tissues to deliver oxygen and nutrients and carry away waste products.

Carcinogen = A chemical, infectious or physical agent that can cause cancer.

Carcinoma = A cancer that arises from epithelial tissue (the lining of an internal organ or the skin).

Caregiver = A voluntary caregiver is a person, usually a family or community member, who looks after a person with a disability or health problem, and who is unpaid.

Cataracts = An eye problem in which the lens or covering of the eye becomes cloudy, mak-

List of Words

ing it more and more difficult to see. The dark, round, center part of the eye (pupil) looks gray or white when a light is shined on it.

Cerebral Palsy (se-reeb-rul pahl-zee) = When injuries to the brain cause damage to the nerves and loss of movement. The injuries happen while a baby is growing in the womb or near the time the baby is born.

Cervix (sur-vicks) = The narrow entryway between the vagina and the uterus. The cervix is the part of the uterus which extends into the vagina. It is the passageway between the uterus and vagina. The cervix serves as a boundary between outside of the body and the inside of the body, keeping substances like sperm out of the uterus.
 The muscles of the cervix are flexible so that it can expand to let a baby pass through when he/she is being born.

Cervix = The opening of the womb at the back of the vagina.

Cesarean section = When it is dangerous for a baby to be born through the vagina, the woman can have an operation in which her abdomen is cut open and the baby is taken out.

Chemotherapy (key-mo-ther-uh-pee) = The use of a chemical or chemotherapeutic agent to treat cancer or to limit its further progress. Treatment with anticancer drugs that destroy cancer cells. Chemotherapy is often known as chemo, a term used for medicines to treat cancer. Cancer happens when cells in the body develop wrong and grow in an uncontrolled way. Since cancer cells tend to divide very fast, chemotherapy works by getting in the way of these cells dividing and trying to stop the cancer from spreading. Sometimes chemo can cure the disease by helping to get rid of all the cancer cells in the body.

Chlamydia (kluh-mid-ee-uh) = The most common sexually transmitted (passed) disease in the U.S. Many women do not have symptoms of chlamydia. Untreated, chlamydia can lead to pelvic infection and infertility (inability to become pregnant). People who are sexually active and who have multiple sexual partners are at the highest risk of getting chlamydia. A doctor can test and treat people for chlamydia. Learn more about this STD.

Cholesterol (ke-leh-ste-ral) = A soft, waxy substance that is present in all parts of the body. It helps make cell membranes, some hormones, and vitamin D. The liver makes all the cholesterol a person's body needs, so eating too much from animal foods like meats and whole milk dairy products can make your cholesterol go up.

Chromosomes = Tiny rod-shaped pieces in the nucleus of a cell that hold the DNA code needed to build a human. Most human cells have 46 chromosomes including 22 pairs of autosomes and the X and Y sex chromosomes. Sperm cells have 23 chromosomes.

Chronic = Refers to diseases and symptoms that continue or occur again and again for a long time without change. Something that lasts for a long time, or that occurs often. Compare with acute.

Chronic Fatigue Syndrome = A very severe and long-term feeling of weakness and being tired, even after getting rest.

Circulation = Blood flowing through the arteries and veins in the body.

Circulatory system = The heart, the blood, and the system of blood vessels that moves blood through the body.

Cleft lip and palate = Abnormal growth of the lip and or roof of the mouth that happens before a baby is born. This can affect the way the lip looks, and also cause problems feeding as an infant and learning to speak.

Clinical breast examination (CBE) -The process of examining the breasts by a carefully trained health professional in order to detect early signs of breast cancer, when potentially still curable.

Clinical depression = Clinical, or major, depression is an illness that involves the body, mood, and thoughts. It affects the way a person functions, eats and sleeps, feels about herself, and thinks about things. Depression is not the same as a passing "down" mood. It is not a sign of personal weakness or a condition that can be willed or wished away. This condition can be treated with medication and counseling.

Clinical trial = A research activity used to evaluate the efficacy and safety of promising approaches to disease prevention and control. Interventional trials determine whether experimental treatments or new ways of using known therapies are safe and effective under controlled environments. Observational trials address health issues in large groups of people or populations in natural settings.

Clitoris = The part of the vulva most sensitive to touch.

Clotting = The process by which the body forms a plug to seal damaged blood vessels and stop bleeding.

Colostomy = A colostomy is a surgical incision into the colon to make an opening to the outside of the abdomen. This opening serves as a substitute anus, allowing the intestines to get rid of bodily waste until the colon can heal. Waste falls into a collection pouch outside of the body.

Colostrum = The yellow-colored milk that comes from the breasts for the first 2 or 3 days after birth.

Community = A collective of people identified by their common values and mutual concern for the development and wellbeing of their group or geographical area.

Community health workers = Health workers who work in the community and may or may not have formal training.

Complementary and alternative medicine [also called CAM] = Forms of treatment that are used in addition to, or instead of, standard treatments. Their purpose is to strengthen your whole mind and body to maximize your health, energy, and well-being. These practices are not considered "standard" medical approaches. They include dietary supplements, vitamins, herbal preparations, special teas, massage therapy, acupuncture, spiritual healing, visualization, and meditation.

Complementary and alternative medicine (CAM) = refers to a broad range of therapies used both to treat and prevent disease that are not considered to be part of conventional medicine.

Complete remission = When a cancer survivor shows no signs or symptoms of cancer.

Complications = Problems or things that go wrong.

Compress = A folded cloth or pad that is put on a part of the body. The compress may be soaked in hot or cold liquid.

Conception = When the egg and sperm join to begin making a baby.

Condom (kon-dum) = Made of thin rubber, designed to cover the penis during sex; also used to prevent the spread of some STDs. Not 100% error proof; A narrow bag of thin rubber that the man wears on his penis during sex. The bag traps the man's sperm so that it cannot get into the woman's womb and make her pregnant. Condoms also help prevent the spread of sexually transmitted infections including HIV/AIDS.

Constipation = When a person has a difficult time passing stool.

Contagious = An illness that can be spread

List of Words

easily from one person to another.

Contraception (birth control) = Any method of preventing pregnancy. See family planning.

Contraceptive gel = A slippery jelly or cream that is put into the vagina before sex to prevent pregnancy.

Contractions (pains, labor pains) = When the womb squeezes and becomes hard. Contractions open the cervix and help push the baby out of the womb.

Conventional treatment [also called conventional therapy] = An accepted and widely used treatment for a certain type of disease. This is based on the results of past research and experience. This term is often used as a contrast to alternative, or complementary, treatment. You usually get conventional treatment from doctors and nurses in a hospital or clinic.

Convulsion = An uncontrolled "fit" or seizure. A sudden jerking of part or all of the body.

Cord (umbilical cord) = The cord that connects the baby at its navel (belly button) to the placenta.

Counseling = Counseling is a general term that refers to a range of services provided by a professional that are designed to reduce emotional distress. The counseling process involves identifying the causes of distress and using specific techniques to relieve and manage distress. When a trained person helps you think about your situation or decisions you need to make. For example, some people are trained especially to help people cope with HIV/AIDS.

Coverage = The proportion of all eligible people screened by a program, calculated as the total number screened divided by the number of those who are eligible.

Crabs = Small parasites that feed on human blood.

Cramps = A painful tightening or contraction of a muscle. Many woman have cramps that begin just before monthly bleeding or just after it starts.

Crude (death) rate = The portion of a defined population that died during a specified period. The word "crude" is used to distinguish this measure from a rate that has been adjusted for differences in the age structure of populations (i.e. an agestandardized rate.)

Cryosurgery = Treatment performed with an instrument that freezes and destroys tissue. It can be used to treat cancer. This is a form of cryotherapy.

Culture Test = Samples of body tissue are taken from an infected area of your body. These samples are used to find out what is causing an infection.

Cyst = A sac or capsule filled with fluid.

Cystic Fibrosis (sis-tick fy-broh-sis) = A disease that causes both breathing and digesting problems. Cystic fibrosis runs in the family.

Cysts = Unlike cancerous tumors which are solid, cysts are fluid-filled masses in the breast. Cysts are very common, and are rarely associated with cancer. Ultrasound is the best way to tell a cyst from a cancer, because sound waves pass right through a liquid-filled cyst. Solid lumps, on the other hand, bounce the waves right back to the film.

D

D&C [also called dilation and curettage] = A procedure that removes the inside lining of the uterus. First the cervix is opened (or dilated) so that a small spoon-shaped instrument (called a curette) can be put into the uterus. Then the curette is used to take out the uterine lining.

Date rape = When a woman is forced to have sex by a man she is dating or courting. Your date forces sex on you while on a date.

DCIS [also called ductal carcinoma in situ or

intraductal carcinoma] = Abnormal breast cells that involve only the lining of a milk duct. These cells have not spread outside the duct into the normal surrounding breast tissue.

Dehydration = When the body loses more liquid than it takes in.

Dementia = When a person has severe difficulty remembering things and thinking clearly.

Denial = Denial is a psychological term that describes an unconscious defense mechanism characterized by the refusal to acknowledge painful realities, thoughts or feelings.

Deoxyribonucleic Acid (DNA) = The material that spells out the code for each gene on a chromosome.

Dependence = When the mind feels an overpowering need for a drug.

Depression = When a person feels extremely sad or feels nothing at all.

Diabetes (dy-uh-bee-teez) = When there is too much sugar in your blood. It can be caused by having not enough of the chemical that monitors blood sugar, called insulin, or by having a resistance in your body to insulin.

Diagnosis = The identification of a disease or health condition, or the name of the disease or condition.

Diagnostic procedure = A method used to see if a disease is present or not. It is also used to figure out what kind of disease is present.

Dialysis = A way to clean the blood when the kidneys are not working properly. (Cleaning the blood is usually the kidneys' job.) The blood passes through a special machine that removes chemicals, waste products, and toxins.

Diaphragm = A family planning method in which a soft rubber cup, usually filled with contraceptive gel or cream, is worn over the cervix during sex.

Diarrhea = Passing 3 or more loose, watery stools in a day.

Differentiation = This term describes how mature the breast cancer cells are compared to normal breast cells. Well-differentiated tumor cells that are mature look a lot like normal breast cells and tend to grow slowly. Undifferentiated, or poorly differentiated, tumor cells do not look or work like normal cells. They grow quickly and have a tendency to spread.

Digestion = When food is broken down by the stomach and intestines to be used by the body or to pass out of the body as waste.

Dilation and curettage (D and C) = To gradually open the cervix and then scrape out the womb. Often used for an abortion or to find the cause of abnormal bleeding from the vagina.

Disability = Physical or mental limitations that affect daily living.

Discharge (from the vagina) = The wetness or fluid that comes out of the vagina.

Discrimination = When people are ignored or treated badly because of who they are (for example, because they are women or old or poor).

Disease-specific survival = The percentage of people in a study who have survived a particular disease since diagnosis or treatment. Only deaths from the disease are counted. Subjects who died from some other cause are not counted.

Disinfection = Cleaning tools and equipment in a certain way to get rid of nearly all the germs.

Dizziness = Feeling lightheaded or unsteady.

DNA (deoxyribonucleic acid) -The biochemical carrier of genetic information; the constituent material of all genes.

Dose = The amount of a medicine you should take at one time.

Douche = Washing out the vagina. This can

List of Words

cause harm because it washes out the natural wetness

Douching (doo-shing) = Douching is rinsing or cleaning out the vagina, usually with a pre-packaged mix of fluids. The water or solutions are held in a bottle and squirted into the vagina through tubing and a nozzle. Health care providers do not suggest douching to clean the vagina. Douching changes the delicate chemical balance in the vagina, which can make a woman more prone to bacterial infections.

Down Syndrome = When an extra copy of a chromosome is present when a baby develops. (A chromosome holds a cell's genetic information for a person.) The extra chromosome usually causes mental and physical abnormalities.

Drug dependence (say: drug dee-pend-ins) = An addiction to drugs, or the inability to stop using harmful substances despite the harmful problems they cause.

Drugs = Substances, like alcohol and cocaine, that can be used in harmful ways to alter the mind.

Duct = A tiny part of the body shaped like a tube or pipe. Body fluids pass through it—for example, tear ducts, bile ducts, and milk ducts.

Ductal carcinoma in situ [also called DCIS or intraductal carcinoma] = Abnormal breast cells that involve only the lining of a milk duct. These cells have not spread outside the duct into the normal surrounding breast tissue.

Durable power of attorney = This document is also called a health care proxy. A durable power of attorney is a form of advance notice that allows an individual to give another individual legal authority to make decisions on his or her behalf. This document is used in situations where a person is not capable of making his or her own decisions.

Dysmenorrhea (dis-men-or-ee-uh) = Painful menstrual periods that can also go along with nausea and vomiting, and either constipation or diarrhea. Dysmenorrhea is common among adolescents.

Dysplasia = Cells that do not look normal under a microscope but are not cancer.

Early detection = The detection of cancer prior to the development of symptoms, or as soon as practicable after the development of symptoms.

E

Eating disorders = An eating disorder is a severe illness that requires help from a health care provider, the sooner the better. Bulimia nervosa is an eating disorder where a person binges, or eats a large amount of food all at once and then purges, or forces themselves to vomit, takes laxatives, or diuretics (water pills). Starving yourself by eating very little or nothing at all is another eating disorder called anorexia nervosa. People who have this condition can have a strong fear of body fat and weight gain. Binge eating disorder happens when a person cannot control her desire to overeat and often keeps the extreme eating a secret. Unlike bulimia, with binge eating disorder, a person does not purge her food. Extreme exercise to control weight is also a type of eating disorder.

Ectopic pregnancy (ek-top-ik preg-nan-cy) = A fertilized egg is implanted outside the uterus, usually in the fallopian tubes.

Effectiveness = The extent to which a specific intervention, procedure, regimen or service, when implemented, does what it is intended to do for a defined population.

Ejaculation (e-jak-yu-la-shun) = When a man reaches his peak of sexual pleasure and his semen comes out.Penis ejects whitish discharge, called semen.

Electrolysis (uh-lik-tral-i-sis) = An electrical current is used to remove unwanted hair.

Embryo = An unborn baby is called an embryo between the second and eighth weeks after conception.

Emotional numbness = Emotional numbness is a symptom of emotional trauma, where an individual becomes detached from others, is unable to react appropriately emotionally or suppresses emotions.

Emphysema (say: em-fuh-zee-muh) = A disease than involves damage to the air sacs (alveoli) in the lungs. The air sacs have trouble deflating once filled with air, so they are unable to fill up again with the fresh air needed to supply the body. Cigarette smoking is the most common cause of emphysema.

Encapsulated = Contained in a specific, localized area and surrounded by a thin layer of tissue.

Endocrinologist = A doctor who specializes in treating problems involving the body's hormone system.

Endometrial biopsy = A test that takes a sample of tissue from the lining of the uterus. Then the tissue is looked at under a microscope to see if it is normal or abnormal.

Endometrial cancer = Cancer of the inner lining of the uterus.

Endometrial = Having to do with the endometrium – the layer of tissue that lines the inside of the uterus.

Endometriosis (en-doh-mee-tree-oh-sis) = A condition where tissue that normally lining the uterus grows in other areas of the body. This can cause pain, irregular menstrual bleeding, and infertility for some women. This can happen in the pelvis or in the abdomen. This is not a cancer. But it can result in cysts, pain, infertility problems, and other symptoms.

Endometrium (en-doh-mee-tree-um) = The lining of the uterus.

Endoscopy -The use of a thin, lighted tube (called an endoscope) to examine the inside of the body.

Endothelial cell -The main type of cell found on the inside lining of blood vessels, lymph vessels, and the heart.

Endurance (en-der-ans) = The measure of your body's ability to keep up an activity without getting tired. The more endurance you have, the longer you can swim, bike, run or play a sport before tiring out.

Enema = A solution of water put up the anus to make a person pass stool or to increase the amount of fluid in the body.

Enriched (ehn-ritcht) = When vitamins or minerals are added to a food to make it more nutritious. An example is calcium-enriched orange juice.

Epidemiology = The study of the distribution and determinants of health-related states or events in specific populations.

Epilepsy (ep-il-ep-see) = A brain disorder that causes seizures, which are uncontrollable body movements.

Equal Employment Opportunity Commission = The EEOC is the federal agency that enforces laws to protect employees from employment discrimination. It also oversees Alternative Dispute Resolution.

Erection = When a man becomes sexually excited and his penis gets hard.

Erythrocytes (er-ith-roh-syts) = Redblood cells.

Esophagus = The tube connecting the mouth and the stomach that food goes down.

Estrogen -Estrogen is a hormone made by the ovaries in women. This hormone helps control a woman's menstrual cycles (periods).
Estrogen plays important roles in puberty, the menstrual cycle, and in reproduction.

List of Words

Estrogen receptor [also called ER] = This is a special type of protein found on some cancer cells. Estrogen attaches to it, and this can cause the cancer cells to grow.

Etiology = The cause or origin of disease.

Evaluation = Assessment of a service or program against a standard. Evaluations can be: (1) formative (informs the development and improvement of a programme); (2) an assessment of the process (describes the program).

Evidence-based medicine = Clinical decision-making based on a systematic review of the scientific evidence of the risks, benefits and costs of alternative forms of diagnosis or treatment.

Evidence-based practice = Practice that is based on scientific evidence that demonstrates effectiveness.

Examination (exam) = When a health worker, nurse, or doctor looks at, listens to, or feels parts of the body to find out what is wrong.

Excisional biopsy -Surgery that takes out an entire lump or suspicious area to be checked under a microscope.

Exhaustion = Extreme tiredness.

Fallopian tube -The Fallopian tube is the tube that connects each ovary to the uterus. This tube is the path that an egg must travel to get from the ovary to the uterus.

F

Fallopian tubes (say: fa-lo-pee-in toobz) = The organs that connect the ovaries to the uterus. There is a fallopian tube on each side of the uterus. When one of the ovaries releases an egg, it travels through the fallopian tube toward the uterus. Fertilization (when a man's sperm and a woman's egg join together) usually happens in the fallopian tube.

Familial cancer risk assessment = The investigation of (1) a reported family history of cancer; (2) an individual who develops cancer at a young age (usually under 50 years) with no family history to assess cancer risk for individuals and/or members of their family.

Family and Medical Leave Act = A federal law that provides job-protected unpaid medical leave for employees who qualify under this law.

Family planning = When a woman uses methods to prevent pregnancy, so that she can have the number of children she wants, when she wants them.

Farsighted = Being able to see things that are far away but not things close by. Often happens after age 40.

Fats = Foods, like oils and butter, that give the body energy.

Fecal = Wastes from the digestive tract; feces.

Female condom = A thin piece of rubber that fits into the vagina and covers the outer folds of the vulva. The condom prevents a man's sperm from reaching the woman's womb.

Fertile time = The time in a woman's cycle when she can get pregnant. For most women, this time starts about 8 days after the first day of the last monthly bleeding and lasts for about 11 days.

Fertility awareness (Natural Family Planning) = A family planning method that teaches a woman how to know her fertile time.

Fertilization = See conception.

Fetoscope = A tool for listening to and counting the heartbeat of the baby inside the mother's womb.

Fetus = The baby growing inside the womb fever When the body temperature is higher than normal.

Fiber = Parts of certain plants that when eaten help the body pass stool.

Fibroadenomas = Fibroadenomas are movable, solid, rounded lumps made up of normal breast cells. While not cancerous, these lumps may grow. And any solid lump that's getting bigger is usually removed to make sure that it's not a cancer. Fibroadenomas are the most common kind of breast mass, especially in young women.

Fibrocystic breast disease = Breast gland tissue build-up or cysts. They can become swollen and painful. They are not cancerous. But some types of fibrocystic changes are associated with an increased risk of breast cancer in the future.

Fibroid [also called leiomyoma] -A type of benign (non-cancerous) tumor. It is usually found in the wall of the uterus or digestive system. Growths in the womb that can cause abnormal bleeding from the vagina, pain, and repeated miscarriage.

Fine-needle aspiration [also called needle biopsy] -This is a test that uses a hollow needle to remove tissue or fluid. Then the material is looked at under a microscope to see if it is normal or abnormal.

Fistula = A hole in the skin between the vagina and the urine tube or rectum that causes urine or stool to leak from the vagina.

Flashback = When a person suddenly remembers something from the past as if it is happening now.

Flexibility = When the muscles and joints can move easily, without stiffness or pain.

Folic acid or folate = A B-vitamin that helps make healthy red blood cells. It is especially important that a pregnant woman get enough folic acid in her diet in order to prevent birth defects in the baby.

Fortified (fore-tih-fyde) = When ingredients are added to foods or drinks to either make them taste better or add nutrients. An example is breakfast cereal fortified with vitamins.

Free radicals = These are the chemicals released in a process called oxidation. Oxidation is when molecules in cells split and become unstable. This unstable activity causes a chain reaction in the surrounding molecules. The resulting free radicals can harm important molecules in the cells, including genes. Free radicals can work both for us and against us: Increased free radical activity might combine with other factors to cause some cancers. On the other hand, radiation therapy works in part by creating free radicals.

G

Gallbladder = A small, muscular sac attached to the liver. The gallbladder collects a liquid that helps digest fatty foods.

Gallstones - Hard material that forms in the gallbladder and can cause severe pain.

Gang rape = When a woman or girl is raped by more than one man.

Gangrene = When skin and tissue dies because of a lack of blood to that area.

Gastrointestinal system = The gastrointestinal system is, essentially, a long tube running through the body that works to digest food and then remove it from the body. This system includes the esophagus, stomach, pancreas, small intestine and large intestine.

Gender role = The way a community defines what it means to be a woman or man.

Gene therapy = Treatment that tries to fix a gene that's causing a cancer or making the cancer grow. It may also help the body's ability to fight the cancer. It may help make cancer cells easier to attack with new treatments.

Generic = The name of the main ingredient in a medicine.

Genes = Genes come from both parents and are responsible for inherited characteristics, such as eye and hair color. Genes are in all body

List of Words

cells. The functional unit of heredity, genes are composed of DNA sequences. They are located within the chromosomes, and determine particular characteristics of an individual.

Genetic mutation =An error in the gene caused by damage. This may result in a faulty or altered protein, or no protein being produced.

Genetic testing = Analyzing an individual's genetic material to diagnose a genetic disease or condition, or to determine a predisposition to a particular health condition.

Genetic testing = Checking a person's genes to see if there are changes that could lead to an increased risk for getting a specific disease.

Genetics = The study of heredity and the variability of inherited traits.

Genital area (jen-ih-tul air-eeh-uh) = The area around the vagina, penis, scrotum, anus, and thigh.

Genital Herpes (jen-ih-tul her-peez) = An STD caused by the herpes simplex virus type 1 (HSV-1) and type 2 (HSV-2). A sexually transmitted infection that produces sores on the genitals or on the mouth.

Genital warts = Growths on the genitals, caused by the HPV virus which is passed during sex.

Genitals = The sexual parts both inside and outside a woman's body.

Genome -The genetic material of an individual.

Germs = Very small organisms that can grow in the body and cause some infectious diseases.

Gingivitis (jin-jih-vyt-is) = Inflammation of the gums, the first stage of gum disease. Gingivitis is caused by plaque deposits, which are made up of bacteria, mucus, and food debris. Injury to the gums from harsh brushing or flossing can also cause inflammation.

Gland = A small sac that produces fluid.

Glands (glanz) = Special groups of cells that do a certain job. The pituitary gland, for example, makes hormones that affect growth.

Glaucoma = A disease of the eye in which too much pressure builds up inside the eyeball and damages vision. Glaucoma can happen slowly (chronic glaucoma) or suddenly (acute glaucoma).

Goal = A high-level strategic action.

Goiter = A swelling on the lower front of the neck (enlargement of the thyroid gland) caused by lack of iodine in the diet.

Gonorrhea (gan-e-re-ae) = An STD caused by a bacteria called neisseria gonorrhoeae, a bacterium that can grow and multiply easily in the warm, moist areas of the reproductive tract, including the cervix, uterus, urethra, and fallopian tubes inside of you. Learn more about this STD.

Gonorrhea = A sexually transmitted infection.

Graft vs. host disease -Graft vs. host disease is a disease that may happen after you receive a bone marrow transplant. When someone going through treatment for cancer receives bone marrow from a donor, it is possible that the donor's white cells will attack parts of the receiver's body. The parts of the body commonly affected by GVHD are the skin, stomach and liver.

Granulocytes (say: gran-you-lo-syts) = White blood cells that are very important in helping the body prevent and fight infections caused by bacteria.

Gray = A gray is a unit of measure for the dose of radiation therapy given to a particular part of the body.

Groin = the very top of the leg where it joins the body in the front, next to the genitals.

Guidelines = A formal statement directing a defined task or function. Examples include clinical practice guidelines and guidelines for the

List of Words

ethical conduct of medical research.

Gynecologic oncologist = A doctor who specializes in treating cancers of the female reproductive organs. These organs include the vulva, vagina, uterus, fallopian tubes, and ovaries.

Gynecological examination (gine-eh-kol-uh-j-kl ig-zam-e-na-shun) = Exam inside vagina to make sure organs are healthy.

Gynecologist (gine-eh-kol-uh-jist) = A special type of doctor that deals with women's health, especially with the health of women's reproductive parts including the uterus, cervix, and vagina.

Gynocologic oncologists = Physicians who treat cancers of the female reproductive organs (i.e. cervix, uterus, ovaries).

H

Halitosis (hal-i-toe-sis) = Offensive or bad breath.

Hallucinations = Seeing strange things or hearing voices that others do not see or hear.

Health care proxy = Also referred to as durable power of attorney, a health care proxy is a form of advance notice that assigns an individual to make decisions for a person who is not capable of making his or her own decisions.

Health care team = A health care team includes any doctors, nurses, social workers, psychologists, nutritionists or other health care providers you depend on for medical service, help and information.

Health centers = Places that provide a middle level of health care, usually in larger towns. Health centers may have trained nurses and doctors.

Health inequality = Differences in health that are unnecessary, avoidable and unjust.

Health promotion = The process of enabling people to increase control over and improve their health.

Health status = A description and/or measurement of the health of an individual or population.

Heart disease = Coronary artery disease, the most common type of heart disease, happens when the heart doesn't get enough blood.

Helper foods = Foods that provide nutrition—like protein, vitamins, minerals, fats, and sugar—that are needed in addition to the main food.

Hemoglobin (heem-oh-glo-bin) = Substance containing iron found in red blood cells, which helps the blood carry and deliver oxygen to body tissues.

Hemophilia (heem-o-feel-ee-ah) = A disease that makes it difficult for the blood to clot, which is how the blood sticks together to stop flowing. Without clots, a simple cut can cause someone to lose a dangerous amount of blood. This disease affects mostly boys.

Hemorrhage = Heavy bleeding.

Hemorrhoids = Small, painful bumps or lumps at the edge of the anus or inside it. They are a type of swollen veins that may burn, hurt, or itch.

Hepatitis = A serious disease of the liver caused by a virus. Some forms of hepatitis can be sexually transmitted.

Hepatitis (hep-uh-tyt-is) = Inflammation of the liver, caused by infections from bacteria, viruses, or toxins such as alcohol or drugs. There are different types of hepatitis, including Hepatitis A, B, C and autoimmune hepatitis. Learn more about this Hepatitis B and Hepatitis C.

Herbal supplements = Herbal supplements are different types of medicines that come in a variety forms, such as teas, vitamin pills, or creams. There has not been a lot of research

List of Words

done on herbal supplements to really know how well they work or how safe they are, so it is important that you ask your doctor before taking anything that he or she has not given you.

Herbicides = Chemicals used to kill unwanted plants.

Herpes = Several diseases caused by different viruses that cause sores on the mouth or genitals.Herpes can be passed through sex.

Herpes zoster (shingles) = A painful rash caused by the chickenpox virus, with blisters on the face, back, and chest.

High blood pressure = When the force or pressure of the blood upon the walls of the arteries and veins is harder than normal.

HIPAA = The Health Insurance Portability and Accountability Act of 1996 (HIPAA) was signed into law on August 21, 1996. This law includes important new protections for millions of working Americans and their families who have preexisting medical conditions or might suffer discrimination in health coverage based on their health.

Histopathological diagnosis -The determination of the nature of a disease by the microscopic examination of cells and tissues.

HIV (H-I-V) = HIV stands for the human immunodeficiency virus, which destroys the immune system that protects the body. This makes it hard to fight infections. People who have HIV may not have any symptoms for up to 10 years, but they can give it to others through unprotected sex and sharing drug needles. HIV leads to full-blown AIDS.

HIV/AIDS HIV, or human immune-deficiency virus = the virus that causes AIDS. We sometimes use the phrase 'HIV/AIDS' since infection with HIV eventually leads to AIDS.

Hives = Hard, thick, raised spots on the skin that itch severely. They may come and go all at once or move from one place to another. A sign of allergic reaction.

Hodgkin's lymphoma (hodj-kinz limf-oh-muh) = A type of cancer that affects the tissue found in lymph nodes (glands that protect the fluids in your body), the spleen, the liver, and bone marrow.

Home remedies = Traditional ways of healing.

Homicide (HOM-uh-side) = The killing of one person by another. Homicide is not legal and is a punishable crime.

Hormonal methods = Family planning methods that prevent the woman's ovary from releasing an egg and keep the lining of the womb from supporting a pregnancy.

Hormonal therapy [also called hormone therapy or endocrine therapy] = Cancer treatment that removes, blocks, or adds hormones.

Hormone = A hormone is a natural body chemical, such as estrogen, that has effects on or controls other parts of the body. Synthetic hormones, such as birth control pills, are drugs similar to human hormones. A hormone is a chemical substance carried throughout the body in the blood where it stimulates or suppresses cell and tissue activity. They circulate in the blood and control the actions of certain cells or organs. For example, estrogen is made in the ovary, travels in the blood to the breast, and can stimulate the growth of breast cells. Estrogen and progesterone are the most important hormones for women.

Hormone replacement therapy [also called HRT] = Hormones (estrogen, progesterone, or both) given to women after menopause. They are used to ease symptoms of menopause.

Hospice = Hospice refers to programs that focus on quality of life for dying persons. Most hospice care is provided in the patient's own home.

List of Words

Bereavement follow-up services are offered to family members in the year after the death of their loved one.

Hospital = A medical center with doctors, nurses, and special equipment for finding or treating serious illnesses.

HPV test = Like a Pap test, an HPV test is done on a sample of cells collected from the cervix. Learn more about HPV.

HPV = A sexually transmitted disease that can cause wart-like growths on the genitals. There are many types of HPV, and some types do not cause growths. Regular pap tests or HPV tests can catch the virus. HPV can lead to pre-cancerous cell changes in the cervix, so detection and treatment are important. Learn more about HPV. Some strains of Human Papilloma Virus cause genital warts, others cause cervical cancer. There is now a HPV vaccine.

Human genome project -An international project designed to identify the totality of the sequences of human genes.

Hydrogen peroxide = A chemical that kills germs, often used for cleaning wounds.

Hymen = A thin piece of skin that partially closes off the vaginal opening. In some communities, a woman is no longer considered a virgin if her hymen is torn, even though it can be torn by activities other than sex.

Hyperthyroidism = Hyperthyroidism is a condition that can happen when your body produces too much thyroid hormone. Some of the symptoms are cramps, diarrhea, chest pain, weight loss and nervousness.

Hypothalamus = The hypothalamus is an area deep in the brain that is part of the limbic system. The hypothalamus controls sex hormones, sperm production, blood pressure, body temperature and more, by making and sending hormones through the bloodstream as messengers to the pituitary gland.

Hypothyroidism = Hypothyroidism is a condition that can happen when your body doesn't produce enough thyroid hormone. Some of the symptoms are weakness, hair loss, constipation and feeling tired all the time.

Hysterectomy = An operation in which the womb (uterus) is removed. In a 'total hysterectomy', the tubes and ovaries are also removed.

I

Imaging = Methods of producing pictures of areas inside the body. Examples of these are X-rays, mammogram, and ultrasound.

Immune system (im-yoon) = A complex system whose job is to protect the body against infection and foreign substances. The immune system works to seek out, identify, and kill invaders.

Immune system = The parts of the body that recognize harmful germs and try to fight off infection.

Immunizations (im-you-niz-a-shuns) = Immunizations keep people from getting sick by immunizing, or protecting, the body against certain infectious diseases. Vaccines contain parts or products of infectious organisms or whole germs that have been changed or killed. A vaccine gets the body's immune system ready to fight off infection by that germ. Most immunizations that prevent you from catching diseases like measles, whooping cough, and chicken pox are given by a shot.

Immunosuppression = This is a way to make the body's immune system weak so it is less able to fight infection or disease. It also makes the body less likely to reject a transplant. Sometimes, if you've had a transplant, your doctor may use special drugs to weaken your immune system. At other times, it's harmful to have a weak immune system. This could happen as a side effect of treatment (like from chemotherapy). Or it can

List of Words

be a part of a disease, like AIDS.

Implantation = When the fertilized egg attaches to the womb wall at the beginning of pregnancy.

Implants = A family planning method in which small tubes containing hormones are put under the skin.

In situ cancer = Early cancer that has not spread into nearby tissue.

In vitro = A process that takes place in the laboratory – outside the body. (This is the opposite of "in vivo," which means in the body.)

In vitro fertilization (IVF) -A woman takes hormones to ripen multiple eggs in her ovaries, which are then taken out with a needle placed through the top of the vagina. In a laboratory, the eggs and sperm are combined to create embryos. These embryos will then be transferred back into the woman's uterus.

In vivo = A process that takes place in the body. (This is the opposite of "in vitro," which means outside the body, or in the laboratory.)

Incest = Sexual relations between family members or relatives.

Incidence rate -The rate at which new cases of cancer occur.

Incidence -The frequency of occurrence of any event or condition in a defined population over a defined period of time.

Incision = A cut made into the body.

Incisional biopsy = Surgery in which a part of a lump or suspicious area is taken out of the body. It is then looked at under a microscope to see if it's normal or abnormal.

Infant formula = Artificial milk for babies used instead of breast milk. Infant formula and other replacement foods do not have the same nutrition or health benefits as breast milk.

Infected (in-fektd) = To have a disease or virus.

Infection = A sickness caused by bacteria, viruses, or other organisms. Infections may affect part of the body or all of it.

Infectious disease = Diseases caused by germs or parasites that can be spread from one person to another.

Infertility (in-fur-til-ih-teeh) = When a couple has problems getting pregnant after one year of regular sexual intercourse without using any birth control methods. Infertility can be caused by a problem with the man or the woman, or both.

Inflammatory breast cancer = A fairly rare type of breast cancer. The breast looks red and swollen and feels warm. The skin of the breast may look like the skin of an orange. Sometimes a lump is also found in the breast.

Injections = When medicine or other liquid is put into the body using a syringe and needle.

Inner folds = The part of a woman's genitals that lie just inside the hairy outer folds of the vulva. The inner folds are soft flaps of skin without hair that are sensitive to touch.

Intervention = A program or series of programs to address a need or concern.

Intestines = The guts or tube-like part of the food canal that carries food and finally waste from the stomach to the anus.

Intramuscular injection (IM) = Injection deep into the muscle.

Intra-uterine device (IUD, IUCD) = A small object that is put into the womb to prevent pregnancy.

Intravenous (IV) = When medicines or fluids are put into a vein.

Invasive lobular carcinoma [also called ILC] = Cancer that starts in the milk glands. It grows into the normal surrounding tissues. Between 10% and 15% of all breast cancers are of this type.

List of Words

Iodine = A mineral found in the ground and some foods that prevents goiter and mental slowness at birth.

Iron = A mineral found in some foods that helps make the blood healthy.

Irradiation = The use of high-energy radiation—from x-rays, neutrons, and other sources—to kill cancer cells and shrink tumors. Radiation may come from a machine outside the body (external-beam radiation therapy) or from materials called radioisotopes. Radioisotopes produce radiation and can be placed in or near the cancer or in the area near cancer cells. This type of radiation treatment is called internal radiation therapy, implant radiation, interstitial radiation, or brachytherapy. Systemic radiation therapy uses a radioactive substance, such as a radiolabeled monoclonal antibody, that circulates throughout the body. Irradiation is also called radiation therapy, radiotherapy, and x-ray therapy.

Irrigation = Irrigation is adding water to flush an area such as the bowel. This stimulates a bowel movement, similar to an enema.

J

Jaundice = Yellow color of the skin and eyes. Jaundice can be a sign of hepatitis or of new-born jaundice.

Joints = Places in the body where bones come together.

K

Kidneys = Two large organs in the lower back that make urine by cleaning waste from the blood.

Killer cells = White blood cells that attack cancer cells and body cells that have been invaded by foreign substances.

L

Labia = Large and small folds of skin that are part of the vulva.

Labor = The work a woman's body does in childbirth, when her womb squeezes or contracts, causes her cervix to open, and pushes her baby down through the vagina and out of her body.

Laparoscope = A thin, lighted tube used to look at tissues and organs inside the abdomen. Also used to remove part or all of the colon through small incisions made in the wall of the abdomen.

Latex = A material like thin rubber. Condoms and gloves are often made of latex.

Latrine = A hole or pit in the ground for passing urine or stool. A toilet.

Laxatives = Medicine used for constipation to make stools softer and more frequent.

Lean = Meat and poultry that has little or no fat, making it healthier to eat.

Legumes (leh-goomz) = Seeds or pods of a certain kind of plant that are used as food. Examples of legumes are different kinds of beans such as black, garbanzo, and pinto, and also lentils.

Lesion -An area of abnormal tissue change. For example, a lump, wound, or area of injury.

Leukocytes (loo-ko-syts) = White blood cells.

Lice = Tiny insects that attach on the skin or hair of people and other animals.

Ligaments (lih-guh-mentz) = Straps that fasten bones to each other. Strong fibers in a person's body that help hold muscles and bones in place.

Limbic system = The limbic system involves various structures of the brain that control emotions, hormonal secretions, mood, motivation, and pain and pleasure sensations.

Literacy = The ability to read and understand written information.

Liver = A large organ under the lower right ribs that helps clean the blood and get rid of

List of Words

poisons.

Living will = This is a form of advance notice that specifies in writing what kind of medical care a person wants or does not want in the event of terminal illness or incapacity.

Lobe = A portion of an organ such as the liver, lung, breast, or brain.

Lobular carcinoma in situ [also called LCIS] = An overgrowth of cells in the lobules of the breast. These cells are not likely to turn into an invasive cancer. But having them means a higher risk of getting breast cancer in either breast.

Local cancer = An invasive malignant cancer confined entirely to the organ where the cancer began.

Localized = Keeping to the site of origin, without any sign of spread to other areas.

Loss of consciousness = When a sick or injured person seems to be asleep and cannot be awakened. Unconscious.

Lubricants = A slippery cream or jelly used to make dry surfaces wet. Lubricants are often used on condoms during sex.

Lumpectomy = A lumpectomy is surgery to remove a tumor and possibly some surrounding healthy tissue. The tissue is examined to determine if cancer cells have spread beyond the tumor.

Lung capacity = Lung capacity is the measure of the amount of air that the lungs may contain at various points in the respiratory cycle.

Lupus (loo-pus) = One of the diseases that causes the immune system, which normally protects the body, to actually attack it. Lupus can cause problems with the skin, joints and organs on the inside of the body.

Lymph fluid = Lymph fluid is the clear fluid that travels through the lymphatic system and carries cells that help fight infections and other diseases. It can also be called lymph.

Lymph glands (limf glandz) = Commonly called, lymph nodes, are a network of vessels that contain white blood cells to help fight infection.

Lymph node dissection = Lymph node dissection is a surgery that removes lymph nodes so they can be examined to see whether they contain cancer. This surgery can also be called a lymphadenectomy.

Lymph node mapping = Lymph node mapping is a procedure to identify lymph nodes that contain tumor cells. Dyes and radioactive substances are usually injected into the area of the tumor to help the surgeon locate the lymph nodes. It can also be called sentinel lymph node mapping.

Lymph nodes = Lymph nodes are small, bean-shaped organs located along the vessels of the lymphatic system. Clusters of lymph nodes can be found in the neck, underarms, chest, abdomen, and groin. Lymph nodes store white blood cells that help fight infection. They also filter lymphatic fluid. Sometimes they are called lymph glands. Small lumps under the skin in different parts of the body that trap germs. Lymph nodes become swollen and painful when they get infected.

Lymph vessel = The lymph vessel is a thin tube that carries lymphatic fluid and white blood cells through the lymphatic system. It can also be called a lymphatic vessel.

Lymphatic system = The lymphatic system is a network of tissues, organs, vessels, and glands that produce, store, and carry cells that fight infection in the human body.

Lymphedema = A condition in which too much lymph fluid collects in tissue. This causes swelling. It can happen in the arm after lymph nodes in the underarm are removed. It can also happen if there is radiation to the lymph nodes

List of Words

or chemotherapy. It can get worse if the arm is hurt in any way.

Lymphocytes (limf-oh-syts) = White blood cells that produce antibodies.

M

Magnetic resonance imaging [also called MRI] = This is a test that looks at areas inside your body. Detailed pictures are made by a magnet linked to a computer. These are read by a radiologist.

Main food = The main food, usually low-cost, that is eaten with almost every meal. This main food usually provides most of the body's daily food needs. For good nutrition, the body also needs helper foods.

Maintenance therapy = Treatment that is given to help a primary (original) treatment keep working. Maintenance therapy is often given to help keep cancer in remission.

Malignancy = An uncontrolled growth of cells. It can spread into nearby normal tissue. It can also travel to other parts of the body.

Malignant = Cancerous; a growth that tends to spread into nearby normal tissue and travel to other parts of the body.

Malnutrition = When the body does not have enough of the foods it needs to stay healthy.

Mammogram = An x-ray picture of the breast.

Mammography = The use of x-rays to create a picture of the breast (mammogram) to help diagnose and localize breast cancer.

Marker = A diagnostic indicator for where disease may develop.

Massage = A way of touching the body to relieve pain, tension, or other signs. Massaging the belly can help the womb contract and stop heavy bleeding after birth, miscarriage or abortion.

Mastectomy = A mastectomy is surgery to remove a woman's breast. It is usually done to treat breast cancer. Sometimes women at high risk for breast cancer get mastectomies because they want to decrease their risk for breast cancer.

Mastitis = See breast infection.

Masturbation = Touching one's own body to bring personal sexual pleasure.

Maternal mortality = When a woman dies due to problems from pregnancy and birth.

Mediation = Bringing in an outside person(s) to help end a conflict.

Medical abortion = Using certain medicines to end a pregnancy.

Melanoma = Melanoma is a type of cancer that begins in the cells that are responsible for the color of your skin, hair and eyes. Melanoma usually shows up as a dark spot on your skin or begins as a mole. Melanoma can also develop in the eye. Advanced melanomas can spread to other parts of the body, like your lymph nodes, lungs or liver.

Membranes = A thin layer of skin or tissue that either covers organs inside the body or lines other parts. An example is the sac that surrounds and protects the baby when it is in the mother's womb.

Menarche (men-r-kee) = The first menstrual period or beginning of menstruation.

Meningitis (men-in-jyt-is) = A dangerous infection that affects the brain and spinal cord.

Menopause (men-o-pawz) = The last menstrual period or end of menstruation. The average age of menopause is 50. After menopause, a woman can no longer become pregnant.

Menopause = When a woman's monthly bleeding stops forever. Menopause is when menstrual periods stop because the ovaries are producing low levels of hormones or almost

List of Words

none at all. Menopause is sometimes called the "change of life."

Menstrual cycle = The monthly cycle of hormonal changes in a woman's body before menopause. A cycle starts at the beginning of one menstrual period and ends at the beginning of the next.

Menstruation (men-stroo-ay-shun) = The monthly period or menstrual bleeding. During menstruation, the extra blood and tissue that built up inside the uterus during the menstrual cycle is expelled through the vagina, usually over a period of 3-7 days.

Metabolism (muh-tab-ul-iz-um) = The different ways that the body makes and uses energy, such as in digesting food.

Metastasis = The spread of cancer to another location in the body.

Metastatic cancer = Metastatic cancer is cancer that spreads to a different part of the body. For example, if lung cancer spreads to the bone, it is called metastatic lung cancer, not bone cancer.

Microscope = An instrument that makes very tiny objects look larger.

Midwife = Someone with special training or experience to help a woman give birth.

Migraines = Severe headaches with blurred eyesight.

Minerals = Substances in foods—like iron, calcium, and iodine—that help the body fight disease and recover after injury or illness.

Miscarriage = When a woman loses a developing baby before it is old enough to survive outside the womb.

Modified radical mastectomy = A modified radical mastectomy is a surgery for breast cancer in which the breast, the lining over the chest muscles, and some or all of the nearby lymph nodes are removed. Sometimes the surgeon also removes part of the chest wall muscles.

Monitoring = The performance and analysis of routine measurements aimed at detecting changes.

Monthly bleeding (menstruation, monthly period) = When a bloody fluid leaves a woman's womb and passes through the vagina and out of her body. It happens about every 28 days and lasts for a few days.

Monthly cycle = The period of time between the beginning of one monthly bleeding and the beginning of the next. About 2 weeks after a woman starts her monthly bleeding one of her ovaries releases an egg, and about 2 weeks after that she starts another monthly bleeding.

Morbidity = Illness.

Mortality = Death.

Mortality rate = The portion of a defined population that dies during a specific period.

Mucous method = When a woman checks the consistency of the mucus of the vagina to determine when she is most fertile.

Mucus = A thick, slippery wetness that the body makes to protect the inside of the vagina, nose, throat, stomach, and intestines.

Multiple myeloma = Multiple myeloma is cancer of the plasma cell. Plasma cells are found in lymphatic tissue and produce antibodies to help fight infection.

Muscular Dystrophy (mus-kew-lar dis-trof-ee) = A group of disorders that causes muscles to be weak and causes loss of muscle tissue.

Natural methods (of family planning) = Methods of preventing pregnancy that do not require any devices or chemicals.

N

Nausea = When a person feels sick to her stomach, as though she wants to vomit. This often happens to women during the first 3 or 4 months of pregnancy. Also called "morning sickness."

Nipple = The center of the dark-colored part on the outside of the breast where milk comes out.

Nutrition = Good nutrition is eating enough food and the right kind of food so the body can grow, be healthy, and fight off disease.

O

Obesity (oh-bee-sit-ee) = Obesity is more extreme than being overweight. A person is thought to be obese when weight is 25 percent (for women) more than the weight she should be for her height. Obesity can be defined using BMI (Body Mass Index). A person with a BMI over 30 is thought to be obese.

Objective = The expected results from an activity or program.

Occupational therapist = Occupational therapists will evaluate the impact of the cancer or its treatment on your activities at home or at work. They can help you learn to manage your daily activities and incorporate any physical changes caused by cancer into your home and work life.

Occupational Therapist = A specialist who works on special activities with patients as part of the treatment of their illness, injury, or other health issue.

Oncologist = A physician who treats cancer. A clinical oncologist or radiotherapist is a doctor who treats cancer with radiation. A medical oncologist treats cancer with drugs.

Oncology = The study, diagnosis, treatment and management of cancerous tumours.

Operation = When a doctor makes a cut in the skin in order to repair damage inside, or to change the way the body functions.

Optimal treatment = Treatment known to provide the best outcome based on current knowledge.

Organ = A part of the body that is more or less complete in itself and does a specific job. For example, the lungs are organs for breathing.

Osteoclasts = Cells in your body that break down bone.

Osteoporosis = Weak, brittle bones that break easily. Osteoporosis is more common in older women, because they produce less estrogen after menopause.

Ostomy = Surgically-created opening to the outside of the body.

Outcomes = All the possible changes in health status that may result from exposure to a causal factor or from the handling of a health problem. The anticipated overall effects of an Intervention or program, especially in relation to whether the overall program goal has been achieved.

Outer folds = The fatty lips of the vulva that protect the outside genitals and close up when the legs are together.

Ovaries (o-var-eez) = Two organs (about the size of an almond or grape), one on each side of the uterus, in the pelvis of a female. The ovaries contain eggs (ova) and make female hormones. When one of the ovaries releases an egg about once each month as part of the menstrual cycle, it is called ovulation. Small sacs about the size of an almond or grape, one on each side of the womb. Ovaries produce eggs that join with a man's sperm to make a baby.

Overactive bladder = Overactive bladder is characterized by involuntary bladder contractions that occur as your bladder is filling with urine. A person will have a sudden, intense desire to urinate.

Overdose = Taking too much of a drug or medicine at one time. This can cause serious

List of Words

injury or death.

Over-the-Counter = Over-the-counter medicines are medicines you can buy at a pharmacy or store with out a prescription, or an order from your doctor. Examples include cold medicine, medicines for stomach pain, or pain relievers.

Ovulation (ov-yoo-lay-shun) = When the ovaries release an egg, about once each month, as part of the menstrual cycle. When an egg is released from one of the ovaries during the middle of a woman's monthly cycle.

P

Palliative care (c) = Palliative care refers to maintaining high quality of life for those living with a serious illness. This type of care is focused on comfort and provides relief from pain and other distressing symptoms. Palliative care also concerns end-of-life care, rather than curing a disease.

Palliative care (a)=An approach that improves the quality of life of patients and their families facing the problems associated with life-threatening illness, through the prevention and relief of suffering by means of early identification and impeccable assessment and treatment of pain and other problems, physical, psychosocial and spiritual.' (WHO 2002).

Palliative care(b) =Palliative care is the active total care of patients whose disease is not responsive to curative treatment. Control of pain, of other symptoms, and of psychological, social and spiritual problems is paramount, to achieve the best possible quality of life for patients and their families.

Pap smear = A screening test to help identify malignant or premalignant changes in the cervix. It is performed by obtaining cells from the exterior of the cervix uterus, staining them with a special technique derived by Papanicolau

(hence the Pap test), and examining them under a microscope. (Alternative name: pap test).

Pap Test = Exam performed inside the vagina to check the cervix for problems. A test in which some skin cells are scraped from the cervix during a pelvic exam and then examined under a microscope to see if there are any early warning signs of cancer.

Paralysis = Loss of the ability to move part or all of the body.

Paraneoplastic syndrome = Paraneoplastic syndrome is a condition that develops as an effect of having a cancer, but is not caused directly by the tumor. It is often caused by the body's immune response against the cancer.

Parasites = Tiny worms and animals that can live in a person (or animal) and cause disease.

Parkinson's disease = Parkinson's disease is a chronic disease of the nervous system characterized by: a tremor of the hands, arms, legs, jaw, and face; stiffness of the limbs and trunk; and bladder problems. These symptoms will grow worse over time.

Partial response = Usually described as a 50% reduction in the size of a tumor after treatment.

Pathologist -A doctor who specializes in the examination of normal and diseased tissue.

Peer counselor = Someone who is trained to talk with another person who is in a similar situation. For example, one young woman may counsel another young woman, or someone who used to drink too much may counsel another person who is trying to quit.

Peer Pressure = Social pressure on somebody to act or dress a certain way in order to be accepted as part of a group.

Pelvic area = Everything between a woman's hips. This is where a woman's reproductive parts are.

Pelvic exam = An examination of a woman's

genitals both inside and outside her body. A pelvic exam sometimes includes a speculum exam.

Pelvic floor muscles = Pelvic floor muscles are the group of muscles surrounding the opening of the bladder and urethra that help with bladder support and closure.

Pelvic Inflammatory Disease (PID) = A general term for infection of the lining of the uterus, fallopian tubes, or the ovaries. Most cases of PID are caused by bacteria that causes STD's such as chlamydia and gonorrhea. The most common symptoms include abnormal vaginal discharge (fluid), lower stomach pain, and sometimes fever.

Pelvic inflammatory disease (PID) = An infection of the reproductive parts in a woman's lower abdomen. Also called pelvic infection.

Penis = The male sex organ, also used to pass urine. The penis gets hard during sex and releases a fluid called semen that contains sperm.

PEP = The short-term use of antiretroviral medicines to prevent health workers accidently exposed to HIV or women who have been raped from getting HIV.

Period = See monthly bleeding.

Permanent methods (of family planning) See sterilization.

Person-centred -Recognition of a person's total wellbeing, including their physical, emotional, spiritual, social and practical needs within the context of family and community. This means recognizing and responding appropriately to a culturally appropriate holistic view of health.

Pesticides = Poisonous chemicals used to kill insects that destroy food crops.

Phosphodiesterase-5 inhibitors (PDE-5 inhibitors) = PDE-5 inhibitors are medicines like Viagra, Levitra or Cialis that can help men get erections by increasing the levels of certain chemicals in the tissues inside the penis. They promote blood flow. In women, PDE-5 inhibitors might help with vaginal lubrication and swelling, especially for women who have low estrogen and do not want to take replacement hormones.

Physical therapist = A physical therapist can help you adjust to the physical changes in your body by teaching you exercises and physical activities that can help condition your muscles and restore strength and movement.

Physical Therapist = A specialist who uses body movements to help treat injuries and other physical health issues.

PID = See pelvic inflammatory disease.

Piles (hemorrhoids) = Swollen veins around the anus, which can itch, burn, or bleed.

Pimple = A spot or small infected swelling that grows, often on the face, due to extra oil on the skin. Common in adolescent girls and boys. Also called acne.

Pituitary (Puh-too-eh-ter-ee) = The pituitary gland is a small gland attached to the brain as part of the endocrine system. A gland is a group of cells that makes and then releases special chemicals called hormones. The pituitary gland makes different hormones that affect how other glands in the system release their hormones. Among other hormones, the pituitary makes growth hormone and endorphins, special chemicals that help provide natural pain relief from within the body.

Pituitary gland = The pituitary gland is a small gland at the base of the brain. It is controlled by the hypothalamus, and in turn sends out messenger hormones that control sperm production in the testicles.

Placenta (afterbirth) = A spongy organ in a woman's womb that passes the baby everything

363

List of Words

it needs to grow during pregnancy. The baby is connected to the placenta by the cord. After the baby is born, the placenta also comes out of the womb.

Plant medicines = Flowers, leaves, roots and other parts of plants that can be used to treat diseases.

Plasma (plaz-muh) = The liquid part of blood, which contains nutrients, proteins, minerals and dissolved waste products.

Platelets (playt-lats) = Small cells floating in the blood that play a key role in blood clotting.

Pneumonia = An infection of the small breathing tubes deep in the lungs.

Polycystic Ovarian Syndrome = PCOS is a mild hormonal imbalance that can cause irregular periods, unwanted hair growth, weight gain, and acne. This is a common condition that begins during the teenage years.

Polyps = Growths found usually in the womb. Polyps are almost never caused by cancer.

Population health = The health of a population, measured by health status. Populations may be defined by locality, biological criteria such as age or gender.

Population-based = Pertaining to a defined population.

Potential years of life lost (PYLL) = PYLL is a measure of premature mortality that represents the number of years of life "lost" when a person dies prematurely from any cause. For example, if one assumes a life expectancy of 75 years, the PYLL for a person dying at age 25 would be 50.

Precursor = A condition or state preceding the overt, pathological onset of a disease. Precursor states may sometimes be detectable by screening, or may be used as a risk marker.

Predictive value = In screening and diagnostic tests, the probability that a person with a positive test is a true positive (i.e. does have the disease) is referred to as the "positive predictive value of the test." The predictive value of a negative test is the probability that a person with a negative test does not have the disease.

Pregnancy in the tube =A pregnancy that grows in one of the fallopian tubes, instead of in the womb.

Premature menopause = Premature menopause is defined as menopause that happens in women before the age of 45. Some chemotherapy medicines, radiation to the ovaries, or surgery to remove both ovaries can put a young woman into sudden, early menopause. Premature menopause can be temporary or permanent. Women in premature menopause due to cancer treatment tend to have more severe hot flashes and vaginal dryness than women who experience a gradual, natural menopause.

Prenatal = The time between when a woman gets pregnant and when she gives birth.

Prenatal care = Checkups during pregnancy, when a midwife or specially trained health worker examines a pregnant woman to make sure the pregnancy is going well.

Pre-seminal fluid = The fluid that comes out of the penis before ejaculation of semen. There may be only a small amount of this fluid, but it can still pass viruses such as HIV. Also called "pre-ejaculate."

Pressure sores (bed sores) = Sores that form over bony parts of the body when a person lies or sits on that part of the body for too long without moving.

Prevalence = The number of cases of disease in a population, at a defined point in time, irrespective of the time of diagnosis. It is usually expressed as the number of cases of disease per 100,000 individuals in the population. It is a measure of the total burden of disease in a population.

List of Words

Prevent = Stopping something before it starts.

Prevention = Actions aimed at eliminating or minimizing the impact of disease and disability.

Primordial follicle -Immature follicles that make up your ovarian reserve.

Principle = A fundamental basis for action.

Privacy = When a person gives information to a health worker, nurse, or doctor and knows it will not be overheard by, or repeated to, others.

Progesterone = A female hormone.

Progestin =A hormone made in a laboratory that is similar to the progesterone made naturally in a woman's body. It is found in some hormonal family planning methods.

Progestin only pill = A method of family planning that contains one hormone—progestin—but no estrogen.

Prolapsed uterus = When the muscles that hold up the womb become weak, causing it to fall or drop down into the vagina.

Prophylactic = Use of medical procedures or treatments to prevent or defend against a disease.

Prostate = The prostate is the gland that surrounds the neck of the bladder and urethra in men. It supplies seminal fluid, the milky liquid that contains sperm, for ejaculation.

Proteins = Body-building foods necessary for proper growth and strength.

Protocol = A defined program for treatment.

Psycho-oncology = The study, understanding and treatment of social, psychological, emotional, spiritual, quality-of-life and functional aspects of cancer as applied across the cancer control continuum.

Puberty = The stage of growth when adult sexual body parts mature and fertility becomes possible. The process of developing from a child to sexual maturity, when a person becomes capable of having children. In a girl, puberty includes a growth spurt, development of breasts and hips, growth of body hair, and the beginning of menstruation (having periods).

Pubic Area = On and around the genitals.

Pubic bone = The front part of the pelvic bones, just beneath the hair on a woman's genitals.

Public health services = Services offered on a population basis. These include all programs, interventions, policies and activities that improve and protect the health of individuals and the community. Public health services intervene at the population or group level, as distinct from individual personal health services.

Public health = The science and art of promoting health, preventing disease and prolonging life through organized efforts of society.

Pulse = The heartbeat, which tells how fast and how hard the heart is working. The pulse can be felt at certain points on the body, like the inside of the wrist or the neck.

Purification = Killing harmful germs in water before drinking it.

Pus = White or yellow fluid that is filled with germs, often found inside an infected tear or wound.

Q

Quality of Life = Quality of life refers to the level of satisfaction that an individual experiences in life. Factors include: economic status, physical and mental health, relationships with others, personal development, and recreation.

Quality-of-life = A measure of the extent a patient is free from pain or disability caused by disease, and the extent he or she is able to perform the normal functions of life unaided.

List of Words

R

Radiation = Rays of energy given off by certain elements. Radiation is harmful because it kills cells in the body. But it can also be used to treat cancer by killing cancer cells.

Radiation oncologist = A specialist in the treatment of cancer using X-ray techniques.

Radiation Therapy = Radiation therapy uses high-energy rays to kill or shrink cancer cells. External radiation is the use of a machine to aim high-energy rays at the cancer from outside the body. Internal radiation therapy is the placement of a radioactive substance, such as cesium, iridium, or iodine, inside the body as close as possible to the cancer.

Radiation treatment = When a machine sends rays of energy into a person's body to kill cancer cells. The rays cannot be seen or felt.

Radical cystectomy = A radical cystectomy is a surgery to remove the bladder or nearby tissues and organs (such as the prostate gland, seminal vesicles and part or all of the urinary tube).

Radical hysterectomy = A radical hysterectomy is a surgery sometimes used to treat cervical cancer. It removes the cervix, the uterus and part of the vagina. A radical hysterectomy sometimes involves removing nearby lymph nodes, ovaries or the fallopian tubes.

Radical prostatectomy = A radical prostatectomy is a surgery to treat prostate cancer by removing the prostate gland and the two small glands behind it called the seminal vesicles. These three glands produce the liquid that makes up a man's semen.

Rape = When a man puts his penis, finger, or any object into a woman's vagina, anus, or mouth without her consent.

Rate = A measure of the frequency of occurrence of a phenomenon. A rate is an expression of the frequency with which an event occurs in a defined population in a specified period of time.

Rectal exam = Checking the rectum for growths or other problems. A rectal exam can also give information about the wall or lining of the vagina.

Rectum = The lower part of the intestine that is connected to the anus.

Red blood cells = Small, hemoglobin-filled blood cells that carry oxygen to the body's tissues.

Registered Dietitian (dy-eht-ish-uhn) = An expert on food health. In the United States, anyone who wishes to become a registered dietician must take certain courses and pass an exam.

Rehabilitation (ree-hab-il-ih-tay-shun) = Training, therapy, or other help given to someone who has a serious injury or illness. This training will help him or her to live a healthy and productive life.

Relative survival = Relative survival is the ratio of the proportion of observed survivors in a cohort of cancer patients to the proportion of expected survivors in a comparable set of cancer-free individuals.

Relaxation techniques = These are techniques, or things that you can do, to help you relax. They are often used for reducing stress. Relaxation techniques include meditation (sitting still, breathing slowly and clearing your mind), yoga, deep breathing, and visualization (closing your eyes and seeing a scene that relaxes you, such as a beach or a mountain lake).

Reproductive health = Health services like family planning services or prenatal care, that help prevent or treat health concerns connected to a woman's reproductive parts.

Reproductive organs = The parts of the

List of Words

body involved in reproduction (producing a baby). In a female, they include the uterus, ovaries, fallopian tubes, and vagina.

Reproductive parts = The parts of a man's and a woman's body that allow them to make a baby.

Resistance = The ability of something to defend itself against something that would normally harm or kill it. Many bacteria and viruses can become resistant to the effects of medicines like antibiotics and antiretrovirals so these treatments no longer work against disease.

Rheumatoid Arthritis (roo-muh-toyd arthrytis) = A painful disease that causes joints, tissues, and sometimes other parts of your body, to swell. It is usually inflammatory and causes pain, swelling, and stiffness.

Rhythm method = A family planning method in which a woman counts the days of her monthly cycle to find out when she is most fertile. She then avoids having sex during her fertile time.

Risk factor = Something that increases an individual's chance of developing a certain disease or condition.

S

Safer sex = Avoiding direct contact with a sexual partner's genitals, blood, semen, or vaginal wetness.

Sanitation = Public cleanliness to prevent disease, such as providing clean drinking water and keeping public places free of waste.

Scoliosis (sko-lee-oh-sis) = When the spine curves either away from the middle of the body or to the side.

Screening = Cancer screening is the early detection of cancer, or precursors of cancer, in individuals who do not have symptoms of cancer. These interventions are often directed to entire populations or to large and easily identifiable groups within the population. A screening test is not intended to be diagnostic; rather, a positive finding will have to be confirmed by special diagnostic procedures.

Screening mammogram =A screening mammogram is an x-ray of the breast used to detect breast changes in women who have no signs of breast cancer. It usually involves two x-rays of each breast.

Scrotum = The bag between a man's legs that holds his testicles or balls.

Self-esteem = How you feel about yourself – how you feel about who you are, the way you act, and how you look and about her role in her family and community.. When a person does not think too highly of themselves, she is said to have low self-esteem.

Semen = The liquid containing a man's sperm, which is released from his penis during ejaculation.

Sepsis = A serious infection that has spread into the blood.

Sequelae = A morbid condition(s) or symptom following a disease.

Sex worker = Anyone who exchanges sex for money or other favors, goods or services.

Sexual assault = Any type of sexual activity that you do not agree to, including touching you or forcing you to touch someone and forcing a body part into your vagina, rectum (bottom) or mouth. Another term for this can be child molestation.

Sexual assault = Unwanted sexual contact.

Sexual contact = Any type of contact during sexual activity between two people, including sexual intercourse, oral sex, and skin to skin contact in the genital area (around the vagina, penis, scrotum, anus, and thigh). STDs such as genital herpes, HPV (warts), and syphilis can be passed by having sexual contact with areas that

List of Words

are not be covered by a condom.

Sexual Dysfunction = Sexual dysfunction is the inability to react emotionally and/or physically to sexual stimulation in a way expected of the average healthy person or according to one's own standards. Sexual dysfunctions may affect various stages in the sexual response cycle - desire, excitement and orgasm. Dysfunction can be caused by a wide range of psychological, physiological, or combined reasons.

Sexual harassment = Unwanted sexual attention from anyone who has power over a woman.

Sexual Health = The World Health Organization defines sexual health as "the integration of the physical, emotional, intellectual, and social aspects of sexual being in ways that are positively enriching, and that enhance personality, communication, and love. Every person has a right to receive sexual information and to consider sexual relationships for pleasure as well as for procreation."

Sexual health = When a woman has control over her sexual life.

Sexual intercourse = Sex involving putting the penis in the vagina.

Sexual intercourse = Sex with the penis in the vagina.

Sexual roles = The way a community defines what it means to be a woman or a man.

Sexually transmitted disease (STD) = Once called venereal diseases or VD - infectious diseases that spread from person to person through sex.

Sexually transmitted infections (STIs) = Infections passed from one person to another during sex.

Shock = A dangerous condition with severe weakness or loss of consciousness, cold sweats, and fast, weak pulse. It can be caused by dehydration, heavy bleeding, injury, burns, or a severe illness.

Side effects = When medicines or hormonal methods cause changes in the body other than those needed to fight disease or prevent pregnancy.

Specimen (spes-e-men) = A sample of body tissue used for testing or examination.

Speculum = A small metal or plastic tool that holds the vagina open.

Sperm = Tiny organisms in a man's semen that can swim up a woman's vagina and fertilize an egg. This is how a pregnancy starts.

Sperm cell = A sperm cell is a cell made in a man's testicles that contains 23 chromosomes (either an X or Y sex chromosome and 22 autosomes). The sperm cell has a tail, which helps it swim through the woman's reproductive system to meet an oocyte. The sperm has an oval head with a special "cap" that contains chemicals that can drill a hole in the oocyte, allowing the sperm to enter and fertilize the oocyte. Only one sperm can fertilize an egg.

Spermatogonia = Spermatogonia are the cells in each testicle, which become active around puberty and start producing sperm cells. It takes about three months to produce a mature, human sperm.

Spermicide = A contraceptive cream, gel or foam that helps prevent pregnancy by killing sperm.

Spina Bifida (spyna bif-id-uh) = A birth defect that stops the bones of the spine from finishing forming correctly. It can cause legs to be paralyzed (unable to move) and cause loss of control over the bladder.

Spiritual distress = Spiritual distress is when an individual is trying to find meaning in life or is questioning or feeling unsure about his or her spirituality. Spiritual distress can cause problems in that person's daily life.

Squeezing exercise = An exercise to help strengthen weak muscles that cause a woman to pass urine often or to leak urine.

Stage = A description of how widely a cancer has spread to adjacent lymph nodes and other parts of the body.

Staging (cancer) -Cancer staging systems describe how far cancer has spread and put patients with similar prognosis in the same group. In overall stage grouping, there are four stages. In general, stage I cancers are small localized cancers that are usually curable, while stage IV usually represents inoperable or metastatic cancer. Stage II and III cancers are usually locally advanced and/or with involvement of local lymph nodes.

Stakeholders = Organizations/groups with a direct interest and involvement in aspects of cancer control.

Statistics = The science of collecting, summarizing, and analyzing numerical data. The term is also applied to the data themselves.

Sterile = When something is completely free from germs.

Sterilization = A permanent way of making a woman or man unable to have children.

Steroids = A class of medicines used to treat many different health problems. Steroids can have serious side effects if used for a long time.

Stethoscope = An instrument used to listen to sounds inside the body, like the heartbeat.

STIs See sexually transmitted infections.

Stomach = The sac-like organ in the belly where food is digested.

Stool = The waste that passes from the anus during a bowel movement.

Strategy = A course of action to achieve targets.

Stress = Any activities or events that put pressure on a woman, causing tension in her body and mind.

Stress incontinence = Stress incontinence is characterized by urine leaks when applying pressure to a full bladder in activities such as coughing, laughing and exercising.

Stroke = A sudden loss of consciousness, feeling, or ability to move caused by bleeding or a clot inside the brain.

Subcutaneous injection = An injection into the fatty tissue under the skin, not into the muscle or vein.

Support and rehabilitation = At the broadest level, the provision of the essential services to meet the physical, emotional, nutritional, informational, psychological, spiritual and practical needs throughout a person's experience with cancer.

Support groups = When people with a common problem meet together to help one another.

Surgery = When a doctor cuts into the body to find out what is wrong or to treat an illness. An operation.

Surveillance = Systematic ongoing collection, collation, and analysis of data and the timely dissemination of information to those who need to know so that action can be taken.

Survivor = You are a survivor from the time you find out you have cancer, through your treatment and for the rest of your life.

Survivorship = Cancer survivorship describes the many experiences and emotions that are part of living life as a cancer survivor.

Syphilis (sif-e-les) = An infection caused by a bacteria called bacterium treponema pallidum. A sexually transmitted infection.

Syringe = An instrument used to inject medicine.

List of Words

Systemic effects = Systemic effects are after-effects of cancer and cancer treatment that can affect many body systems and organs rather than being contained in one area or organ.

T

Tamoxifen = Tamoxifen is a hormone medicine used to prevent or treat breast cancer. It protects breast cells from the hormone estrogen. However, tamoxifen also acts like a weak estrogen in the vagina and uterus. Tamoxifen does not interfere with women's desire for sex and may actually add some vaginal lubrication for women who are in menopause.

Taxanes = Taxanes are a group of chemotherapy drugs that includes paclitaxel (Taxol) and docetaxel (Taxotere). These drugs are used to prevent the growth of cancer cells.

Tendons = Bands of tough tissue that connect a muscle with a bone or other part.

Testicles = The part of the male genitals that is inside the scrotum and makes the sperm.

Testosterone = Testosterone is a hormone made in men's testicles and in women's ovaries and adrenal glands. Testosterone is released into the bloodstream where it travels to many parts of the body. It helps men and women feel desire for sex. A woman's body naturally produces less testosterone than a man's body.

Testosterone (teh-stass-tuh-rone) = A hormone made mostly by the testes. This hormone causes many of the changes males deal with during puberty—deeper voices, body and facial hair, and the making of sperm.

Tetanus = A serious disease caused by a germ that lives in the stools of people or animals. Tetanus enters the body through a wound.

Thermometer = An instrument used to measure how hot a person's body temperature is.

Thrombocytes (throm-boh-syts) = Platelets, which are in your blood.

Thrush = A fungal infection that causes white patches and soreness on the skin inside the mouth, on the tongue, and the tube that connects the mouth with the stomach.

Thyroid = The thyroid is a gland located at the base of the neck. The thyroid produces hormones to regulate metabolism and calcium balance in the body.

Thyroid gland = A gland in the front of the throat that makes hormones that affect growth and development. The thyroid needs iodine to work properly.

Tissue = The material making up the muscles, fatty areas, and organs of the body.

Toxemia = A dangerous condition during pregnancy, which can lead to seizures (convulsions).

Toxic = A harmful substance that can cause disease or death when it enters the body is said to be toxic.

Toxic Shock Syndrome = A very rare but dangerous illness that affects the whole body. TSS is caused by bacteria that make toxins (poisons) in the body. Tampon use can make it easier for bacteria to enter the body. Symptoms include high fever that comes on suddenly, dizziness, rash, and feelings of confusion.

Toxicity = When a person takes too much medicine and it builds up to a dangerous level in the body.

Traditional healers = Healers who use methods based on beliefs that have been passed down from generation to generation.

Transmitted = To give to someone else; to spread.

Trauma = When something horrible happens to a person or to someone the person is close to.

Trend = The general direction (for example, rising falling or stable) of change over time.

List of Words

Trichomonas = A disease of the genitals that is passed during sex.

Trichomoniasis (trik-e-me-ni-e-ses) = A common STD that affects both men and women, although symptoms are more common in women.

Tubal ligation = An operation in which the fallopian tubes are cut or tied so the egg cannot travel to the womb to be fertilized.

Tuberculosis = A serious infection caused by a germ that usually affects the lungs.

Tumor = A new and abnormal formation of tissue, as a lump or growth. Tumors may be benign (rarely life-threatening) or malignant.

U

Ulcer = A chronic open sore of the skin, the stomach, or the intestines.

Ultrasound = A machine that uses sound to take a picture of the inside of the body without cutting it open. It is often used during pregnancy to see the baby inside the womb.

Unsafe sex = Direct contact with a sexual partner's genitals, blood, semen or vaginal wetness—if there is any chance you or your partner has a sexually transmitted infection (STI).

Urethra = The tube that carries urine from the bladder to the outside of the bodyr; in the male, also serves as a passage for the release of semen from the body.

Urethra = A short tube that carries urine from the bladder to the hole a person urinates from.

Urge incontinence = Characterized by the frequent and sudden need to urinate.

Urinary Tract Infection (UTI) = An infection that happens in the bladder or tube leading to the bladder. It is usually caused by a type of bacteria.

Urine Test = A strip of special paper is dipped in the urine after urination. This will show if there are any abnormal problems in the urine.

Urologist = A urologist is a physician specializing in treating problems involving male and female urinary functions or the male reproductive organs.

Uterus (yoo-ter-us) = Also called the womb. The uterus is a pear-shaped, hollow organ in a female's pelvis where a baby develops during pregnancy. The uterus is made up of muscle with an inside lining called the endometrium. The endometrium builds up and thickens during the menstrual cycle to prepare for a possible pregnancy each month. But if no pregnancy occurs, the extra tissue and blood are shed during menstruation. See womb.

V

Vaccinations or vaccines = Medicines that are injected to give protection against specific diseases like tetanus.

Vagina (vah-jye-na) = Sometimes called the birth canal. The vagina is a muscular passage that leads down from the cervix, (the lower part of the uterus) to the outside of a female's body. During menstruation, menstrual blood flows from the uterus through the cervix and out of the body through the vagina.

Vaginectomy = A vaginectomy is a surgery to remove part or all of the vagina. Total vaginectomy is usually a treatment for vaginal cancer or advanced cancer of the cervix. Parts of the vagina may be removed as part of surgery to treat bladder or colorectal cancer. Vaginal reconstruction is often done at the same time.

Varicose veins = Abnormally swollen veins—often blue, lumpy, and winding—on the legs of older people, pregnant women, and women who have had a lot of children. Pregnant women also sometimes have varicose veins in the genitals.

Vasectomy = A permanent method of pre-

List of Words

venting pregnancy, in which the tubes that carry sperm from the testicles to the penis are cut.

Veins = Thin-walled blood vessels that receive blood from capillaries and return it to the heart.

Vinca alkaloids = Vinca alkaloids are anticancer drugs that slow down cancer cell growth by stopping cell division. They are made from the periwinkle plant.

Virgin = Someone who has never had sex.

Virus = Germs smaller than bacteria, which cause some infectious diseases.

Vitamins = Vitamins and minerals are drugs that replace or fix low levels of important natural substances in your body. You get vitamins and minerals from food. Some types of food have more of these good substances than others. If you need extra vitamins and minerals, you may have to take pills that have them. Foods that the body needs to work properly, to fight disease, and to get better after a sickness or injury.

Vomiting = Throwing up the contents of the stomach through the mouth.

Vulva (vul-vuh) = The vulva covers the entrance to the vagina and has five parts: mons pubis, labia, clitoris, urinary tract opening, and vaginal opening.

W

White blood cells = Blood cells that are involved in fighting infection and helping to heal wounds.

Withdrawal = The period of time in which the body gets used to being without a drug or alcohol to which it is physically addicted.

Withdrawl = Penis is pulled out of the vagina during sex, before ejaculation.

Womb (uterus) = A sac of strong muscle inside a woman's belly. Monthly bleeding comes from the womb, and the baby grows inside the womb during pregnancy.

X

X-rays = Pictures of parts of the inside of the body, like the bones or the lungs, which are created by rays sent through the body. The body does not need to be cut open.

Y

Yeast infection = A vaginal infection with white, lumpy discharge, itching, and burning. These infections are common during pregnancy and when taking antibiotics.

My Wellness Journey Notes

Tips for Talking to your Health Care Provider

- List your questions and concerns. Before your appointment, make a list of what you want to ask. When you're in the waiting room, review your list and organize your thoughts. You can share the list with your health care provider.

- Describe your symptoms. Say when these problems started. Say how they make you feel. If you know, say what sets them off or triggers them. Say what you've done to feel better.

- Give your health care provider a list of your medications. Tell what prescription drugs and over-the-counter medicines, vitamins, herbal products, and other supplements you're taking. Some people find it easier to just bring in all of their medicines for the health care team to see.

- Be honest about your diet, physical activity, smoking, alcohol or drug use, and sexual history. Not sharing information with your health care provider or nurse can be harmful!

- Describe any allergies to drugs, foods, pollen, or other things.

- Don't forget to mention if you are being treated by other doctors, including mental health professionals, alternative medicine providers and traditional healers.

- Ask questions about any tests and your test results. Get instructions on what you need to do to get ready for the test(s). Ask if there are any dangers or side effects. Ask how you can learn the test results. Ask how long it will take to get the results.

My health concerns:

Signs and symptoms:

The medicines I currently take:

My diet, habits and behaviors:

My Allergies:

Other health care providers I am seeing or Treatment I am having:

Questions I have about treatment:

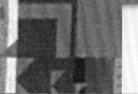

Tips for Talking to your Health Care Provider

Information about my condition:

Pregnancy plans

My treatment options & coverage:

New medicines:

Other questions I have for my health care provider:

• Ask questions about your condition or illness. If you are diagnosed with a condition, ask your doctor how you can learn more about it. What caused it? Is it permanent? What can you do to help yourself feel better? How can it be treated?

• Tell your health care provider if you are pregnant or intend to become pregnant. Some medicines may not be suitable for you. Other medicines should be used with caution if you are pregnant or about to become pregnant.

• Ask your health care provider about any treatments he or she recommends. Be sure to ask about all of your options for treatment. Ask how long the treatment will last. Ask if it has any side effects. Ask how much it will cost. Ask if it is covered by your health insurance.

• Ask your health care provider about any medicines he or she prescribes for you. Make sure you understand how to take your medicine. What should you do if you miss a dose? Are there any foods, drugs, or activities you should avoid when taking the medicine? Is there a generic brand of the drug you can use? You can also ask your pharmacist if a generic drug is available for your medication.

• Ask more questions if you don't understand something. If you're not clear about what your health care provider is asking you to do or why, ask to have it explained again.

• Bring a family member or trusted friend with you. That person can take notes, offer moral support, and help you remember what was discussed. You can have that person ask questions, too!

Women's Screening Test Checklist

Talk to your health care provider about your results and write them down here. Ask when you should have the next test and write down the month and the year.

Test	Last Test (mo/yr)	Result	Next Test Due (mo/yr)	Questions for my Provider
Weight & BMI				
Cholesterol total				
HDL (good)				
LDL (bad)				
Blood Pressure				
Mammogram				
Clinical Breast Exam				
Pap Smear				
Colorectal cancer				
Diabetes				
Sexually Transmitted Infections				
HIV Infection				
Bone Density				
Depression (for some)				

All ages:
Weight and BMI (body mass index)

Age 21 or after becoming sexually active:
Clinical Breast Exam
Pap test
Sexually Transmitted Infections test
HIV Infection test

Age 40
Mammograms

Age 45
Cholesterol, HDL, LDL

Age 50
Colorectal Cancer

Age 65
Bone Density

Other tests at various ages, talk to your health care provider:
Diabetes
Depression